A Handbook of Children and Young People's Participation

Perspectives from theory and practice

**Edited by
Barry Percy-Smith
and Nigel Thomas**

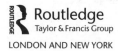
Routledge
Taylor & Francis Group

LONDON AND NEW YORK

First published 2010
by Routledge
2 Park Square, Milton Park, Abingdon, Oxon, OX14 4RN

Simultaneously published in the USA and Canada
by Routledge
270 Madison Avenue, New York, NY 10016

Routledge is an imprint of the Taylor & Francis Group, an informa business

Typeset in Baskerville by
Bookcraft Ltd, Stroud, Gloucestershire
Printed and bound in Great Britain by
CPI Antony Rowe, Chippenham, Wiltshire

British Library Cataloguing in Publication Data
A catalogue record for this book is available from
the British Library

Library of Congress Cataloging-in-Publication Data
Percy-Smith, Barry.
A handbook of children and young people's participation : perspectives
from theory and practice / Barry Percy-Smith and Nigel Thomas.
   p. cm.
   1. Children's rights. 2. Participation. I. Thomas, Nigel, 1950–
   II. Title.
HQ789.P374 2009
323′.042083–dc22   2009009796

ISBN10: 0-415-46851-5 (hbk)
ISBN10: 0-415-46852-3 (pbk)
ISBN10: 0-203-87107-3 (ebk)

ISBN13: 978-0-415-46851-0 (hbk)
ISBN13: 978-0-415-46852-7 (pbk)
ISBN13: 978-0-203-87107-2 (ebk)

A Handbook of Children and Young People's Participation

A Handbook of Children and Young People's Participation brings together key thinkers and practitioners from diverse contexts across the globe to provide an authoritative overview of contemporary theory and practice around children's participation. Promoting the participation of children and young people – in decision-making and policy development, and as active contributors to everyday family and community life – has become a central part of policy and programme initiatives in both majority and minority worlds. This book presents the most useful recent work in children's participation as a resource for academics, students and practitioners in childhood studies, children's rights and welfare, child and family social work, youth and community work, governance, aid and development programmes.

The book introduces key concepts and debates, and presents a rich collection of accounts of the diverse ways in which children's participation is understood and enacted around the world, interspersed with reflective commentaries from adults and young people. It concludes with a number of substantial theoretical contributions that aim to take forward our understanding of children's participation.

The emphasis throughout the text is on learning from the complexity of children's participation in practice to improve our theoretical understanding, and on using those theoretical insights to challenge practice, with the aim of realising children's rights and citizenship more fully.

Barry Percy-Smith is Reader in Childhood and Participatory Practice at the SOLAR Action Research Centre, University of the West of England, Bristol, UK. He has extensive experience using participatory and 'whole system' action inquiry approaches in research, evaluation and development projects with children, young people, practitioners and policy makers. He is Coordinator of the Children's Participation Learning Network, an international forum for critical debate about children and young people's participation, and has published and presented numerous papers on the subject.

Nigel Thomas is Professor of Childhood and Youth Research at the University of Central Lancashire, UK, and Co-Director of The Centre, which exists to promote and research children and young people's participation, inclusion and empowerment. He has twenty years' experience of social work practice and has taught and researched extensively in the field of children's welfare, rights and participation.

Contents

PART II
Learning about children's participation in practice   51

Illustrations

Figures

Plates

Tables

Boxes

Contributors

Lalatendu Acharya is a management and communications professional with experience working in corporate, government and development sectors and has extensive experience working with children as a Communications Officer for UNICEF. He is currently pursuing a PhD in health communication at Purdue University exploring issues concerned with development, participation and empowerment as they relate to building a voice for children.

Priscilla Alderson is Professor of Childhood Studies, Social Science Research Unit, Institute of Education, University of London. Her interests include rights and ethics, children's competence and consent, living with long-term illness or disability, respectful education, health and social services, and research about children in broader economic, ecological, evolutionary and ethical contexts. She teaches on the MA in the Sociology of Childhood and Children's Rights course. Details of over 300 publications are on www.ioe.ac.uk/ssru.

Sara L. Austin is Director of the President's Office of World Vision Canada and has worked on programme and policy initiatives in a variety of national contexts. Sara has particular expertise in international human rights law, with a particular focus on children's rights. She serves on the Board of Directors of the Canadian Coalition on the Rights of the Child, and is a member of the Advisory Council for the UN Study on Violence Against Children.

Tom Cockburn is Senior Lecturer at the University of Bradford. He has undertaken research into children and young people with various voluntary and public sector organisations in the UK. He has published on a wide variety of issues concerning children and young people including: citizenship, theorising participation in public spaces, utilising feminist theory, and research methods with practitioners. Currently his research interests include theorising children and young people's participation in Europe.

Yolanda Corona Caraveo and **Carlos Pérez** are professors at the Autonomous Metropolitan University, Mexico. Yolanda researches on young people's participation in resistance movements and indigenous children's participation in their communities. She has edited several books and journal issues on children in vulnerable situations, participation, and politics. Carlos's research interests include social and resistance movements, political culture, and epistemology.

Julián Hernández is studying for a Master's degree in social and political studies at the National Autonomous University of Mexico. Current interests include youth and citizenship, traditional indigenous people and participation rights in Mexico and the emergence of youth as social and political agents.

Anne Crowley was until recently Assistant Director with Save the Children UK and is currently studying for a PhD at Cardiff University, exploring the impact of children and young people's participation in public decision making. Prior to becoming involved in policy and research, Anne worked with young people as a social worker and probation officer. **Anna Skeels** is manager of the Participation Unit in Wales, hosted by Save the Children, leading the strategic development of children and young people's participation. Anna previously worked with young people 'at risk' in Cardiff and has a strong commitment to inclusion, participation and children's rights.

Ann Dadich is Research Fellow at the Centre for Industry and Innovation Studies (CInIS) at the University of Western Sydney. She is a registered psychologist and member of the Australian Psychological Society. Ann's research expertise is in the related fields of health and mental service systems, social policy, community psychology, and youth mental health. Her work in government and third sectors with young people and people who support them continues to inform her approach to conducting research that is both empirical and respectful.

Clare Feinstein is currently the Advocacy and Child Protection Specialist for War Child Holland. She has many years of experience working on children's participation and child protection issues. **Annette Giertsen** has been working on children's participation in Latin America, Africa, Asia and Eastern Europe for the last 10 years as an adviser for Save the Children Norway. **Claire O'Kane** has 15 years of children's participation and protection experience in Asia, Africa and Europe. She is currently the Child Protection in Emergencies Adviser for Save the Children in Burma.

Robyn Fitzgerald is a researcher at the Centre for Children and Young People at Southern Cross University, Lismore, Australia. **Anne Graham** is Professor of Childhood Studies and Director of this Centre. Emeritus Professor **Anne Smith**, formerly Director of the Children's Issues Centre, is now based at the University of Otago College of Education. **Nicola Taylor** is Senior Research Fellow at the Centre for Research on Children and Families at the University of Otago, New Zealand. The authors' shared research interests include children's participation and citizenship; ethical considerations in child- and youth-related research; children's well-being and rights in families, education and legal systems, and in other everyday contexts.

Lucy Jamieson is the Senior Advocacy Coordinator at the Children's Institute, University of Cape Town. Her work focuses on facilitating the participation of civil society in law-reform processes affecting children; this includes children on the street, children in alternative care and (through projects such as Dikwankwetla) children affected by HIV. **Wanjirũ Mũkoma** holds a PhD in psychiatry and mental health. She was the HIV/AIDS Programme Manager at the Children's Institute (where the Dikwankwetla – Children in Action project was housed), and is currently working in Kenya at Liverpool VCT Care and Treatment.

Vicky Johnson is Co-director of Development Focus Trust, which delivers participatory training, evaluation, children's rights and participation, and action research. She has worked as an adviser and consultant in environment and social development for over 15 years with government and non-governmental organisations internationally and in the UK. Her publications include *Listening to Smaller Voices* (1994) and *Stepping Forward* (1998). She is currently completing a PhD at the University of Central Lancashire.

Perpetua Kirby is an independent research consultant and Director of PK Research Consultancy. Her research focuses primarily on children and young people's participation across different sectors within the United Kingdom, including within health, education, local and national government departments, and non-governmental organisations. **Sophie Laws** is Policy and Research Manager for Coram, a London-based charity working for better chances for children, with a particular interest in children and young people's participation. She is co-author of *Research for Development: a practical guide* (Sage 2003) and *So you want to involve children in research?* (Save the Children Sweden 2004).

Renate Kränzl-Nagl is Professor of Sociology and Empirical Social Research at the Upper Austria University for Applied Social Sciences in Linz. Her main areas of interest are childhood, youth and family research and policies, and participatory research. **Ulrike Zartler** is a sociologist at the University of Vienna, Department of Sociology. Her main research and teaching fields are sociology of childhood and family, transition processes in families, children's participation, and qualitative research methods. Both authors were researchers at the European Centre for Social Welfare Policy and Research (research area Childhood, Youth and Families) for many years.

Gerison Lansdown is an international children's rights consultant who has published and lectured widely on children's rights, both nationally and internationally. She was actively involved in the drafting of the Convention on the Rights of Persons with Disabilities. She is currently Vice-chair of UNICEF-UK, an Associate of the International Institute for Child Rights and Development in Victoria, and Co-director of CRED-PRO, an international initiative to develop child rights educational programmes for professionals working with children.

Jack Lewars first became formally involved with Student Voice at the age of 15 via the launch conference of the English Secondary Students' Association in February 2005. He was subsequently elected onto ESSA's Executive Council, a post which he held until 2007. He then went on to become ESSA's National Student Support Officer during his gap year. Jack is currently studying Classics at university, and keeps in touch with Student Voice through occasional work for ESSA.

Karen Malone is Associate Professor at the University of Wollongong, Chair of the Child-Friendly Cities Asia-Pacific Network and Asia-Pacific Director of the UNESCO Growing Up in Cities project. She has extensive project experience with young people and has published widely on child and youth environments, environmental education and participatory research methodologies. **Catherine Hartung** is a PhD candidate at the Child and Youth Interdisciplinary Research Centre at the University of Wollongong, concerned with the theoretical deconstruction of children's participation in the field. She has worked as a teacher, designer, and as a researcher on a Communities for Children project in Melbourne.

Greg Mannion is a Senior Lecturer at the Stirling Institute of Education, University of Stirling, Scotland. Greg first worked as a primary teacher and adult educator in Ireland. He completed a doctorate at Stirling in 1999 on children's participation. His research interests relate to socio-spatial and ecological dimensions of learning, child–adult relations, outdoor learning, education for sustainable development/global citizenship, post-16 education, literacies for learning and the use of visual and participatory research approaches.

Kate Martin is Senior Development Officer for the Council for Disabled Children in the UK, leading on a national project promoting the active participation of disabled children, and is undertaking a part-time PhD. Kate has worked in a range of voluntary and statutory organisations, promoting disabled children's inclusion and participation. **Anita Franklin** is Senior Researcher at the Children's Society in the UK, managing projects with disabled children. She has extensive experience working with vulnerable children and young people, including work with the University of York, where she authored a number of publications concerning the participation of disabled children.

Jan Mason is Professor of Social Work and **Natalie Bolzan** is Associate Professor at the University of Western Sydney (UWS), Australia. Jan and Natalie are both members of the Social Justice and Social Change Research Centre at UWS. The other researchers in the network who contributed to the chapter are: Usha Nayar, Anil Kumar (TATA Institute for Social Sciences, Mumbai, India); Qing Ju, Chen Chen, Zhao Xia (China Youth and Children Research Centre, Beijing, China); Swarna Wijetunge (National Education Research and Evaluation Centre, University of Colombo, Sri Lanka); Nittaya Kotchabhakidi, Dalapat Yossatorn, Athiwat Jiawiwatkul and Nithivadee Noochaiya (National Institute for Child and Family Development, Mahidol University, Bangkok, Thailand).

Brian McGinley is Lecturer and Director of the Post Graduate Community Education Programme at the University of Strathclyde, Co-director of the Scottish Centre for Youth Work Studies and joint editor of the *Scottish Youth Issues Journal*. He has extensive experience of youth work practice and research, with interests in inclusion and equality issues in marginalised communities. **Ann Grieve** is a lecturer in Educational and Professional Studies in the Faculty of Education, University of Strathclyde. Her areas of research interest are in communication, relationships and behaviour, linked to concepts of inclusion, participation and social justice, and continuing development of education professionals.

Kirrily Pells is completing her PhD at the Centre for International Human Rights of the University of London. Her thesis focuses on rights-based approaches with children and young people in post-conflict situations, with a case study on Rwanda. In addition to fieldwork conducted in Rwanda, Kirrily has carried out consultancies for CARE International and Save the Children. She has also worked with organisations operating at the community level in both Rwanda and Bosnia.

Patricia Ray is a medical doctor who worked as a clinician in the UK and in Mozambique during the civil war. In the 1990s she lived in South East Asia, engaged with child-centred health and development programming. She joined Plan in 1995 and undertook roles in programme management and strategic planning at country, regional and international levels. She now works as an independent consultant, providing technical services and writing on child-centred development programming.

Fahriye Hazer Sancar is a professor and **Yucel Can Severcan** a PhD student in the College of Architecture and Planning at the University of Colorado. Both are associates of the Children, Youth and Environments Centre. Dr Sancar has degrees in Architecture and her PhD is in Man–Environment Relations. Her research interests include environmental aesthetics, sustainable and healthy communities, and collaborative methods in planning and design, with special emphasis on children and youth. Yucel Severcan has degrees in City and Regional Planning and Urban Design. His current work centres on place attachment and the design of public open spaces.

Harry Shier worked in England for 25 years on adventure playgrounds and playwork training. In 1988 he founded Playtrain, an independent training agency specialising in children's rights, play, and creativity. In the 1990s he worked extensively on children's participation, developing the Article 31 Children's Consultancy Scheme. Since 2001 he has worked in Nicaragua as an education advisor with a local community education organisation, supporting child workers on the region's coffee plantations in defending their rights.

Tiina Sotkasiira is a doctoral student at the Karelian Institute, University of Joensuu. She is currently researching cultural identification and the experiences of everyday racism among minority youth in Russia. **Lotta Haikkola** is a doctoral student at the Department of Sociology, University of Helsinki. Her research concerns second-generation immigrant children's transnational networks and their impact on identities. **Liisa Horelli** is Adjunct Professor at the Center for Urban and Regional Studies, Helsinki University of Technology. She conducts action research on community informatics-assisted participatory planning and community development with young and elderly people.

Joachim Theis has worked for over 20 years in international development in Africa, the Middle East and Asia. He currently works in the UNICEF Regional Office for West and Central Africa as regional child protection adviser. He has previously worked in East Asia and the Pacific on rights-based approaches, participation and child and adolescent development. In Vietnam he carried out participatory poverty assessments, research on child labour, and developed poverty reduction strategies.

E. Kay M. Tisdall works at the University of Edinburgh. She is Programme Director of the MSc in Childhood Studies (www.childhoodstudies.ed.ac.uk) and Co-director of the Centre for Research on Families and Relationships (www.crfr. ac.uk). Recent collaborative publications include the book *Research with Children and Young People* and a special issue on children's participation for *The International Journal of Children's Rights*. She previously was Director of Policy and Research at Children in Scotland, a non-governmental organisation.

Alan Turkie has a background in community development and group psychotherapy. His primary interests are in supporting diverse communities to work effectively together and in enabling marginalised groups, particularly young people, to participate in decision making. Alan has led workshops on participation and social inclusion in the UK and overseas and published extensively on these subjects. He formerly worked as a senior lecturer in higher education and now acts as a consultant adviser to organisations.

Afua Twum-Danso is a lecturer in the Sociology of Childhood at the University of Sheffield. Her recently completed PhD thesis from the University of Birmingham is entitled 'Searching for a middle ground in children's rights: The implementation of the convention on the rights of the child in Ghana'. The thesis moved beyond the universality and relativity debate in order to identify a middle ground in children's lives which can be used to engage local communities in dialogue.

Sarah C. White is Director of the Centre for Development Studies, University of Bath, UK. Her teaching and research explore how social identities, culture, and relationships figure in development processes. She has worked on gender, child rights, participation, race, religion, and well-being. Her main research location is Bangladesh. **Shyamol A. Choudhury** works for Save the Children. Over the last 16 years he has been engaged in the specialised field of child rights – namely child protection, child participation, child rights programming and children in emergencies.

Hiromi Yamashita and **Lynn Davies** are both based at the Centre for International Education (CIER), School of Education, the University of Birmingham, UK. CIER engages in research and teaching in the areas of global justice internationally. Hiromi's interests include issues of participation (at all ages), democratic decision making, environmental risk communication, sustainable development, global citizenship and education in coastal regions. Lynn's interests include educational management internationally, particularly concerning democracy, citizenship, gender, and human rights. A specific interest is in education and security, and how education contributes to conflict or to peace and civil renewal.

The editors

Barry Percy-Smith is Reader in Childhood and Participatory Practice at the SOLAR Action Research Centre, University of the West of England, Bristol, UK. He has extensive experience working with children, young people, practitioners, and policy makers using participatory and 'whole system' action inquiry approaches in research, evaluation, and development projects in organisations and communities. He was a contributor to the UNESCO Growing Up in Cities programme, co-editor of the *Children, Youth and Environments* special issue on participation and coordinates the Children's Participation Learning Network.

Nigel Thomas is Professor of Childhood and Youth Research at the University of Central Lancashire, UK, and Co-director of the Centre, which exists to promote and research children and young people's participation, inclusion and empowerment. He has 20 years' experience of social work practice and has taught and researched extensively in the field of children's welfare, rights, and participation. His publications include *Children, Family and the State* (Macmillan 2000; Policy Press 2002), *Social Work with Young People in Care* (Palgrave 2004), and *Children, Politics and Communication* (Policy Press 2009). He is co-editor of the journal *Children & Society*.

Foreword

Martin Woodhead

PROFESSOR OF CHILDHOOD STUDIES, THE OPEN UNIVERSITY

Exactly 100 years ago, in 1909, a book was published with the bold title *The Century of the Child*. The author, Swedish feminist and social reformer Ellen Key, set out her vision for the transformation of childhood during the twentieth century. The title of the first chapter boldly asserted 'The Right of the Child to Choose his Parents', by which she meant that every child was entitled to quality care at home as well as a sound education, rather than literally to choose their parents! Her child-centred pedagogy also anticipated other themes in this handbook. Ellen Key recognised the balance to be struck between protecting children and enabling them to participate, famously captured by the assertion that: 'At every step the child should be allowed to meet the real experience of life; the thorns should never be plucked from his roses.'

Ten years later, in 1919, Eglantyne Jebb responded to the suffering of children in the defeated nations of Europe in the wake of the First World War by setting up the first overseas relief agency for children – the Save the Children Fund. The core mission of Save the Children already had a long history in the work of nineteenth-century social reformers and philanthropists, which she had studied as a student at Oxford University. Jebb's contribution was in establishing Save the Children as an international (and increasingly global) mission to improve the health and well-being of all children. But she was also pioneering in her insistence that compassion towards suffering children was not enough. She formulated simple principles based on respect for the individual child, notably, that every child had the right to life, to food, to care and protection, to normal development, and (interestingly in light of subsequent international child labour conventions) the right to be in a position to earn a livelihood without exploitation. Five principles were formalised in the original 'Declaration of the Rights of the Child' which was endorsed by the newly established League of Nations (forerunner of the United Nations) in Geneva in 1924.

One of the original signatories of the Geneva Declaration (as it is commonly called) was the Polish doctor, pedagogue and children's writer Janusz Korczak. He is best remembered for setting up an orphanage in the Polish ghetto during the Second World War and in 1942 insisting on accompanying the children in his care to their deaths in the Treblinka extermination camp. By coincidence, 2009 marks another anniversary relevant to the themes of this handbook. One of Korczak's final books was published in 1929 under the visionary title of *The Child's*

Right to Respect, and included a proclamation that is just as radical now as it was 80 years ago:

> Children are not the people of tomorrow, but are people of today. They have a right to be taken seriously, and to be treated with tenderness and respect.

The ninth year in each decade continued to serve as a milestone in the development of childhood policy during the second half of the century, with the UN Declaration of the Rights of the Child in 1959, and the International Year of the Child in 1979.

This brings us to 1989, which is unquestionably the most significant milestone for development of current child policies, globally, and the foundation for many of the participation initiatives discussed in this handbook. Until 1989, the concept of children's rights had most often been framed in terms of beliefs about their nature and needs, and the responsibilities of adults to provide the best possible care and education, and protection from harm. The United Nations Convention on the Rights of the Child (UNCRC) redefined the status of children and young people by also acknowledging their civil and political rights, notably through Article 12, on the right to express views freely, and the right to be heard in any judicial and administrative proceedings affecting the child. Less commonly cited are Articles 13, 14, 15 and 16, which give the child the right to freedom of expression, freedom of thought, conscience and religion, rights to peaceful assembly and rights to privacy. These rights are carefully qualified by recognition of the duties of parents to provide direction to the child, in accordance with the child's 'age and maturity' and 'evolving capacities'. Even so, they mark a radical departure from earlier rights frameworks, in establishing that the child may have separate interests, views and feelings from their family, and other sources of authority, and that the child has the capacity (under guidance) to think about, communicate and make decisions. The UNCRC is also much more comprehensive in its scope than the earlier Declaration of 1959 and places much greater emphasis on the responsibilities of governments to ensure children's best interests are protected and promoted. Moreover, implementation of the UNCRC is overseen by the requirement on governments to report regularly to the UN Committee on the Rights of the Child in Geneva.

The UNCRC set out the foundational principles on which much child participation practice, research and theory is now built, supported by the full authority of an international human rights convention. Since 1989, this most extensively ratified Convention has required a fundamental re-evaluation of the status of children and young people, at least in theory, and increasingly in practice. The individual child is no longer to be viewed merely as an object of concern, care and protection, whose life and destiny are shaped and regulated by laws, institutions, parents and professionals, acting in what they judge to be the child's interests. Henceforth, children are also to be recognised (and supported towards recognising themselves) as active in the process of shaping their lives, learning and future. They have their own view on their best interests, a growing capacity to make decisions, the right to speak and the right to be heard. This very different image of the participating child has recently been reaffirmed by the UN Committee on the Rights of the Child, with particular reference to the young child:

> The Convention requires that children, including the very youngest children, be respected as persons in their own right. Young children should be recognised as active members of families, communities and societies, with their own concerns, interests and points of view.
>
> (General Comment 7, 2005)

Embracing the child-centred, child-enabling and child-empowering values underlying participation is one thing. Putting these values into practice is quite another. While some projects were from the beginning spectacularly successful, this has not always been the case. Enthusiastic participation projects have not always used appropriate methods, nor been based on a sufficiently elaborated conceptual framework, with over-reliance on compelling but ultimately simplistic models, notably the participation ladder. For example, recognising that the right to participation applies to all children, of all ages and capabilities, is fundamental, but applying that universal principle in ways that are sensitive and appropriate has proved less straightforward. Listening to a 6-month-old means something very different from listening to a 6-year-old, or a 16-year-old. But the fact that a 6-month-old is not yet able to communicate through the conventions of spoken or written language does not mean they cannot communicate their feelings, ideas and wishes. Also, children's participation does not diminish adults' roles and responsibilities. On the contrary, it increases the challenges to scaffold children's participation effectively and appropriately in respect to their situation and capacities.

It is encouraging that promoting 'children's participation' has emerged as an explicit goal for numerous rights-based organisations, innovative programmes and research projects, including those reported in the chapters that follow. If anything, there can sometimes be a misleading (and potentially dangerous) tendency to elevate participatory rights over and above provision and protection rights, and imply that children's rights are all about participation rights. This neglects the important principle within the UNCRC of the interdependence of rights. By contrast, and more commonly, lip service is paid to participatory principles, but effective implementation is patchy, frequently tokenistic and with notable variations between different institutional settings, between different sectors of government and especially between different political and cultural contexts. The same variability of uptake applies within child research, with some areas of inquiry still strongly adhering to an unqualified positivist paradigm, within which children are objectified as human potential, moulded and shaped by positive and negative influences, with little scope for acknowledging their subjectivity, activity and agency, at least on the face of it. More encouragingly, recent decades have also seen the emergence of an increasingly influential field of interdisciplinary child research, premised on the recognition that children are active agents in constructing their childhood and should be active participants in child research.

One of the biggest challenges for progressing children's and young people's participation is the concept of 'participation' itself. It is attractively all-encompassing, but at the same time far too bland. There is a world of difference between the cosy image of young children's social participation in everyday settings under the benign guidance of respectful parents and teachers, compared with the more challenging image of young people taking to the streets to protest against an oppressive political regime, impending military action, or the impact of climate change. In other words, participation isn't just about adults 'allowing' children to offer their perspectives, according to adults' view of their 'evolving capacities', their 'age and maturity' or their 'best interests'. It can also involve young people confronting adult authority, challenging adult assumptions about their competence to speak and make decisions about issues that concern them. If we are to develop fully the potential for children and young people to participate in society, we may need to move beyond 'listening' and 'giving children a say', and to focus more directly on the meaning of participation in everyday life and on how young people can live 'active citizenship'. As the editors and some contributors note, this may mean moving beyond the UNCRC – or at least, beyond Article 12.

Finally, promoting children's participation can seem somewhat empty rhetoric in authoritarian settings, where respect for elders is demanded, and enforced by fear of (as well as actual) beatings, which are still commonplace in homes and schools throughout many regions of the world. Equally, projects to empower children in contexts where many adults are disenfranchised and have little power to improve their lives can at best seem idealistic, and at worst may be counterproductive, or even exploitative. All of which highlights the inseparability of promoting children's rights and responsibilities from promoting adults' rights and responsibilities, and the inseparability of participation rights from protection and provision rights.

Huge progress on these issues has been made between 1989 and 2009, as the following chapters illustrate. One of the strengths of this comprehensive handbook is that most of the chapters take the practice of participation as the best starting point for building an adequate conceptualisation of the subject. Taken together, they encompass a vast array of types of participation, contexts for participation and models for participation. The Handbook will be an essential resource for anyone embarking on a child participation initiative as well as for students and scholars in childhood research and children's rights.

One final thought. When Ellen Key published *The Century of the Child* in 1909 she believed she was setting out an agenda that would transform twentieth-century society, centred on valuing the child. What she may not have foreseen was that the core concept of 'child centredness' has itself come under scrutiny, not least because it seems to objectify children and set them apart from society. Recognition of children's participatory rights has been the catalyst for a serious review of children's multiple contributions to society. At the same time, numerous challenges lie ahead in ensuring implementation of participatory rights in meaningful ways, for all children and young people, as citizens in the twenty-first century.

Introduction

Nigel Thomas and Barry Percy-Smith

When it was first suggested to us (by Martin Woodhead, author of the Foreword) that the time was right for a substantial edited collection of writing on children and young people's participation, the example of Bob Franklin's *Handbook of Children's Rights* (Franklin 1995; 2002) immediately came to mind. Those two volumes, it seems to us, were very influential in extending thinking on the subject of children's rights, and they have continued to be an invaluable resource for students and practitioners at all levels. So we decided to call this a 'Handbook' too, and to ask Routledge if they would like to publish it. We were delighted when they agreed to do so, and we are grateful for the commitment that Grace McInnes and her team have given to this project.

We think the time is right for such a book, not only because of the wealth and variety of activity that now takes place under the umbrella of children and young people's participation, but also because it is a field, to use a resonant phrase, 'in search of definition'. We do not claim to offer any conclusive answer to this quest, but we do hope that, with our many contributors, we have assembled something that will assist in that process of definition. Our aim has been to achieve a better understanding of the diverse ways in which the participation of children and young people is understood and enacted across the world.

As Gerison Lansdown reminds us in the opening chapter, there has been a huge growth of activity under the heading of children and young people's participation in the past 20 years and, of all the factors that have come together to produce this upsurge, the most obvious is the influence of the United Nations Convention on the Rights of the Child (CRC). The CRC encompasses an extensive range of rights, social and economic as well as civil and political, the implications of which vary in different countries. Unlike earlier declarations, the CRC asserts children's right to have a voice in decision making, as well as rights to freedom of thought and expression, and states that have ratified the CRC (that is, nearly every state in the world) are committed to implementing those rights and are accountable for doing so.

Another factor in promoting the interest in children's participation has been the development of social theories that see children as social actors in their own right, not simply as objects of socialisation. Such theories also remind us that childhood is not a universal given, but varies in its construction, interpretation and enactment across different cultures and contexts. The same, we think, applies to children's participation. For children in the minority or 'Western' world, subject to the discipline and segregation of schooling and living in increasingly commodified and 'virtual' worlds, 'participation' offers the possibility of realising a sense of citizenship and inclusion through active involvement in local decision making, although such processes are sometimes distant from children's everyday lives. For children in the majority world, 'participation' is often as much about survival, meeting their basic needs and contributing to their family and community, as it is about choice and self-realisation; at the same time, as we see in the following pages, some of the most striking examples of young people's empowerment and capacity for leadership emanate from the majority world.

Both majority and minority worlds offer examples of 'participation' work that can be seen as a real force for change, enhancing the effectiveness of projects and services, improving communities and promoting inclusion and citizenship. Equally, both worlds have seen critiques of 'participation' as providing a masquerade of political accountability, a smokescreen for inaction and an illusion of empowerment. Participation seen as consultation or 'having a say' has often resulted in little changing, as adults continue to make decisions without taking real account of children's views or giving them an effective part in decision-making processes.

Article 12 of the CRC reads:

1   States Parties shall assure to the child who is capable of forming his or her own views the right to express those views freely in all matters affecting the child, the views of the child being given due weight in accordance with the age and maturity of the child.
2   For this purpose, the child shall in particular be provided the opportunity to be heard in any judicial and administrative proceedings affecting the child, either directly, or through a representative or an appropriate body, in a manner consistent with the procedural rules of national law.

Apart from the moot points around 'the child who is capable of forming his or her own views' and 'given due weight in accordance with the age and maturity of the child', which have been much discussed, this statement has two possible limitations as a foundation for children and young people's participation. First, the phrase 'the child', and the formulation of Part 2 of the Article, may be taken to imply that only individual and private matters are concerned. Some (e.g. Nigel Cantwell) have argued that this was the intention of the drafters, and that it is illegitimate and unwise to seek to extend its meaning. Others (e.g. Gerison Lansdown) counter that the article is clearly open to a wider interpretation, and that it should be used positively to support public and collective forms of participation. Although we incline to the latter view, we also see the difficulty. Second, Article 12 only talks about 'views'; it is arguable – indeed, it is argued in this Handbook – that participation involves more than simply expressing 'views', and that it also encompasses various forms of action. We argue in the Conclusion that, while Article 12 provides an essential foundation for participatory initiatives of all kinds, it is not by itself a sufficient basis for the kind of development which we, and many of our contributors, want to see in the future.

Although there have been immense advances in the practice of children's participation (some of them displayed in this volume), we still lack a credible and coherent body of theory to inform this practice. As Karen Malone and Catherine Hartung point out in their chapter, the practice of participation has been informed by a wide range of theoretical sources, yet participation lacks its own distinctive theoretical framework, and the theories that have been drawn upon are often not especially child centred. In some ways, practice has outstripped theory. In part, this is the result of the diverse contexts and realms in which children (and adults) seek to participate, but equally it is a consequence of the divergence of views about how children's participation is, or should be, interpreted and enacted. Recently a number of writers have been working to address this gap, and some of the contributions to this volume attempt to take this process further. However, there is some way to go before a comprehensive theory of children's participation can be advanced.

Amid the ambiguity and uncertainty about what we mean by participation, there is a growing awareness that it is most meaningful when it is rooted in children's everyday lives. As demand grows for evidence of the impacts and benefits of children's participation in decision making, attention turns towards the individual and social processes involved, as much as the formal 'political' effects. We see in some of the following chapters that the need for participation is often a response to 'structural violence' – abuse, neglect, discrimination and conflict. The conclusion we draw, along with many contributors to this volume, is that relying on adults to take account of children's views is insufficient to ensure children's participation rights. If children are to achieve real benefits in their own lives and their communities, and create a better future, they can only do this by being active citizens, articulating their own values, perspectives, experiences and visions for the future, using these to inform and take action in their own right and, where necessary, contesting with those who have power over their lives.

Our intention in this text is not to provide definitive answers to all these contested issues, and certainly not to produce a definitive theory of children's participation. Rather, as we struggle to untangle the contradictions and paradoxes in our own thinking, we hope to contribute by drawing together thinking and practice from different settings and contexts, to enable some collective consideration of where we have come from, where we are now, and where we may be heading. The task we set ourselves was threefold:

1   to open a window, as wide as possible, on some of the practice currently taking place;
2   to give a platform to some of the critical work currently being done to theorise participation;
3   and to create a space for dialogue – between theory and practice, between what we may call the majority and minority worlds, and between adults and young people.

The process of planning the book was as open and collaborative as we could make it. At an early stage in the planning process, after informal discussion with the publishers, we issued an open call for proposed contributions, via personal contacts and email distribution lists, as well as approaching a few contributors directly. In the five weeks during which the call was open, we received 150 initial offers of contributions from all over the world. Each potential contributor was invited to provide a 150-word abstract, and in total some 70 did so. From these we identified 42 contributions whom we either definitely wanted to include or who we considered to have potential. These contributors were invited to produce fuller outlines of their proposed chapters. Other colleagues were asked to amend their abstracts, or asked whether they would provide commentaries (see below). When all responses had been received a further selection was made, and a formal proposal was put to the publisher.

The reason for planning the book in this way was both to reflect our belief in participation as a method and approach, and also to create a space in which those working in the field of children and young people's participation could engage in dialogue over its meaning and purpose. We were delighted to receive such a strong and enthusiastic response; from the beginning it gave us a high degree of confidence, which we hope others will share, in the quality and range of the contributions. The offers which we did not accept were in many cases of equal quality, but of less direct relevance to the project. We excluded many from the UK, partly because we did not want the book to be dominated by UK concerns. We also took an early decision that the book would *not* be about children and young people's participation in research. In part, this was because there were so many potential contributions in this category that it was clear to us that the topic merited a separate book. (Although there are a few chapters which are based on participatory research projects, the focus is always on wider notions of participation as developmental practice.)

We think that the range of material, from theory, and especially from practice, that we have collected here is reflective of the range of work being done around the globe. That is not to claim that it is comprehensive. There is much work of significance that is not represented here, often because people did not hear about the project in time, or because it did not suit them to contribute for a variety of reasons. In the spirit of collaboration and dialogue that has governed our work on the Handbook, we invited other colleagues to contribute commentaries on particular sections of the book. These include a significant number of young people, which helps to redress the predominance of adult authors in the main chapters. We later invited contributions from children and young people in non-written forms, and as a result are able to include the work of the young consultants of Santa Martha which follows chapter 20. Finally, we invited authors to exchange drafts and discuss their chapters during the editing process, particularly those who were contributing to the same sections of the book, and we are glad that some, at least, were able to take up this opportunity, within the constraints of time and workload which affect us all.

Outline of the Handbook

Caesar divided Gaul into three main parts, to make it more easily governable. We have done the same with this book, in order to make it easier – for us as editors and for you as readers – to manage its size and complexity.

Part I sets the context, with three chapters whose aim is to reflect critically on the current state of play in children and young people's participation, on what has been achieved and on the challenges that remain. Gerison Lansdown takes the CRC as her starting point and considers what is needed in order to make the Article 12 rights a reality for children in all settings and all nations, and to overcome the political and ideological barriers that lie in the way. Karen Malone and Catherine Hartung explore the different theoretical frameworks and models that underlie thinking about children's participation, and look at some examples of actual practice by young people that may test accepted views of the subject. Sarah White and Shyamol Choudhury begin with a story from a children's organisation in Bangladesh, and use this to question the meaning of children's agency in particular structures and cultures – in this case, one characterised by violence.

Part II is a very substantial bringing together of reflections on practical experiences of *doing* participation. Because of its size (23 chapters in total) we further divided and subdivided it according to the themes that characterise the chapters. For each subsection we also invited one commentator (or group of commentators) from the minority world and one from the majority world to provide critically reflective commentaries. (Not all of the latter were able to contribute in the time available.) Where possible these included perspectives from young people. The first section looks at different *contexts for practice*. The first subsection, 'Working in particular situations', includes an account of children's participation in peace building in Bosnia-Herzegovina, Guatemala, Nepal and Uganda by Clare Feinstein, Annette Giertsen and Claire O'Kane (with contributions from children and young people); Patricia Ray's reflections on participation of children living in particularly difficult situations; and an analysis by Lucy Jamieson and Wanjirũ Mũkoma of children's participation in the law reform process in South Africa. The commentary is by Fran Farrar, Talha Ghannam, Jake Manning and Ellie Munro from England's National Youth Agency. The second subsection, 'Working with particular groups', features Priscilla Alderson's reflections on individual participation by younger children; a critique by Kate Martin and Anita Franklin of disabled children's participation (or lack of it); Ann Dadich's account of participation among young people with mental health issues in self-help groups; and an examination of children's participation in 'family group conferences' by Perpetua Kirby and Sophie Laws. The combined commentary is by Alessandro Martelli, Rita Bertozzi and Nicola De Luigi from Italy and Anita Mathew from India. The third subsection, 'Working in particular cultural contexts', begins with a snapshot of a very large project by Jan Mason and Natalie Bolzan in Australia with colleagues in China, India, Sri Lanka and Thailand, looking at understandings of children's participation in different cultures. The other chapters are by Afua Twum-Danso, on the construction of childhood and CRC rights in Ghana; and by Yolanda Corona Caraveo, Carlos Perez and Julián Hernández on participation in indigenous traditional communities in Mexico. The commentary is by Manfred Liebel and Iven Saadi from Germany, who also work in Latin America.

The second section is about *approaches to practice*. The first subsection, 'Methods and frameworks', includes chapters by Vicky Johnson on promoting rights through children's involvement in evaluation in Nepal, South Africa and the UK; Renate Kränzl-Nagl and Ulrike Zartler on a cross-European project to promote children's participation in schools and communities; Tiina Sotkasiira, Lotta Haikkola and Liisa Horelli on a learning-based network approach to youth participation in Finland; and Anna Skeels and Anne Crowley on attempts to measure the impact of participation in Wales. The commentary is by Janet Batsleer from England. The second subsection, 'Strategies and practices', features a reflection by Kirrily Pells on ways to challenge obstacles to the participation of children and young people in Rwanda; an account by Lalatendu Acharya of the 'child reporters' phenomenon in Orissa; Harry Shier's report of the work of young 'promotores' and 'promotoras' in Nicaragua; and an analysis by Hiromi Yamashita and Lynn Davies of how students acquired status as 'professionals' in some English secondary schools. The combined commentary is from two groups of young people facilitated by Rachel Henderson in England and Maha Damaj in Lebanon. The third subsection, 'Spaces and structures', begins with Sara Austin's account of children's participation in citizenship and governance in India, Latin America and the Philippines. This is followed by no fewer than three critiques of 'official' youth participation in the UK: Brian McGinley and Ann Grieve on youth councils in Scotland, Alan Turkie on the UK Youth Parliament and Jack Lewars on the weaknesses of 'student voice' in schools. The section concludes with Fahriye Sancar and Yucel Severcan's inspiring account of participation in a youth organisation in Turkey. Our final commentary is by Colin Williams, Jessica Edlin and Fiona Beals from New Zealand.

Part III of the Handbook explores new ways of thinking about children and young people's participation, with five chapters that in different ways aim to offer fresh theoretical perspectives on the subject. Robyn Fitzgerald, Anne Graham, Anne Smith and Nicola Taylor explore children's participation as a *struggle over recognition*, using this as a theoretical tool to foreground the importance of dialogue and reflect 'the complex interplay between agency and power'. Tom Cockburn and Kay Tisdall each explore the relationship between participation, governance and democratic processes, from different but complementary angles: Cockburn's focus is on children's engagement with deliberative democratic mechanisms, and on the potential and the limitations of this approach, while Tisdall uses theories of governance to consider the potential of schools as deliberative spaces for children and young people. Greg Mannion also focuses on ideas of space and dialogue, using geographical and post-structuralist theories to understand how relations between children, young people and adults can be improved through changes to the spaces they inhabit. Finally, Joachim Theis brings theory back to practice, and makes a powerful argument for a children's *citizenship* that encompasses both civil rights and civic engagement.

We would like to express our gratitude to all our contributors and to those who assisted them, to the many other friends and colleagues who supported us in this enterprise, and to our partners and families. All royalties from the book will be invested in a fund to support the participation of young people in dialogue and debate.

References

Franklin, B. (1995) *Handbook of Children's Rights*, London: Routledge.
Franklin, B. (2002) *The New Handbook of Children's Rights*, London: Routledge.

Note

Many contributors refer to Roger Hart's 'ladder of participation' for children and young people, originally published in Hart, R. (1992) *Children's Participation: from tokenism to citizenship*, Florence: Unicef. This is out of print but can be downloaded from www.unicef-irc.org.

Many contributors also refer to the United Nations Convention on the Rights of the Child. This is reproduced in many sources, but an authoritative version is available on the website of the Office of the United Nations High Commissioner on Human Rights at www.unhchr.ch/html/menu3/b/k2crc.htm (accessed 4 July 2009).

Part I
Children's participation
Progress and challenges

1 The realisation of children's participation rights

Critical reflections

Gerison Lansdown

Children's participation has been one of the most debated and examined aspects of the Convention on the Rights of the Child since it was adopted by the UN in 1989. Books have been written, research has been undertaken, thousands of initiatives have been introduced, and spaces for children's voices have been created, from the school to the global community. Children have been engaged in advocacy, social and economic analysis, campaigning, research, peer education, community development, political dialogue, programme and project design and development, and democratic participation in schools. The last 20 years have been a period of both advocacy to promote and legitimate the concept of participation, and exploration of strategies for translating it into practice. Indeed, for many people, children's rights have become synonymous with participation. What is now needed is a stronger focus on the application of that learning to embed participation as a sustainable right for all children, in all areas of their lives. In order to achieve this goal, we need to go back to the Convention on the Rights of the Child and analyse carefully the rights it embodies and the specific obligations it therefore imposes on governments. Child participation will never become a reality without holding governments fully to account for introducing the necessary legislation, policy and practice to ensure that children are enabled to claim their right to be heard and be taken seriously in all decisions affecting them. We also need to reflect on the learning from the considerable body of experience gained over the years since the Convention was adopted, to address challenges that are unique to children's participation and to explore how they can be met.

The need for clarity of definition

Despite its widespread usage, there remains considerable lack of clarity about what is actually meant by participation in the context of children's rights. The problem is in part triggered by the fact that the term 'participation' is widely used, at least in the English-speaking world, to describe forms of social engagement. Children participate in a conversation, in games, in cultural activities, in contributing to the economic security of the family. Participation is part of belonging within a family or community. However, in the context of the Convention on the Rights of the Child, it has come to be applied as a shorthand for the right embodied in Article 12 to express views freely and have them taken seriously, along with the other key

civil rights to freedom of expression, religion, conscience, association and information, and the right to privacy. In other words, its meaning is much more specific.
And if advocacy to promote children's right to participation is to be effective, it is
imperative that it is grounded in a clear understanding of the scope of the relevant
rights in the Convention and the obligations they impose on governments.

Article 12 applies to every child 'capable of forming his or her own views'.
Children from the very youngest ages are able to form views, even where they
are not able to communicate them verbally. There should be no lower age limit
on the right to participate, and it should not be limited to the expression of views
in 'adult' language. Research reveals that tiny babies speak a complex 'language'
and that adults who can 'read' it can provide more sensitive and appropriate
care.[1] Implementation of Article 12 requires recognition of and respect for non-
verbal forms of communication such as play, body language, facial expression, or
drawing and painting, through which very young children make choices, express
preferences and demonstrate understanding of their environment.

Children have the 'right to express those views freely'. Children, particularly
girls, younger children and children with disabilities, are often denied opportunities to express their views freely. Free expression of views by children necessitates
a commitment to a cultural change, in which adults begin to recognise the importance of listening to and respecting children. In order to contribute their views,
children need access to appropriate information and to safe 'spaces' where they
are afforded the time, encouragement and support to enable them to develop and
articulate their views.

Children are entitled to express their views 'in all matters affecting' them. Most
aspects of decision making, from the family to the international level, have either a
direct or an indirect impact on children and can therefore be defined as legitimate
matters of concern: for example, schooling, transport, budget expenditure, urban
planning, poverty reduction or social protection.

The views of the child must be 'given due weight in accordance with the age and
maturity of the child'. It is not sufficient to listen to children. It is also necessary
to give their views serious consideration when making decisions. Their concerns,
perspectives and ideas must inform decisions that affect their lives. By requiring
that attention is given to both age and maturity, Article 12 makes clear that age on
its own should not be used to limit the significance accorded to children's views.
Children's level of understanding is far from uniformly linked to age. Considerable
evidence exists to indicate that information, experience, social and cultural expectations and levels of support all contribute to the development of children's capacities (Lansdown 2005). Maturity, which implies the ability to understand and assess
the implications of a particular decision, must therefore be considered.

In addition, Article 12 addresses the right to be heard in 'judicial and administrative proceedings affecting them'. This applies to court proceedings such as
custody or child protection proceedings, as well as administrative proceedings
dealing with, for example, education appeals, public planning or social security. It
applies both to proceedings which are initiated by the child, such as a complaint
against ill-treatment, or appeal against a school exclusion, as well as to those
initiated by others in which the child has an interest, such as parental separation

or adoption. Children are also entitled to be heard 'either directly or through a representative or appropriate body'.

Overall, then, Article 12 elaborates the child's right to be involved and taken seriously in decision making, and it requires governments to *assure* the realisation of this right to every child. Four levels of involvement can be identified in the decision-making process: to be informed; to express an informed view; to have that view taken into account; to be the main or joint decision maker (Alderson and Montgomery 1996). Article 12 implies that all children capable of forming a view are entitled to the first three levels; it does not extend rights to the fourth level. In other words, it embodies the presumption that adults retain responsibility for the actual decision, while being informed and influenced by the views of the child.

However, although most of the discourse to date has focused on Article 12, it is necessary to look at other articles in the Convention in order to gain a real understanding of the concept of participation as a human right. Article 5 elaborates the status of children in relation to the adults who have responsibility for them. It emphasises that any direction and guidance provided by parents or other caregivers must be 'in accordance with the child's evolving capacities' and support the 'exercise by the child of his or her rights'. This provision is significant in two respects. It introduces the recognition that it is the child who exercises his or her own rights. It also emphasises that the level of adult support needed to enable the child to do so must take account of the capacities of the individual child. In other words, it implies a transfer of responsibility for decision making from responsible adults to children, as the child acquires the competence, and of course willingness, to do so. It therefore entitles children to engage at the fourth level of decision making. The rights to freedom of expression, religion, conscience and association can also be exercised directly by the child once they have the capacity to do so.

Taken together, these rights, together with the right to information, can be understood as constituting the right to participation. Participation is a fundamental human right in itself. It is also a means through which to realise other rights. It recognises children as citizens entitled and – with differing degrees of capacity according to their environment, age and circumstances – able to contribute towards decisions that affect them, as individuals, as specific groups of children such as girls or working children, and as a constituency. Any advocacy to promote children's participation must be rooted in a clear understanding of how the Convention on the Rights of the Child elaborates the concept and the explicit obligations it imposes on governments.

The need to hold governments to account

The realisation of children's participation rights involves the transition of children from the status of passive recipients to respect as active agents. It necessitates a transfer of greater power for children to have influence in their lives. However, despite the many initiatives that have evolved in all regions of the world, this shift in status continues to be an unfulfilled aspiration for most children. It cannot be realised through piecemeal initiatives on the ground, however innovative and radical. Projects and programmes which create spaces for children's participation are important but not sufficient. On their own, they are not sustainable, they rarely engage very young children, they do little to address the rights of individual children to exercise their right to be heard and they can only ever engage a small proportion of the children in any society. Furthermore, the opportunity to participate is usually dependent on the goodwill of the adults involved in the child's life – an initiative within a local authority or NGO, willingness on the part of a school to establish a school council, an enlightened doctor willing to provide a child with information and listen to and respect their views. Meaningful and sustained realisation of children's participation rights requires the introduction of a wide range of legislative, policy and practice provisions which establish both entitlement and the opportunity to hold governments and others to account to realise that entitlement. This would include, for example:[2]

*   *Legal entitlements* – for example, complaints mechanisms, access to the courts and to legal aid, definition of parental responsibilities in family law, entitlement to establish school councils, introduction of ages of consent, prohibition on early marriage or female genital mutilation, lowering of voting ages.
*   *Systematic provision of information on rights for children of all ages and abilities* – for example, human rights education in schools, child-friendly information on what to expect in hospital, child-friendly consultative documents from governments. Children cannot exercise their rights unless they have access to information in a form which they can use and understand.
*   *Sensitisation and awareness raising of adults* – pre- and in-service training on the rights of children for all professionals working with and for children, and parent education programmes.
*   *Systemic mechanisms for influencing public decisions at all levels* – development of child-friendly and collaborative public services, support for child-led organisations, peer education, access to the media, community mobilisation, child representation on local and national policy-making bodies, and consistent access to government to enable dialogue on all relevant aspects of policy development.
*   *Mechanisms for remedy and redress* – children need to be able to challenge violations of their rights through complaints procedures or through access to the courts when necessary.

Of course, one of the challenges facing advocates for children's participation is the lack of opportunities for meaningful participation for any citizens in many countries. Where there is no freedom of the press, no multi-party system, no independent judiciary, limited access to the courts, no devolution of power from the centre, no independence for women, no political accountability or transparency, weak civil society institutions and no history of any form of consultative democratic processes at national or local levels, it is difficult to establish mechanisms for sustained or meaningful participation of adults. And the barriers are usually far greater for children. In many cultures, children, and more particularly girls, are expected to be silent in the presence of adults. They are not encouraged to express their views at home, in school or in community gatherings. Asking questions or challenging adult opinions is strongly disapproved of. It may be possible to achieve *ad hoc* meetings with government, or small-scale initiatives to give children a voice, but these processes do little to change the fundamental status of children or provide them with any realistic avenues through which to challenge violations or neglect of their rights. In these contexts, little will change unless considerable investment is made in working with adults to sensitise them to children's participation rights and the positive impact of their realisation. Furthermore, in addition to continuing to create opportunities for children's participation, it is also important to build partnerships with other social movements and human rights initiatives to ensure that children's rights are reflected in, and are a part of, any broader advocacy for greater democracy and participation.

The need to face the challenges in realising children's right to participation

The presumption of children's incapacities

Beyond the lack of recognition of children's right to be heard is a lack of understanding that children have the capacities to contribute to decision making. Too often, adults underestimate children's capacities or fail to appreciate the value of their perspectives, because they are not expressed in ways which would be used by adults.

Our knowledge, to date, as to children's capacities for informed and rational decision making in their own lives remains limited. A very considerable body of research has been undertaken to identify predetermined physiological or psychological factors linking age with the acquisition of competencies. However, it is important to acknowledge that this research is undertaken almost exclusively in North America and Europe, and largely in laboratory conditions, away from children's day-to-day lives.[3] Significantly, even within these parameters, there is wide-ranging variation in findings across the research. And there are inadequate comparative data looking at the contrasting competencies of children in differing social, economic and cultural environments. Indeed, a growing body of recent research suggests the need for extreme caution in drawing conclusions on age-related competencies, arguing instead that a wide range of other factors influence how children function. To date, developmental psychology has failed to provide scientifically valid prescriptive yardsticks against which children's evolving capacities can be evaluated (Woodhead 1997). Bronfenbrenner, for example, has urged the need to look at the environment or setting in which a child develops, as well as at the child him- or herself, and has criticised research which studies children only briefly, in strange situations and with unfamiliar people (Bronfenbrenner 1979).

Recent research into children's own perspectives and experiences indicates that adults do consistently underestimate children's capacities. This failure takes different forms in different cultural contexts. In many developing societies, children are acknowledged as having the capacity to take on high levels of social and economic responsibility. However, their rights to negotiate those contributions or to exercise autonomous choices are likely to be more restricted. In most Western societies, on the other hand, while, in theory, a high premium is placed on civil and political liberties and autonomy, children are denied opportunities for participation in decision making and the exercise of responsibility in many areas of their lives, because of extended social and economic dependency and an enhanced perception of the need for protection. This, in turn, reduces opportunities for developing the capacities for emerging autonomy, which then serves to justify their exclusion from decision making. A downward spiral is thus created.

Obviously, many children's physical immaturity, relative inexperience and lack of knowledge do render them vulnerable and necessitate specific protections. However, it seems clear that children are widely denied opportunities for decision making in accordance with their evolving capacities. Neither legal frameworks nor policy and practice in most countries throughout the world give sufficient consideration to the importance of recognising and respecting the real capacities of children. Given these widespread adult perceptions of both children's status and their capacities, there is a great deal of work to be done to strengthen awareness and build skills in children's participation. Initiatives often fail because the adults working with children do not recognise or promote children's potential contribution and, consequently, fail to relinquish their control over children in favour of an approach based on partnership or collaboration. It is not enough to work with children. Investment needs to be made with adults if children's participation is to be attainable as a goal.

Participation and the nature of childhood

The fact of children's childhood status does impact on the nature of their participation. In general, once the members of a community feel empowered, they can advocate for themselves in claiming their rights. However, the same is not true of children. Although children can be powerful and effective advocates for their own rights, given appropriate access to information, space and opportunity, their youth and their relatively powerless status mean that they can only sustain this role where there are adults to facilitate the process. In a recent study of child participation across South Asia, for example, children involved in projects and programmes, even those led by children themselves, highlighted a continuing need for support from adults in respect of access to information, administrative help, access to policy makers, maintaining a skills base and counselling and advice (UNICEF ROSA 2004). Autonomous activity on the part of children is not, in most instances, a realistic goal and therefore necessitates a longer-term commitment on the part of supporting adults, and recognition that, without their continued involvement, the activity will not be sustained. This continuing dependence on adults, and children's lack of power and relative vulnerability, does expose them to a greater potential for exploitation or manipulation. It places a greater onus of responsibility on agencies working with children to guarantee adherence to ethical principles, monitored by children, to protect against such abuse.

In addition, whereas other marginalised groups, for example, ethnic minorities or indigenous peoples, remain part of that constituency throughout their lives, children do not. They grow up and cease to be children. Women, for example, can continue in self-advocacy on behalf of women throughout their lives. But children can only advocate for themselves during the limited period of their childhood. As soon as they reach adulthood, many of the factors contributing to their vulnerability to abuse, such as the lack of franchise or legal capacity, diminish. If they are also, for example, members of an indigenous community, they can continue to press for their rights in that capacity, but not from the perspective of children. Because the specific rights violations associated with childhood are time-limited, there is a constant process of haemorrhaging of older children, and newly emerging cohorts of younger children needing support. This pattern has major implications for the ongoing investment to support children's participation.

Building sustainable, community-based participation

Much of the emphasis in child participation has involved facilitating children's access to high-level events in order that their views can be heard by those in a position to take action. The critique of the frequent failure to build sustainable links between these activities and the children's own local communities has been well rehearsed. It is a phenomenon which is probably unique to the situation of children. Comparable difficulties are less likely to arise with adults, because it is easier for them to organise themselves from the grassroots and form their own associations and networks. It raises three key, linked issues of concern. First, it can lead to a lack of legitimacy. Selecting children to participate in these events engenders a tension between, on the one hand, a commitment to creating opportunities for participation and, on the other hand, the obligation to ensure that the development process is locally owned by children themselves. It is important to ensure that children have access to politicians and policy makers. Yet creating this access through locally owned routes is difficult when children do not, in the main, have their own organisations or networks through which this can happen. Children experience greater challenges in forging the necessary building blocks to ensure a continuity of dialogue between themselves as individuals and their peers, and consequent legitimacy for their involvement. There is a need, therefore, to support the development of child-led initiatives at local level which can serve to generate cohorts of children able and mandated to speak on behalf of their peers.

The second challenge is to avoid replicating existing power structures. Children's participation provides opportunities for them to challenge power elites and structures which serve to oppress them and, in so doing, to render them more accountable. The pattern of plucking children from their local environment and offering them access to national, regional and global policy arenas risks creating groups of children who are equally unaccountable to the constituencies from which they come. Where this happens, participation is serving to *replicate* rather than *challenge* those power structures. This process is not inevitable: there are some very positive examples of building structures from which children can contribute from a mandated base, such as the child clubs in Nepal (Save the Children Norway/Save the Children US 2002). However, there are also examples of the creation of 'child professionals' who have no sustained links with local, regional or national networks of children. At the same time, it is also important not to demand from children a level of accountability and representation which is not equally demanded of adults. Children are more vulnerable to such criticisms because the legitimacy of their presence in those arenas is less well established.

Finally, without grassroots structures, children are sometimes used to comply with adult agendas. The pressure on organisations to be seen to be promoting children's participation in public arenas can and does sometimes lead to an inappropriate precedence being given to involving children in high-level events, at the expense of building sustainable participation within local communities. In such cases, there is a danger that it is the organisation's agenda that is being prioritised, with children as passive recipients of adult manipulation, rather than as social actors empowered to claim their rights.

Providing appropriate protection

The struggle for justice and respect for human rights, in which marginalised members of the community begin to challenge traditional power bases, can expose those people to risk. When women tackle their lack of economic or political power, it can be perceived as a threat by those who currently hold power. This can and often does lead to retaliation. For children, who are usually the most vulnerable members of society, the risks are even greater, particularly in social environments where there is little or no acceptance of children expressing their views. It is also necessary to recognise that there can be unintended and negative consequences to involving children as social actors engaged in claiming their rights. It is possible that children may lose as much as they gain. Some of these risks are inevitable and unavoidable. There can be no change without risk, no struggle without costs.

Nevertheless, it is important to acknowledge that there is a higher duty of care than when working with adults. For example, whereas adults can make informed choices for themselves as to the nature of risk that they take, children, particularly younger children, may be less able to do so. It is necessary to balance the right to participation with the right to protection, recognising that it can be as harmful to make excessive or inappropriate expectations of children as to deny them the right to take part in decisions they are capable of making (for example, Harper and Marcus 1997; WCRWC 2001).

Erring too far on the side of protection denies children the right to be heard, inhibits opportunities to develop their capacities for participation and, indeed, can serve, perversely, to heighten risk. For example, much research testifies to the failure of many adult-designed strategies for protecting children (Boyden and Mann 2000). Denying policy makers the benefits of children's experience and expertise can and does lead to poor decisions, which may themselves expose children to harm. Furthermore, excluding young people from access to information (for example, on reproductive health) on grounds of 'protection' is more likely to increase their chances of vulnerability to pregnancy and HIV/AIDS. Over-protection can serve to heighten vulnerability by failing to equip children with the information and experience they need so as to make informed choices in their lives. Protective approaches that make children dependent on adult support leave children without resources when those adult protections are withdrawn (Myers and Boyden 2001). And the scale of many national crises is undermining traditional family and community networks that served to protect children's well-being and development. In these environments, there is an acute need to harness children's own potential strengths in order to maximise their opportunities for survival and development. It is worth bearing in mind that the vulnerability of children derives, in some part, not from their lack of capacity, but rather, from their lack of power and status with which to exercise their rights and challenge abuses.

Of course, children are entitled to protections associated with their youth and relative vulnerability. Promoting opportunities for participation, without appropriate recognition of the potential risks involved, may lay children open, for example, to harmful exposure in the media, to government retribution, or to punishment or retaliation by their family or employer. The obligation, in Article 3 of the Convention, to ensure that in all actions 'the best interests of the child shall be a primary consideration' is often applied as the basis on which to assess how the balance should be judged. However, it is important to acknowledge that the application of the concept of 'best interests' is not an unmitigated benefit for children. Any overview of the history of adult treatment of children reveals the extent to which adults have repeatedly acted towards children, in the name of their best interests, in ways which have been harmful – for example, severing children's contact with 'guilty' partners on marriage breakdown, placing children in large institutions, using physical and humiliating punishments and imposing female genital mutilation have all been defended as acceptable and beneficial treatment of children by adults with responsibilities for their care. The best interests principle does not 'trump' other rights in the Convention and so should not be used to override the child's right to express views. Indeed, consideration of the child's views must be an integral part of determining the child's best interests, and in any decision made by adults as to the best interests of the child due weight must be given to the child's expressed wishes in accordance with his or her age and maturity. Without explicit recognition that assessment of children's best interests must be directed towards the realisation of their rights and take serious account of children's own views, it can be used as a powerful tool in the hands of adults to defend any action or decision made on behalf of children.

There is growing evidence that children are capable of exercising agency and utilising their own resources and strengths in developing strategies for their protection. Furthermore, active recognition of and support for children's engagement enhances their developmental capacities. Achieving an appropriate balance between participation and protection in any programme will necessitate assessment of a range of factors, including the capacities of the child, the levels of risk involved, the degree of support available, the child's level of understanding of the nature of the risks involved and, of course, the child's own views.

The need for indicators to measure participation

Two approaches to measurement of children's participation are needed, if it is to be possible to evaluate progress and realise their active and effective engagement in the decisions that affect them as individuals, as groups and as a constituency. First, it is important to identify key indicators or benchmarks against which to evaluate evidence of a cultural climate in which the right of children to be heard and taken seriously is firmly established. The measures outlined earlier in this chapter as needed to hold governments to account provide a comprehensive starting point for these benchmarks.

Second, it is necessary to be able to measure the extent, quality and impact of the actual participation in which children are engaged (Lansdown 2004). Without such measurement, it is not possible to engage in any critical appraisal of what is being done in the name of participation or, indeed, of whether it is actually impacting on the lives of children. Most significantly, children themselves must be directly involved in any processes to evaluate what participation is taking place.

The *extent* of children's actual engagement can be assessed by considering the level of their involvement alongside the point at which they become involved. For example, children's participation can be broadly classified at three levels.

- *Consultative participation.* This is where adults seek children's views in order to build knowledge and understanding of their lives and experience. While it is adult led and managed, and does not involve sharing or transferring decision-making processes to children themselves, it does recognise that children have expertise and perspectives which need to inform adult decision making. Consultation is an appropriate means of enabling children to express views, for example, when undertaking research, in planning processes, in developing legislation, policy or services, or in decisions affecting individual children within the family, in health care or in education, or as witnesses in judicial or administrative proceedings.

- *Collaborative participation.* This provides a greater degree of partnership between adults and children, with the opportunity for active engagement at any stage of a decision, initiative, project or service. Children can be involved in designing and undertaking research, policy development, peer education and counselling, participation in conferences, or in representation on boards or committees. Individual decisions within the family, in education and in health care can also be collaborative rather than consultative, and involve children more fully in decision-making processes. Collaborative participation provides opportunity for shared decision making with adults, and for children to influence both the process and the outcomes in any given activity.

- *Child-led participation.* This takes place when children are afforded the space and opportunity to identify issues of concern, initiate activities and advocate for themselves. Children can initiate action as individuals, for example, in choosing a school, seeking medical advice, pressing for the realisation of their rights through the courts, or utilising complaints mechanisms, or as a group through establishing and managing their own organisations for the purposes of policy analysis, advocacy, awareness raising, through peer representation and education, and use of and access to the media. The role of adults in child-led participation is to act as facilitators to enable children to pursue their own objectives, through provision of information, advice and support.

All three levels are appropriate in different contexts, and initiatives which begin at a consultative level can evolve to enable children to take more control as they acquire confidence and skills. For example, a local authority may decide to consult children on a regular basis on aspects of policy and planning. As the children become more familiar with the governmental processes, they may seek to establish their own council or local parliament through which to take a more proactive and representative approach to bringing issues of concern to the notice of politicians. In respect of public participation, all three levels can also engage children at different points of decision-making processes. Whether children play an active role in situation analyses, planning, programme design, implementation or monitoring and evaluation will have a significant impact on the degree of influence they are able to exert. Overall, therefore, in order to measure the extent of children's engagement, these two dimensions relating to the level of participation and the point of entry need to be considered.

Second, the *quality* of children's participation must be assessed against a set of indicators relating to the principles or standards that are widely agreed to represent appropriate practice when working with children. Participation of children must be transparent, accompanied by appropriate information, voluntary, respectful, relevant, child friendly and enabling, inclusive, safe and sensitive to risk and accountable. The Save the Children Alliance practice standards provide a useful starting point in elaborating these principles (Save the Children 2005).

Finally, the *impact* of children's participation needs to be measured. In any individual initiative or activity, the indicators of effectiveness will need to be determined by the children, together with the relevant adults involved. They may include indicators of impact directly on the children themselves (for example, in terms of confidence, skills building or self-esteem), on the project or programme outcomes, on staff, parents or attitudes towards children within local communities, as well as on the broader realisation of the rights of children.

Conclusion

Achieving meaningful participation of children was never going to be easy. Even in democratic countries, the barriers are significant. Children are not generally viewed as citizens – and even for adults, opportunities for real engagement in active participatory democracy are limited. Creating space for children to be genuinely involved in decisions that affect them, therefore, does necessarily involve a long and continued struggle. The challenges are multiple. The legitimacy of children as social actors, entitled to be involved, has to be established. Attitudes towards recognition of children's capacities need to be reformed. New forms of, and opportunities for, democratic engagement have to be constructed, from the family, the school and the local community to the national political level. Entitlement to participate has to be embedded in legislation, policy and practice as the right of every child. This will all take time. During the first 20 years of the existence of the Convention on the Rights of the Child much of the investment by the child rights community focused on making the case for children's participation and seeking to render children visible in decision-making processes – involving them in projects and programmes, developing models of practice through which children can begin to influence the issues that matter to them in their daily lives, and demanding a place for children at national, regional and global events.

The most positive outcome of these multiple initiatives, from every region in the world, is that they do provide powerful testimony as to the capacities and desire of children to be more involved. There is now significantly greater recognition of the expertise and wisdom that children contribute to policy making. However, the numbers of children able to be involved in these processes have been extremely limited. The vast majority of the world's children have yet to have their participation rights realised. It is now time to reflect on the lessons learned from these experiences, analyse the most effective strategies for addressing the barriers and collaborate with children to capitalise on what we know to be the most effective approaches to achieving participation. However, most importantly, it is imperative that advocacy begins to focus more directly on holding governments to account to fulfil their obligations under the Convention, to build the infrastructure necessary to ensure that the right to participation is systematically upheld for all children, and in all areas of their lives. Fragmented, piecemeal initiatives instigated under the auspices of individuals or agencies are not enough. Real participation does involve a transfer of power to children. Achieving that transfer can only be achieved through the introduction of legal rights, means of redress and wide-ranging cultural change towards respect for children as rights holders, entitled to active participation in all the decisions that impact on their lives.

Notes

1 General Comment No. 7, Implementing Child Rights in Early Childhood (2005) CRC/C/GC/7.
2 UNCRC General Comment No. 12, Article 12 (forthcoming).
3 Although most of the research is still located in the North, there is increasing interest in these issues in developing countries and a corresponding emergence of informal studies, papers and booklets produced by both academics and NGOs.

References

Alderson, P. and Montgomery, J. (1996) *Health Care Choices: Sharing decisions with children*, London: Institute of Public Policy Research.
Boyden, J. and Mann, G. (2000) 'Children's risk, resilience and coping in extreme situations', background paper to the consultation on Children in Adversity, Refugee Studies Centre, Oxford, 9–12 September.
Bronfenbrenner, U. (1979) *The Ecology of Human Development: Experiments by nature and design*, Cambridge, MA: Harvard University Press.
Harper, C. and Marcus, R. (1997) *Child Poverty in Sub-Saharan Africa*, London: Save the Children.
Lansdown, G. (2004) 'Criteria for the evaluation of children's participation in programming', in Bernard van Leer Foundation (ed.), *Early Childhood Matters*, The Hague: Bernard van Leer Foundation.
Lansdown, G. (2005) *The Evolving Capacities of the Child*, Florence: UNICEF Innocenti Research Centre and Save the Children.

Myers, W. and Boyden, J. (2001) *Strengthening Children in Situations of Adversity*, Oxford: Refugee Studies Centre.

Save the Children (2005) *Practice Standards in Children's Participation*, London: Save the Children.

Save the Children Norway/Save the Children US (2002) *The Children's Clubs of Nepal: An assessment of national experiment in children's democratic development* , Kathmandu: Save the Children.

UNICEF ROSA (Regional Office of South Asia) (2004) *Wheel of Change: Children and young people's participation in South Asia*, Katmandu: UNICEF ROSA.

WCRWC (Women's Commission for Refugee Women and Children) (2001) *Against all the odds, surviving the war on adolescents: Promoting the protection and capacity of Ugandan and Sudanese adolescents in Northern Uganda*, New York: WCRCW, 2001.

Woodhead, M. (1997) *Is there a Place for Child Work in Child Development?*, Milton Keynes: Radda Barnen/Centre for Human Development and Learning, The Open University.

2 Challenges of participatory practice with children

Karen Malone and Catherine Hartung

Playing with power: children's participation in theory

> The politics of culture is not pre-determined. Culture is pliable; it is how it is used that matters.
>
> (Duncombe 2002: 2)

The culture of participation, and the role that theories have had in influencing thinking within the field of children's participation, are important to consider if we are to move forward in our approach to their participation. Theories and models are often used interchangeably in the discourse and practice of children's participation. Yet there are substantial differences that are often not distinguished in the literature. What we find is an overemphasis on 'what we did' stories and not much critique of 'why we did it' or 'what were the implications'. Without a theoretical framework, models or 'how to' guides have flourished, and it is not always clear what has informed their construction. Shier (2001) cites research by Barn and Franklin (1996) in the UK which found that Hart's ladder was regarded as the most influential model in framing thinking, along-side the theories of Paulo Freire. But they also commented that respondents said their work was based on 'general principles such as empowerment and respect for young people, rather than specific models or theories' (Shier 2001: 108).

We are talking here of the intellectual work that should reflect these very successful and innovative developments in practice. Theories drawn on from a variety of disciplines to inform the field of children's participation have mostly been adult- or community-based theories adapted to work with children. In fact this could be said for the majority of 'models' – including Hart's ladder, which originated from Arnstein's community participation model. Table 2.1 provides a quick survey of the variety of disciplines and theories drawn on to inform children's participation.

The majority of the theories draw on the structural organisation of children's participation within a formal setting. However, one area less theorised and evident in the literature is the notion of *child-initiated participation*. To ensure that children have the opportunity to participate in society in truly authentic ways, as 'active citizens', we need to reflect upon how formal participatory processes can inhibit children's organic participation. To understand this, it is helpful to consider Antonio Gramsci's notion of the 'organic intellectual' (1971). This refers to the development of individuals who, within the context of their community and through active struggle, obtain the expertise

Table 2.1 Theories informing children's participation

Discipline	Theories / conceptual frameworks	Examples of authors applying the theories
Child development	New sociology of childhood Social cognitive theory	James, Jenks and Prout (1998) Chawla and Heft (2001)
Cultural and social psychology	Social constructivism	Mason and Urquhart (2001)
Environmental psychology	Affordance Behaviour settings Ecological systems theory	Heft (1988) Chawla and Heft (2002) Kytta (2004)
Human geography	Geographies of exclusion Place attachment Geography of childhood Hybridity theory	Malone and Hasluck (2002) Holloway and Valentine (2000) Percy-Smith (2002) Nabhan and Trimble (1994) Malone and Tranter (2005)
Community development	Critical theory Pedagogy of oppressed Participatory action research	Crimmens and West (2004) Hart (1992) Malone (1996) Kruger (2000)
Environmental education	Ecological literacy Empowerment theory Nature deficit disorder Outdoor learning	Moore and Wong (1997) Hart (1992) Louv (2006) Malone (2007)
Educational sociology	Post-structuralism Critical theory	Gallagher (2008) McKendrick et al. (2000)
Urban planning	Learning by design Transformative theory	Moore and Wong (1997) Driskell (2002)

and consciousness to mobilise communities in actions for social change.[1] Gramsci argues that while all individuals have the intellectual and rational capacity to become 'intellectuals', not all are given this function by society. Alongside our 'traditional' intellectuals, he suggests there are 'organic' intellectuals within society who naturally emerge as the 'thinkers' within particular cultural groups. Through the 'spontaneous philosophy' of everyday existence, these organic intellectuals play a vital role in cultivating strategies for empowering their particular communities. He writes:

> There is not a human activity from which every form of intellectual participation can be excluded: *Homo faber* (man the maker) cannot be separated from *Homo sapiens* (man the thinker). Each man [or woman] outside of his professional activity, carries on some form of intellectual activity, that is, he [she] is a 'philosopher' … he [she] participates in a particular conception of the world, a conscious line of moral conduct, and therefore contributes to sustain a conception of the world or to modify it, that is, to bring into being new modes of thought.
>
> (Gramsci 1971: 9)

Another recent example is the work of Gallagher, who utilises the work of Michel Foucault and post-structural theory to unpack some of the myths around 'empowerment'. Gallagher (2008) points out that power dynamics in children's participation are much messier than is often explicated, and that power isn't something that children either possess or do not possess, but something that is fluid, dynamic, negotiated and contextual.

Such theoretical positions can offer insight into current conceptions of participatory projects with children. More specifically, the notion that participatory projects are only recognised when adults initiate them needs to be questioned, and recognition given to 'spontaneous inquiry' by children during their everyday cultural practices. As children are increasingly recognised as a legitimate cultural group in their own right, it is possible to see how they also produce their own thinking 'organically'. To foster children as organic intellectuals, we need to recognise that they have different criteria for what it means to participate, and that simply mimicking adults is not always the most authentic, empowering or beneficial type of participation. In order to provide, maintain or support participatory processes that are social, challenging and entertaining for children, we believe adults need to recognise the inherent power in the popular, networked and 'viral' everyday settings that children are currently constructing and reconstructing. A theory of children's participation should reflect this, and be generated from the field rather than applied from adult-centred theory building.

Roaming the realms: children's participation in practice

> Children are marginalised in adult-centred society. They experience unequal power relations with adults and much of their lives is controlled and limited by adults. The main complications do not arise from children's inabilities or misperceptions, but from the positions ascribed to children.
>
> (Alderson and Goodey 1996: 106)

Childhood is a social construction that varies over time and space. Historically, views of the 'Western' child have tended to see the child as lacking agency and in need of protection. In contrast 'majority world' children demonstrate significant abilities as capable citizens able to take on responsibilities and active roles in their communities. In the West this has given rise to a situation where children are often constrained by adults in their ability to be active in shaping their lives and communities, as adults seek to act in what they perceive as the best interest of the child.

Models of children's participation that emerge from a foundation of these 'images' of children are evident in the way many consultants try to design and regulate the involvement of children in their projects. Children's participation is often defined in terms of the roles that adults ascribe to children, as though children cannot participate in decision making or contribute to society unless they are formally engaged through adult-initiated projects. This undermines the capacity of children and positions them as lacking agency, in contrast to children who are capable and competent, who replicate and appropriate aspects of their culture through their talk and interaction with others and actively participate in the construction of their own social situations (Danby and Farrell 2004).

Although there is no universal definition of children's participation, several are commonly offered in the literature. Chawla (2001: 9) defines it as 'a process in which children and youth engage with other people around issues that concern their individual and collective life conditions'. Hart (1992: 5) defines it as a

> process of sharing decisions which affect one's life and the life of the community in which one lives. It is the means by which a democracy is built and it is a standard against which democracies should be measured.

Upadhyay et al. write that in the Asia-Pacific region the term is still contested and is used for a diverse range of activities, so that there is still no clear agenda for participation:

> Much of the practice of children's participation is loosely based on children's right to expression in all matters affecting the child (CRC Article 12), rather than on children's unconditional right to expression (CRC Article 13) and other civil rights included in the CRC. As a result, children's participation continues to be dominated by one-off processes, rather than by a clear set of commitments and actions of children's civil rights.
>
> (Upadhyay et al. 2008: 21)

They also believe that there are limits on the scope of children's participation which mean that projects rarely have enough momentum to generate real changes, particularly changes reconstituting how power is managed between children and adults. Adult resistance is often at the root of this lack of change, and cultural barriers are often cited as the reason for this – that is, children's participation is not part of traditional culture, or the political arena is not a space where children should be present. Arguments are also often presented that, by engaging children in public affairs, we are 'robbing them of their childhood'. Add to this an ongoing lack of capacity among adults and children to promote and support children's participation, due to the wide range of skills and experience it requires (ibid.).

Models of children's participation

One of the first attempts to problematise the issue of children's participation came from Hart, with his 'ladder of children's participation' (1992).[2] Still considered to be the most influential model within the field, the ladder distinguishes possible types of adult–child interaction represented in participatory practice. Adapted from Arnstein (1969), the model is comprised of eight rungs, with the bottom three, 'manipulation', 'decoration' and 'tokenism', representing forms of non-participation. The top five rungs represent varying degrees of participation, from projects which are assigned to children but with informed roles, to those which are initiated by youth who then share decisions with adults. In his explanation of the model, Hart cautions that it does not imply children should always be operating at the highest rung; that a child may work at whatever level they choose, at any stage of the process (1997: 41). According to Hart, what the model offers is simplicity of form and clarity of goals that enable a wide range of professional groups and institutions to rethink ways of engaging with children. By providing a means for understanding and evaluating current ways of working, the model can help workers to devise a strategy appropriate to their particular context (Hart 2008: 23). Shier (2001) considers that one of the most useful contributions is the identification of the lowest ladder rungs of non-participation, as this has led to real improvements in practice.

The ladder is commonly criticised as implying that participation occurs in a sequence (Reddy and Ratna 2002: 18; Kirby and Woodhead 2003: 243); that different forms of participation can be placed in hierarchical order (Treseder 1997); or conversely, that 'child initiated and directed' should be the highest level of participation, rather than 'child initiated, shared decision making with adults' (Ackermann et al. 2003; Melton 1993). Hart himself has also criticised the model for cultural bias (being conceived primarily from his experience in America and the United Kingdom) and its current misuse as a comprehensive tool for understanding and evaluating projects. He has encouraged a move beyond the ladder:

> from my perspective, I see the ladder lying in the long grass of an orchard at the end of the season. It has served its purpose. I look forward to the next season for I know there are so many different routes up through the branches and better ways to talk about how children can climb into meaningful, and shall we say fruitful, ways of working with others.
>
> (Hart 2008: 29)

The recognition of the model's limitations has led to the emergence of alternative typologies, many of which are similar to, or extensions of, the ladder metaphor rather than reflecting an entirely new framework of children's participation. Five key alternatives are presented by Westhorp (1987), Rocha (1997), Jensen (2000), Shier (2001) and Reddy and Ratna (2002). While the above offer valuable suggestions and additions to Hart's ladder, the fundamental sequential and hierarchical nature of the model remains the same, reflecting a limited and fragmented conceptualisation of children's participation. As Bridgland Sorenson states:

> It is no longer adequate to see participation simply in terms of the 'components of participation' repeated in various publications and embraced over the past twenty or so years. Fundamentally, the means and modes of communication of young people have changed.
>
> (2006: 135)

As an alternative to the ladder, and after a review of three decades' worth of children's participation in practice, Francis and Lorenzo (2002: 161–2) have identified seven realms under which they believe most projects can be categorised – 'romantic', 'advocacy', 'needs', 'learning', 'rights', 'institutionalisation' and 'proactive' (Box 2.1).

We will now use these key realms to describe the different perspectives on the role of children as participants in participation projects. Projects dating back to the 1960s and

---

Box 2.1 The seven realms of children's participation

1 **Romantic realm** Projects dating back to the 1960s and 1970s which promote an image of children as able to envision and create their own environments without the involvement of adults.
2 **Advocacy realm** Projects where children are predominantly planned for, with their apparent needs advocated through adults.
3 **Needs realm** Predominantly projects by urban planners that are increasingly moving towards more 'research based' approaches that can be identified with the social science of children.
4 **Learning realm** Projects which involve teachers and environmental educators without necessarily utilising research knowledge. The focus is on the process of changing perceptions and skills rather than physical places.
5 **Rights realm** Projects are closely related to the United Nations and similar international organisations, where the focus tends to be on children's rights rather than on environmental needs.
6 **Institutionalisation realm** An increasingly popular approach, it relates to international child advocate organisations and city officials who have been forced to involve children.
7 **Proactive realm** This is children's participation with vision, relating to projects that strive to find a balance between focusing on empowering children through spontaneous and child-centred modes of participation, and focusing on making substantial changes.

(Francis and Lorenzo 2002)

1970s are often related to the 'romantic' realm. Such approaches typically promote an image of *children as planners and futurists*. Conversely, within the realm of 'advocacy', children are predominantly planned for, with their apparent needs advocated through adults – *children are viewed as resources*. However, the urban planners who took such an approach started to move more towards the role of *children as co-researchers*.

Unlike 'needs', the realm of 'learning' represents those projects more specifically involving teachers and environmental educators, where settings such as schools and community centres engage primarily with *children as learners*. These are unlike projects associated with global organisations such as United Nations, Save the Children etc., where the focus tends to be on children's rights rather than on environmental needs and the view of *children as active citizens*.

'Institutionalisation' is also an increasingly popular approach to children's participation, and is often used to describe the work by various international child advocate organisations and city officials who 'train' children in adult roles within their organisations (youth council etc.). While projects may encourage planning 'by' children, this is restricted by the institutional boundaries set by adults. In this sense, 'institutionalisation' presents a view of children as mini-adults.

A recent example of building on this model has been the work at Open University, with its focus on training children in formal research methods (Kellett 2005). The essential premise here is that, in order to empower children through participation, they need to be trained in adult ways of acting and researching:

While children's knowledge and understanding of childhood and children's lives is evident, a genuine barrier to children engaging in research is their lack of research knowledge and skills, not least because of issues about validity and rigour ... This is the focus of a large action research study ... interim findings are extremely positive about the ability of children as young as ten to undertake rigorous, empirical research and the impact of such participation on child self-development.

(Kellett 2005: 9)

However, by focusing on what children are lacking, Kellett adopts a deficit approach when viewing children's participation. As Prout asserts, 'Too often children are expected to fit into adult ways of participating when what is needed is institutional and organisational change which facilitates children's voices' (2002: 75). This model of participation has the potential and privileges of 'adult' agendas and undervalues or does not recognise children's own cultural practices. The need to include children through an understanding of their unique cultural practices is further reinforced by the Scottish Youth Parliament's (SYP) manifesto, which states:

We want to be *different*. We want to make the views of young people heard to those people who *should be listening* to us, but we want to do it in a thoroughly innovative way. We recognise that traditional models don't always work and it is our belief people should be able to *make a difference* in a way *that suits them* – we think it's possible to make the whole process interesting and exciting!

(SYP 2003, cited in Hill et al. 2004: 92)

In the seventh and final realm identified by Francis and Lorenzo (2002), 'proactive' refers to participation with vision. Within this realm we begin to see the starting point of a view of children as competent and able to construct their own cultural practices outside the adult domain. Given the everyday practicalities and challenges of participatory projects, though, this more idealistic approach may not always be achievable. Children are cast in the role of *children as social actors*. Children are viewed as being competent in relation to experience and recognised as being 'experts' in their own lives and, most importantly, as capable of being 'change agents' or active citizens in transforming their world.

Children as change agents

Fuelled by the introduction of the child rights movement and these many models of participation, some innovative child researchers started to work with children in more collaborative ways, based on the view that 'the best people to provide information on the child's perspective, actions and attitudes are children themselves' (Scott 2000: 99). With a focus on authentic and meaningful children's participation in research, this led to action research projects carried out *with* children for social change. This shift in focus allowed projects and children to be a catalyst for transformative practices to directly improve their lives. The international UNESCO Growing Up in Cities project has often been cited as one of the key international projects to operationalise this practice on a large scale. David Driskell (2002: 17), in his manual derived from the experiences of the Growing Up in Cities revisitation, wrote:

> one of the most effective strategies for creating better cities is through the actual process of participation: helping young people to listen to one another, to respect differences of opinion, and to find common ground; developing their capacities for critical thinking, evaluation and reflection; supporting their processes of discovery, awareness building, and collective problem-solving; and helping them to develop the knowledge and skills for making a difference in their world.

The role of children as social agents and active citizens has been in some part also driven by minority-world children's global awareness of world issues and the realisation that they, in comparison to the vast majority of children in developing nations, live lives of enormous privilege. This awareness has led to many young people taking up social activist positions around racism, children's rights and the environment. Although their actions are often viewed suspiciously as being the product of their baby-boomer parents and therefore tokenistic, rather than a meaningful activist position, it is clear these young people are more astute in their political campaigning and their view of authentic participation than those young people of the sixties. Rather than T-shirt slogans of 'make love not war', these young people are using the internet and mobile phones and other media to 'culture jam', beating many unwitting multinationals and global organisations at their own game. An example of this was the 1999 campaign by UNICEF Canada that asked children to vote on the top ten principles from the Convention on the Rights of the Child. What organisers weren't prepared for was the backlash it created when a highly articulate children's community demanded that the vote be abandoned because it was patronising and demeaning. Many youth organisations banded together via a network of email lists and issued a joint release saying they wanted to participate in *real* political processes and that adults would never be asked to choose between their basic rights in the same way that UNICEF was asking them to do (McDonnell 2005). This generation is also often labelled as more altruistic than previous generations. According to McDonnell (2005: 183), a survey in 1999 of 5,000 young people in eleven countries showed that they had high levels of altruism, were optimistic about their future and tended to be critical of their self-absorbed, workaholic parents:

> A convergence of forces in modern life – including such factors as television, the Internet and changing child rearing patterns – has resulted in the erosion of the wall of enforced ignorance that has surrounded childhood in Western society for the past several hundred years.
>
> (McDonnell 2005: 190)

When considering children's participation, and particularly children as change agents and active citizens, we believe it is important to acknowledge children as capable and competent agents who, with adults, can imagine and create projects around their lives, instead of the projects that adults imagine and design for them.

The future of children's participation: key challenges and issues

> There is an urgent need to critically reflect on children's participation in social change processes; why change so often does not happen and therefore what needs to happen beyond 'having a say' to make children's participation more meaningful.
>
> (Percy-Smith 2007)

There is evidence, when reflecting on some of the challenges experienced through children's participation in practice, that any 'one size fits all' model will fail to account for the very contextualised and unique ingredients that make up any children's participatory project within a community. Understanding these nuances and being transparent about the positive and negative outcomes of projects is a key element often overlooked, although, as Naker et al. explain, it could be one of the richest outcomes evolving from a project:

> openness to grappling with tensions and contradictions of child participation in practice, and to questioning even enlightened assumptions, is likely the most important ingredient in this work.
>
> (Naker, Mann and Rajani 2007: 102)

Nevertheless, it is becoming clear that children's involvement in single participatory projects is not enough. Unfortunately, much current practice in monitoring and evaluating participatory projects is limited to specific project activities (Hart et al. 2004). While some of the most important outcomes of the projects may be intangible (Chawla et al. 2005), a good starting point is the structure provided by Hart et al. (2004), which divides evaluation of children's participation into four 'realms of impact' – personal, familial, communal and institutional. All of these must be reviewed for a holistic and broader view of participation in practice.

> Participation in practice has moved a long way in the past decade but, as is often the case in new ventures, each step forward alerts us to how much more we need to learn and understand to be effective whether as researchers, practitioners or policy-makers ... the challenge for the next decade will be how to move beyond one-off or isolated consultations to a position where children's participation is firmly embedded within organisational cultures and structures for decision-making.
>
> (Sinclair 2004: 116)

Yet the challenge still exists to evaluate children's participation beyond a success or failure model – not asking did a project 'get participation right' or meet programme targets, but thinking about 'whether, by being critically reflective and learning from the experience, the achievement of a culture of children's participation may become more realisable' (Percy-Smith and Malone 2001: 18).

Through our critical discussions and exploration of the literature we have identified some key challenges for consideration for the field of children's participation. These include: the narrow definition of children's participation; a focus on educational, not transformative outcomes; contestation over child-initiated projects; and last, linked with the first three, the effect of the field being under-theorised and over-practicalised. We will conclude with a short discussion on each of these points.

1   Narrow definition

> Child participation must be authentic and meaningful. It must start with children and young people themselves, on their own terms, within their own realities and in pursuit of their own visions, dreams, hopes and concerns. Most of all, authentic and meaningful child participation requires a radical shift in adult thinking and behaviour – from an exclusionary to an inclusionary approach to children and their capabilities.
>
> (UNICEF 2003)

When one reviews the literature on children's participation and the critique of the various models, it is clear that children's participation – as a field of study in academia, or as a descriptor of a consultancy process with children – is often narrowly defined as only existing if it is named and operated by adults in their domain. Even if adults work very hard to relinquish their power within the 'process', it is within the adult-centric structure that all children's participation comes to be recognised, so that any participatory project, however politically resistant may be its intent, is eventually drawn into the status quo.

2   Focus on educational not transformative outcomes

> Planning with young people is not just about changing or designing physical forms or structures for them. It is about understanding the culture of a community and young people's role with it.
>
> (Malone and Hasluck 2002: 107)

In the late 1970s Pearse and Stiefel (cited in Chawla and Heft 2001) noted that one of the key issues for community involvement in planning was that 'some political leaders expect participation to be 'systems maintaining' while others believe that it should be 'systems transforming'. This issue still holds true for children's participation some 30 years later. So what is the purpose of children's participation? There are plenty of examples of research that claim that children's participation has all types of benefits for children: it increases a child's self-esteem; personal and collective efficacy; greater self-control; greater sensitivity to the perspectives of others; greater hope for the future; it prepares young people to be democratic decision makers and active citizens (Adams and Ingham 1998; Chawla 2001; de Winter 1997; Hart 1997; Sutton 1985); and the list goes on. These personal and sometimes collective changes may be beneficial for the child's future well-being, but the question is, is it enough? Iacofano (1990) believes that citizen involvement in environmental decision making can be rated along a scale with two axes: the *degree of interactivity* – learning about the environment and political structures – and the *degree of actual influence* – what actual changes have been made that will transform (culturally and politically) the places where people live. He states that 'many projects rate high on the axis of education but fail to influence entrenched structures of decision-making'. We believe that for many children's participation projects, even though the intention may be transformative, change mainly occurs as mere 'awareness raising', sometimes moving to actual physical changes, but rarely contesting the dominant political and cultural hegemony. A park may get built, a graffiti wall erected, but these symbols of young people's contribution can act as mere markers of a cultural context that belongs to adults and allows the occasional interference of the child's input a kind of 'tolerance' in order to fulfil the rudimentary requirements of being, say, 'child friendly'. Cultural shifts are far less easy to achieve, but this does not mean the challenge should be ignored.

3   Contestation over child-initiated projects.

Projects entirely initiated and carried out by children are only likely to flourish in areas that don't interfere with adults' interests.

(Chawla and Heft 2001: 4)

Craig Kielburger was only 12 years old when he read a newspaper article about the murder of a Pakistani boy, Iqbal Masik, who was also only 12. What shocked Craig about this boy's death was that Iqbal was murdered for trying to free children from being slaves. Craig, growing up in middle-class Toronto, was outraged that children should be suffering such a life and, along with his classmates, decided to initiate the Free the Children organisation. The organisation was funded by the children through garage sales, pop sales, car washes and bake sales run by them. Craig and his classmates signed petitions and faxed world leaders, and even went to countries to speak with enslaved children, often participating in police raids to free them. Although his actions were comparable with those of adult 'child activists', because he was a child himself he came under a lot of public attack. Beyond the accusation, made by the Canadian magazine *Saturday Night*, that he was a puppet for ambitious parents, many believed 'he was too young to be telling adults and politicians, much less entire countries what they should or should be doing' (www.peaceheroes.com, accessed 4 April 2008). McDonnell writes of the adult reaction to Kielburger's activism in the following way:

Many of the jaded media types covering Free the Children felt Kielburger was just too goody-goody to believe. It was as if they didn't know what to make of a kid who didn't fit the stereotype of disaffected youth hanging out in shopping malls. Many protested he should be doing kid (i.e. inconsequential) things instead of campaigning on world issues.

(2006: 184)

But not all child activists are of the clean-cut superstar variety like Kielburger. At recent anti-globalisation rallies many young activists used more violent means and 'culture-jamming' techniques to illustrate the impact of ever-expanding multinationals. Spray-painting Nike ads, setting up weblogs and MySpace sites, they use more militant tactics to voice their opinions. Other examples of child-initiated action, working outside the domain of adults, are the child-initiated 'pocket park' research projects in Setangaya in Tokyo and the Nepal Children's Clubs often discussed by Hart. What these projects illustrate is that children are able to organise themselves from a very young age to engage in activities that draw on their own interests and expertise in parallel to the adult world around them.

These children-initiated political acts are woven into the everyday cultural frameworks of being and adding to the world that exist in their own child/youth realities, not the world structured and organised by adults who offer a space for children to 'participate' along with them. With expertise in new communications technology, an unprecedented political sophistication, due to their access to global knowledges, and the camaraderie to see themselves as connecting at a global cultural level, children are able to participate at a level outside the reach of adults.

4   Under-theorised and over-practicalised?

In 1992 Hart cautioned that his ladder of participation 'should not be considered as a simple measuring stick of the quality of any programme', and yet its impact in the field as an evaluative tool continues relentlessly. The question is, why the ladder has had such an influence on the field, and how has it managed to maintain that influence for so long, even though, as we have seen, it has been critiqued and revised extensively by many, including Hart himself. One reason may be that it arrived at a time when the emerging field of children's participation had a void of 'intellectual capital'. The ladder was a significant foundation for creating a field of study around children's participation. The weakness, then, is its focus on being a 'practical tool' rather than a theoretical framework; while it has served well for practitioners in the field, we believe there is now a need to develop a theory that will capture the complexities of that field.

Conclusion

The aim of this chapter has been to sketch a map of the state of play in children's participation, in order to open up consideration of ways forward that may include roads less travelled in our thinking and practice; in particular, the road that leads to children's participation defined not by our imposing of a framework on children but by acknowledging that children are participating every day through their own cultural practices and their remaking of themselves and their environments.

What we believe is needed in the field of children's participation is to entice practitioners, children and researchers to be more playful and creative in the relationships they form, to acknowledge that children's culture exists independently of adults, and to think of new ways to interact with children where we are opening up rather than closing down dialogue, and so building an environment that includes all the possibilities of children's participation, even those we haven't thought of. To quote Percy-Smith and Malone (2001: 18):

> authentic participation involves *inclusion* – wherein the system changes to accommodate the participation and values of children – rather than *integration* – wherein children participate in predefined ways in predefined structures.

This is where our theorising of children's participation needs to head, if we are to celebrate and value the role of children as participants both in our projects and in their own right.

Notes

1   See Budd Hall (1981: 11) for further discussions on the relationship between 'organic intellectuals' and researchers in participatory research.
2   While Hart's ladder became most influential after the 1992 publication of *Children's Participation: From tokenism to citizenship*, the model was first published in the *Childhood City Newsletter* in 1980 by the City University of New York.

References

Ackermann, L., Feeny, T. et al. (2003) *Understanding and Evaluating Children's Participation: a review of contemporary literature*, London: Plan UK/Plan International.

Adams, E. and Ingham, S. (1998) *Changing Places: Children's participation in environmental planning*, London: The Children's Society.

Alderson, P. and Goodey, C. (1996) 'Research with disabled children: How useful is child-centered ethics?', *Children & Society* 10: 106–16.

Arnstein, S. (1969) 'A ladder of citizen participation', *American Institute of Planners Journal* 35: 216–24.

Barn, G. and A. Franklin (1996) 'Article 12 – issues in developing children's participation', in E. Verhellen (ed.) *Monitoring Children's Rights*, The Hague: Martinus Nijhoff.

Bridgland Sorenson, J. G. (2006) 'Constraints to youth participation in the current federal political environment'. Master's degree dissertation, Faculty of Community, Education and Social Science, Edith Cowan University.

Chawla, L. (2001) 'Evaluating children's participation: Seeking areas of consensus', *PLA Notes* 42 (October): 9–13.

Chawla, L. and Heft, H. (2002) 'Children's competence and the ecology of communities: A functional approach to the evaluation of participation', *Journal of Environmental Psychology* 22(1–2): 201–16.

Chawla, L., Blanchet-Cohen, N. et al. (2005) '"Don't just listen – do something!" Lessons learned about governance from the Growing Up in Cities Project', *Children, Youth and Environments* 15(2): 53–88.

Crimmens, D. and West, A. (2004) *Having Their Say: Young people and participation: European experiences*, London: Russell House Publishing.

Danby, S. and Farrell, A. (2004) 'Accounting for young children's competence in educational research: new perspectives on research ethics', *The Australian Educational Researcher* 31(3): 35–49.

de Winter, M. (1997) *Children as Fellow Citizens*, Oxford: Radcliffe Medical Press.

Driskell, D. (2002) *Creating Better Cities with Children and Youth*, London: Earthscan/UNESCO.

Duncombe, S. (ed.) (2002) *Cultural Resistance Reader*, New York: Verso.

Francis, M. and Lorenzo, R. (2002) 'Seven realms of children's participation', *Journal of Environmental Psychology* 22: 157–69.

Gallagher, M. (2008) 'Foucault, power and participation', *International Journal of Children's Rights* 16: 395–406.

Gramsci, A. (1971) *Selections from Prison Notebooks*, London: Lawrence and Wishart.

Hall, B. (1981) 'Participatory research, popular knowledge and power: A personal reflection', *Convergence* 14(3): 6–19.

Hart, J., Newman, J. et al. (2004) *Children Changing Their World: understanding and evaluating children's participation in development*, London: PLAN UK/ PLAN International.

Hart, R. (1992) *Children's Participation: From tokenism to citizenship*, Florence: UNICEF.

Hart, R. (1997) *Children's Participation: The theory and practice of involving young citizens in community development and environmental care*, New York: UNICEF/Earthscan.

Hart, R. (2008) 'Stepping back from "the ladder": Reflections on a model of participatory work with children', in A. Reid, B. Jensen, J. Nikel and V. Simovska (eds) *Participation and Learning: Perspectives on education and the environment, health and sustainability*, Netherlands: Springer, pp. 19–31.

Heft, H. (1988) 'Affordances of children's environments: A functional approach to environmental description', *Children's Environments Quarterly* 5: 29–37.

Hill, M., Davis, J. et al. (2004) 'Moving the participation agenda forward', *Children & Society* 18: 77–96.

Holloway, S. L. and Valentine, G. (eds) (2000) *Children's Geographies: Playing, living, learning*, London: Routledge.

Iacofano, D. (1990) *Public Involvement as an Organisational Development Process*, New York: Garland Publishing.

James, A., Jenks, C. and Prout, A. (1998) *Theorising Childhood*, Cambridge: Polity Press.

Jensen, B. B. (2000) 'Participation, commitment and knowledge as components of pupils' action competence', in B. B. Jensen, K. Schnack and V. Simovska (eds) *Critical Environmental and Health Education: research issues and challenges*, Copenhagen: Danish University of Education.

Kellett, M. (2005) *Developing Children as Researchers*, London: Paul Chapman.

Kirby, P. and Woodhead, M. (2003) 'Children's participation in society', in H. Burr, K. and M. Woodhead (eds) *Changing Childhoods: Local and global, Vol. 4, Childhood*, Chichester: Open University Press.

Kruger, J. (2000) *Growing Up in Canaansland: Children's recommendations on improving a squatter camp environment*, Pretoria: HSRC Publishers.

Kytta, M. (2004) 'The extent of children's independent mobility and the number of actualized affordances as criteria for child-friendly environments', *Journal of Environmental Psychology* 24: 179–98.

Louv, R. (2006) 'Leave No Child Inside', *Sierra* 91(4): 52.

Malone, K. (1996) 'School and community partnerships in socially critical environmental education: Research as activism education', PhD thesis, Geelong, Victoria, Australia: Deakin University.

Malone, K. (2007) 'Environmental education researchers as environmental activists', in A. Reid and W. Scott (eds) *Researching Education and the Environment: Retrospect and prospect*, London: Routledge.

Malone, K. and Hasluck, L. (2002) 'Australian youth: Aliens in a suburban environment', in L. Chawla (ed.) *Growing Up in an Urbanising World*, London: Earthscan/UNESCO, pp. 81–109.

Malone, K. and Tranter, P. (2005) '"Hanging out in the school ground": A reflective look at researching children's environmental learning', *Canadian Journal for Environmental Education* (school ground special issue) 10(1): 196–212.

Mason, J. and Urquhart, R. (2001) 'Developing a model for participation by children in research decision making', *Children Australia* 26(4): 16–21.

McDonnell, K. (2005) *Honey, We Lost The Kids: Re-thinking childhood in the multi-media age*, Melbourne: Pluto Press.

McKendrick, J. H., Bradford, M. G., and Fielder, A. V. (2000) 'Kid Customer? Commercialization of playspace and the commodification of childhood', *Childhood* 7(3): 295–314.

Melton, G. (1993) 'Review of "children's participation: from tokenism to citizenship"', *The International Journal of Children's Rights* 1: 263–6.

Moore, R. C. and Wong, H. H. (1997) *Natural Learning: The life history of an environmental schoolyard*, Berkeley, CA: MIG Communications.

Nabhan, G. and Trimble, S. (1994) *The Geography of Childhood: Why children need wild spaces*, Boston: Beacon Press.

Naker, D., Mann, G. et al. (2007) 'The gap between rhetoric and practice: Critical perspectives on children's participation', *Children, Youth and Environments* 17(3): 99–103.

Percy-Smith, B. (2002) 'Contested worlds: Constraints and opportunities growing up in inner and outer city environments of an English Midlands town', in L. Chawla (ed.), *Growing Up in an Urbanising World*, London: Earthscan.

Percy-Smith, B. (2007) '"I've had my say, but nothing's changed!": Where to now? Critical reflections on children's participation', EBS Seminar Abstracts, accessed 1 December 2007 from www.arch.usyd.edu.au/research/env_seminars_abstracts.shtml.

Percy-Smith, B. and Malone, K. (2001) 'Making children's participation in neighbourhood settings relevant to everyday lives of young people', *PLA Notes* 42 (October): 18–22.

Prout, A. (2002) 'Researching children as social actors: An introduction to the children's 5–16 programme', *Children & Society* 16: 67–76.

Reddy, N. and Ratna, K. (2002) *A Journey in Children's Participation*, Vimanapura: The Concerned for Working Children.

Rocha, E. (1997) 'A ladder of empowerment', *Journal of Planning, Education and Research* 17: 31–44.

Scott, J. (2000) 'Children as respondents: the challenge for qualitative researchers', in P. Christensen and A. James (eds) *Research with Children: Perspectives and practices*, London: Falmer Press, pp. 98–119.

Shier, H. (2001) 'Pathways to participation: Openings, opportunities and obligations', *Children & Society* 15: 107–17.

Sinclair, R. (2004) 'Participation in practice: Making it meaningful, effective and sustainable', *Children & Society* 18: 106–18.

Sutton, S. E. (1985) *Learning Through the Built Environment*, New York: Irvington Publishers.

Treseder, P. (1997) *Empowering Children and Young People: Training manual*, London: Save the Children and Children's Rights Office.

UNICEF (2003) 'The state of the world's children 2003', www.unicef.org/sowc03/presskit/summary.html, accessed 12 July 2007.

Upadhyay, J., Ennew, J. et al. (2008) *Children as Active Citizens: A policy programme guide*, Bangkok: Inter-Agency Working Group on Children's Participation.

Westhorp, G. (1987) *Planning for Youth Participation: A resource kit*, Adelaide: Youth Sector Training Council of South Australia.

3 Children's participation in Bangladesh

Issues of agency and structures of violence

Sarah C. White and Shyamol A. Choudhury

'Mar kheye boro hoyecche' – He has grown up being beaten.

20 November 2000

The meeting begins ordinarily enough. Mainly the younger boys are present, so Bhaiya,[1] the adult who works with them, asks them why they joined the group and what they like and dislike about being in Amra.[2] Then it comes out. What we dislike, one of them says, is when the older boys beat us. It is a shock, because a ban on beating is one of the strictest rules of Amra. So we ask what he means, and the story of the previous day tumbles out.

At the end of the meeting a game started, hiding each other's shoes. Most of the shoes were soon found, but Salim's were still missing. At last Alam and another of the younger boys admitted they had seen Kashem hide Salim's shoes in the drain. Salim was furious, and so was Kashem. Losing his temper completely, Kashem attacked the younger boys and yelled that Amra was finished, he would tell everyone what rubbish it was, he would see that it was destroyed.

As the story ends, everyone falls silent. Then Bhaiya speaks. This is something serious, what are we going to do about it, how will we sort it out? We can't just let it go, or Kashem might go on and beat someone else again another time. How do they generally deal with it, when one of the members breaks one of their rules? The answer comes readily: they hold a *bichar*, a hearing among themselves to decide the rights and wrongs of the case and determine punishment. Alam is visibly upset. It is already bad enough, and he doesn't want Kashem to get into any more trouble because of him. 'If I did wrong and my elder brother beat me', Alam explains, 'would I call for a *bichar*?'

The group talk over what they should do. Kashem isn't there, but they could do a mock *bichar*, with someone standing in for Kashem, as a way of working out what should be done. Salim has been quiet, distancing himself from the process, so Bhaiya asks him directly: 'Is a *bichar* needed?'

Salim's answer is equivocal: it is needed and not needed. And then he goes on to explain: 'Kashem', he says, '*mar kheye boro hoyecche*,' he has grown up being beaten.

Bhaiya takes this up. He asks the group: do we need to know what Kashem has been through if we are to judge what he has done?

So they talk about Kashem. How he was arrested and kept in prison on a false charge for more than two months. His continuing chest problems since then, and how, when he first returned to the group, his leg was still swollen following a bad beating in prison; how the case is still ongoing; his difficult home situation.

As they talk, Kashem enters. The greatest issue of all, Bhaiya says, is trust. He knows a game to explore this – would they like to play? Everyone agrees. Bhaiya explains. Two people are to stand opposite each other, three or four paces apart, with one person in the middle, between them. They settle on just one group, with Bhaiya and the oldest boy rocking Kashem from one side to the other, a stiff, inert figure, given into their hands. Everyone watches in silence, arrested.

When they finish Bhaiya asks Kashem: Were you anxious that we might drop you?

Kashem: No.
Bhaiya: But you know what happened yesterday, and that hearing about it, of everyone here I was the most angry, of everyone here I was most strongly against you?
Kashem: But even so, I know you wouldn't do anything to hurt me.
Bhaiya: Would you have the same confidence with everyone here?
Kashem: No. Maybe three or four of them might let me fall.

Others in the group chip in: 'Because they are small and couldn't bear your weight?'

Kashem: No.
Bhaiya: If I had asked the same question a few days ago, would you have given me the same answer?
Kashem: No. A few days ago I would have had confidence in everyone.
Bhaiya: So it is about what happened yesterday?
Kashem: Yes.
Bhaiya: Then we should sit and sort it out together.

They talk a bit and Kashem breaks down. He had a row with his mother and she still wouldn't let him back in the house. When the incident happened, he had been three days on the streets, without hot food or shelter. Bhaiya gives another boy money to go and buy hot food and Kashem eats.

As they talk more, it becomes more complex. Because Kashem had been away from the group on a training course, he wasn't in touch with what was going on. They were doing a role-play of what happens when they are trying to teach literacy and the local kids are being disruptive. All of them were joining in, enjoying acting up. When Kashem came in part way through, he was disgusted at their behaviour. Was this any way to conduct training? He got furious, feeling that they were wrecking Amra and everything it stood for.

When Kashem returns to the group, they discuss the options for punishment. Kashem picks one and makes a pledge: he will neither beat anyone again nor allow any beating to happen.[3]

This event is an example of children's participation. Aside from Bhaiya, all the protagonists are children. The issue was raised by children, and it concerned their own business – how they would conduct their being together. However, it is not typical of the kind of event that goes under the name of 'children's participation' in Bangladesh.[4] There was no 'event', no show, no 'product,' no children's statement, no audience, no pictures to represent the issues. If an evaluation had not happened to be going on, the event would have been unrecorded, just one more meeting in the course of daily work, leaving no trace beyond those particular children's memories. Set up in 1995, Amra was designed not to be a project for children's participation, but to be a children's organisation in which street and working children would get together to work on literacy and consciousness raising with other children like themselves. As the external agenda for children's participation has grown, however, Amra has increasingly been drawn into its slipstream. This chapter asks what the event described above tells us about violence and children's agency. It then reflects on the contrast between Amra in its early years and its more recent history, in order to consider what questions this raises for the theorisation and practice of 'child participation' in international development.

The story of this chapter is one in which we have both shared. Shyamol Choudhury was facilitator of Amra from 1995 to 2001. The chapter draws significantly on his MSc dissertation (Choudhury 2003).[5] Sarah White conducted a review of Amra in 2000 as part of broader research on street and working children.[6] We then undertook a joint follow-up study in 2004–5, looking at how Amra had developed, the style of participation followed, and the implications of this.[7] The fieldwork was undertaken by Shyamol, involving intensive group and individual interviews, consultation and field visits with different categories of members,[8] making up over 100 children in all. It also involved interviews with some of their parents, and staff in the international agency that sponsored Amra and some other non-governmental organisations (NGOs). Shyamol was well known to all the respondents. We believe that this prior relationship gave the interviews a foundation of trust that allowed the children to speak openly and with confidence. It does mean, however, that we write here very much as people implicated in what we are describing.

Children's participation in Bangladesh development

Children's participation in development in Bangladesh takes many forms. In a previous paper (White and Choudhury 2007) we classified these as *presentation, consultation* and *advocacy*. *Presentations* range from street theatre, to child survivors' testimonies, to 'cultural programmes' of singing and dancing. *Consultation* spans children being targeted as survey respondents for inclusion within project-cycle reference groups. *Advocacy* includes children's media, journalism and video projects and lobbying in national and international forums. Common to all these, however, is an underlying positioning of the child as informant, even, at times, as expert. Adult and professional knowledge is downgraded as insufficient and partial. Instead, it is the child who must be teacher: 'You understand your situation much better than we do. We must learn from you.'

This special knowledge that children are said to possess is the predominant justification for advocating their participation. This links into a broader set of arguments for participation in international development. The first is *efficiency*: that only if the beneficiaries are involved will appropriate and sustainable projects be designed. The second is *efficacy*: that when children speak for themselves in national and international meetings the impact is much greater than if the same argument were made by an adult on their behalf. The third is *justice*: that people have a right to speak on and be represented in matters that concern them (cf. UNCRC Article 12). The fourth, which Hart (2007: 2) terms *self-realisation*, claims that through participation children's self-confidence and capabilities will increase. Finally, participation is justified in more radical terms as leading to *empowerment* and *transformation*, whereby young people can challenge underlying structures of domination.

The notion of special knowledge turns on two fundamental ideas: authenticity and distinctive autonomy. The power of these lies in part in their invocation of older, suppressed images of children as innocent and pure, unsullied by the established order. In practice, however, children's participation activities in Bangladesh development are highly performative, characterised by a strong sense of flourish, of theatre, of show. As the list above suggests, they are often, quite literally, staged. They are also deeply hybrid. Even the term for the 'child' of child rights in Bengali (*shishu adhikar*) has undergone a transformation. Originally meaning an infant or very young child, it has been transformed in development-speak into a comprehensive category, such that adolescents linked to development agencies are happy to claim it for themselves.

Living with violence

Since violence was 'their issue', we explore how this affects children's expression of agency and the meaning of participation in their lives. Perhaps the simplest point that the younger boys were making is the importance of the very real differences *within* the group. In a literature that has tended to stress the axis of power between adult and child, drawing attention to power relations among children, even within a self-selected group committed to solidarity, offers an important corrective.

The statement, '*mar kheye boro hoyecche*', he has grown up being beaten, may be interpreted in a number of different ways. In the first place, as Bhaiya took it up, it referred to Kashem's personal story and the need to locate this particular action in relation to it. The complexity of this, and the fact that even those who saw Kashem regularly knew only fragments of what was going on in his life, may give pause for thought to a development policy and programme world that likes to work through national and even global models. It also raises questions for those who like to identify agency with fully conscious individual subjects. While Kashem may have been able to reconstruct in retrospect what was going on, it is very unlikely that he was fully conscious of all those elements as he raised his hand to strike Alam. In fact, it is probable that there were further factors in his personal history and broader context which fuelled his rage, of which he remained unaware.

Second, this statement also points to the wider context of all those children's lives. Street working[9] children in Dhaka are constantly exposed to violence. For

Kashem, over the previous few months this had meant being thrown out of his home and arbitrarily arrested, beaten up and imprisoned. Among Amra members as a whole it has meant the loss of parents through death and abandonment; the death of sisters and brothers through accidents, disease and murder; chronic poor health, stunted growth and disablement through malnutrition and accidents; being made homeless through fire and state-sponsored slum eviction; harassment by police; coercion into criminal activity by neighbourhood gangsters; and being verbally abused, beaten and cheated by employers, clients, passers-by and even teachers. This violence is at once random and systematic: embodied in and beyond particular violent acts is the structural violence of poverty and exploitation.

Galtung (1990) describes a 'triangle of violence' in which direct acts of physical aggression are essentially linked to the 'structural violence' of exploitation and the 'cultural violence' of values, attitudes or imagery that rationalise or legitimate violence. It is easy to see how Kashem's 'agency' of beating the younger boys is related to the structural exploitation and brutality he had experienced and the culture that legitimates those in dominant positions being physically violent towards those 'below': 'If I did wrong and my elder brother beat me, would I call for a *bichar?*'

Culture, context and personal history come together in Salim's intention in making the statement that Kashem had grown up being beaten – it was an ironic comment on the business of the meeting itself. His point was that Kashem – like Salim himself – had grown up in spite of – or even because of – the beating he had received.[10] What, then, was the big deal? Compared with the 'everyday violence' (Scheper-Hughes 1992) in which they lived, how much did Kashem's assault on Alam really matter?

That it did matter was a testimony to the achievement of Amra, that they had established a space together governed by a different norm of relationship that the younger ones felt able to claim against when it was violated. This shows how Galtung's triangle may also work the other way: it is possible to create counter-cultural 'liberated zones' (Connell 1987) in which the normal rules of gender or age-based hierarchy are suspended. This points to the transformatory potential of groups such as Amra, that together they may be able to establish ways of being beyond the capacity of any of the individuals within them to carry through alone. That the rule they had set themselves was violated emphasises the vulnerability of such 'zones' and the power of social structure in shaping agency and normalising certain ways of being. On a personal level, this means that children immersed in violence experience it as normal, and come to reproduce it towards and among themselves. Analytically, it raises serious questions with regard to those approaches that see children as being somehow outside the social system, so that their participation can bring radically new insights untainted by the structures of society that restrict adults' view.

For academics and agencies in the child rights field, that children are actors or subjects in their own right is something of an article of faith. This is a valuable corrective to over-dichotomised models of power, and in development practice it presents an important challenge to default assumptions that 'adults know best', providing an impetus to create spaces in which children can take the initiative. There is, however, a danger of overcompensation: of ignoring the structures through which agency arises; overestimating individuals' autonomy; and under-playing the real constraints that men and women, young and old, face.

Nick Lee's (2001) discussion of the assemblage/actor network approach offers a useful way of exploring this further. Following his reading of Deleuze and Guattri, Lee rejects the idea that the capacity for agency is a property of sovereign (adult) (male?) individuals. Instead, persons are composite *assemblages* that are constantly 'borrowing' from others and from their environments. Once we see agency as deriving from the relations between people and their environment:

> We can ask what a given person, whether adult or child, depends upon for their agency. So ... instead of asking whether children, like adults, possess agency or not, *we can ask how agency is built or may be built for them* by examining the extensions and supplements that are available to them.
>
> (Lee 2001: 131, emphasis added)

For the study of child participation, this means moving away from the fetish of seeking the 'pure', 'true' or unmediated 'voice of the child'. Instead, it means looking at what kinds of (conscious and unconscious) resources children draw on in expressing agency, and how these shape their participation in different ways.

Changing patterns with participation

Kashem's *bichar* exemplifies the group process that lay at the heart of Amra in its early years. It was always very small – in 2000 it had a core group of eight to ten boys working with around seventy children in street-level groups and supported by around thirty others, including formerly active members who still wanted to support the organisation. Its 'field' was the slum environment in which the boys had grown up. Its various initiatives – trying to promote literacy and health, to set up children's fun days, and planning a monitoring cell to report child rights abuses – were all addressed to that immediate context. However, the prevalence of violence and the threat of violence in the lives of the children seriously compromised Amra's capacity to pursue any coherent programme. As on the day of Kashem's *bichar*, 'normal' work constantly had to be suspended to fire-fight an immediate crisis. Much of its energy was internally directed, addressing the problems of its members and building up the group identity as a source of solidarity and a 'liberated zone'. Beyond this, any programme in the slums has to engage with the highly complex and potentially violent formal and informal political structures in the locality. The slums are governed by *mastaans*, godfathers who operate through a mixture of patronage and fear to mediate access to all key resources (Khan 2000). To work there means walking a tightrope between establishing sufficiently good relations to be allowed in, and avoiding capture by particular local factions. The challenge to vested interests presents major difficulties for *any* initiative that seeks to bring about significant change. Thus, when Amra managed to enlist support within the local administration to set up a network of NGOs to address the unhealthy environment of the slums, the demonstration effect of the boys calling and managing community meetings was powerful. What undermined the network was not resistance to children's participation, nor hostility from the local community, but internal contradictions within the NGOs.

Nor did all problems arise from relations with adults: one of the most serious threats to Amra came from its attempt to foster links with the youths who lived near its office. At first things went well – work in the slums was much easier, with such a strong group supporting them. But then others became interested in using Amra as a point of entry for drugs and other illicit businesses in the slum, and tried to use the youths to take it over. Meanwhile the leader of Amra grew closer to those youths, himself becoming almost a proto-*mastaan*. In the midst of this, the Amra members were made homeless by eviction from the slum where they lived. As adolescent boys on the streets face great danger of being picked up by the police, many Amra members left their families and went to live in the office. Then the neighbourhood youth moved in, wanting to use the office as a kind of club where they could drink, smoke, take drugs and show videos. They bullied the younger Amra members, who were afraid to resist. The facilitator received death threats and the neighbours were ready to close the office down. The situation was only resolved by the facilitator's stepping in to negotiate with the neighbours and get the youths to withdraw. This incident was extreme, born out of several risk factors coming together at one time. But the elements that constituted it are all everyday aspects of the structural violence noted above.

Gradually, however, the focus of Amra changed. This began before 2000, as other organisations saw its potential to reach slum-based children and invited Amra to join their vaccination campaigns, research programmes or child consultation activities. These demands built up as the focus on child participation grew and child rights NGOs felt increasing pressure to 'produce' children's participation, particularly in their advocacy activities, to demonstrate their own internal and external legitimacy. The implications of this for Amra were quite contradictory. On the one hand, it gave the core group powerful opportunities to express their views and concerns. On the other hand, the visibility of advocacy/media occasions, the big names they attract, the exposure and personal recognition they offer, the food and expenses they provide, were all quite seductive. Added to the fact that such events have specific times and deadlines, these factors combined to make attendance at these events a priority, rather than maintaining the difficult, uncomfortable, low-profile work with the street-based groups. Over time, therefore, their orientation gradually shifted: from action to advocacy; from the group to the individual; from the slums to the agencies.

Their personal experience of poverty, training in group formation and daily active relationships with other poor children made Amra members highly effective advocates, and this is clearly an important complement to their programme activities. The danger, however, is that this model of children's participation itself dissociates the participants from the children they supposedly represent. Changes in the structures of incentives are reflected in the culture of Amra. In the 2004 interviews with Amra members and their families comments from both core and other members were predominantly commodity and consumption focused. What it was all about, for them, was not lofty talk of children's activism, but the tangible gains of stipend, fancy food, travel expenses, per diems and, above all, relationships with high-status people which might lead to jobs in the longer term. For two or three individuals the experience of participation has been empowering: they have attained a kind of celebrity status. The longer-term effects of this, whether it can be sustained beyond their special status as 'child activists,' and how they will re-adapt to life beyond the 'bright lights' of the global development industry, or indeed find some continuing niche within it, are yet to become clear. What is evident is that differences of power among the children have become more marked. There is alienation of the core from the wider group. Special opportunities, such as for international travel, are hoarded within a tight central group. Smaller children and slum children no longer feel free to come to the Amra office, nor to speak in meetings. If they do try, they risk taunting or humiliation. Amra, they say, has become a '*borolok*' (rich people's) organisation.

Adults and agencies

Amra was unique in the development landscape of Bangladesh as an organisation run by and for children. Despite this, however, the most obvious factor shaping the character of Amra through its different phases is the agency not of children, but of the adults who supported it. It is these adults who, in Lee's terms, supplied the critical 'supplements and extensions' that enabled the boys to express particular forms of agency. Their first programme, of waste management (1995–97), reflected the environmentalist enthusiasm of key officers in the international organisation that supported them. The account of Kashem's *bichar* demonstrates clearly the significance of the facilitator in the second phase (up to 2001), providing a security in which conflict could be expressed without harm, individuals were assured of personal regard, and practical intervention was given when needed. This reflected his background in socialist organising. The adult assigned to Amra from 2002 had a background in acting and the performance arts. He encouraged Amra to develop the acting they already did as part of their literacy and awareness-raising work into 'theatre for development'. To recognise this agency of adults is not to reinstate children as simply passive objects. The boys clearly enjoy working in drama, for example, and two or three of them have subsequently fulfilled a common childhood dream by gaining work in films. What recognising the significance of adults does, however, is to break down the notion of children's agency as somehow autonomous. Its character depends critically on the opportunities and forms of support available.

If children's agency is shaped by structures, so too is the agency of adults. The power of the adults to shape the course that Amra took itself depended on a series of 'supplements and extensions'. Being adult in a hierarchy structured by age is one part of this, but so are other advantages – of class, education and, for some, race. These 'personal' factors were consolidated by their positions within the powerful institution of an international aid agency. Beyond all this, however, the changes in Amra were part of a broader trend in international development which distrusted direct intervention as paternalism and fostering dependency and saw advocacy as more empowering and strategic. Such changes in policies are associated with shifts in the collective consciousness, in which large numbers of people identify with them as their own. Policy change is also associated with change in structures of incentive, and most people adjust their behaviour to align with these. The adults, just like the children, are only partially aware of what is going on in and through them. Nevertheless, it is easy to see that in material terms there are clear advantages for NGO staff in the agency-centred model of participation. The office-centred nature of advocacy work means efficient use of time and a minimum of discomfort. The work is high exposure, the many meetings satisfy the bureaucratic demand of demonstrable activities, the production of media outputs – videos, publications, dramatic performances etc. – gives tangible high-value outcomes to show. Producing these outputs also offers opportunities to bestow lucrative contracts and bring in friends as consultants and, for some at least, to take a cut of the deals for themselves. The attractions of such approaches over the hard, low-capitalised, relatively invisible and highly uncertain work at street level are very clear.

Personal benefits for staff are matched by institutional incentives. If 'child rights' defines the field for development agencies working with children, and participation is seen as the key to other rights, then being able to demonstrate children's participation becomes critical to an agency's legitimacy. 'Made by children' becomes the equivalent of a designer label, adding value to a diverse range of products from project documents, to calendars, to videos, to international statements.

This has both material and symbolic value – it shows the credibility of the agency that promotes it and is effective for fundraising. The relatively high financial cost of producing outputs with such high added value means that large funds can be disbursed with relatively low administrative overheads, providing a model of bureaucratic efficiency. The upward and outward trend in the direction of participation is also indicative. Despite the rhetoric of bottom-up development and the importance of local responsiveness, in the world of development the major financial and esteem rewards, both corporate and individual, derive not from the local but from the global 'community'.

What governs participation?

Child participation is generally posited in terms of politics – the extension of citizenship, democracy, and challenging of entrenched power. The face of politics that is presented is the public face, the 'front-stage', in Goffman's (1990) terms, of negotiated conventions, set-piece debates and the securing of formal pledges from politicians. But as Lukes (1974) and others warn us, this is only one of the many faces of power. There is also Goffman's 'back-stage', the realpolitik of secret deals and hidden alliances that are not discussed even in the boardroom, let alone in a press release. That the public and the private are related is not to be doubted: *how* they are linked, on the other hand, is very difficult to say. This makes it almost impossible to judge the efficacy argument for child participation: how much difference the children's performance really makes.

What, then, does it achieve? As stated above, the children and their parents identified the programme primarily in terms of tangible benefits: foreign travel, stipend and potential job possibilities. The symbolic goods which they perceived were those not of adult–child power reversals, but of material wealth and prestige.

The 'rules of the game' of development construct these as incidental, mere tools required to get the job done, but for those outside the industry, as for many inside, these are not the means to the end, but the end itself. As shown above, the outcomes of participation for Amra are disturbingly close to the market ideal: commodity and consumption focused; individualist; competitive; and differentiating. This seems unlikely to be a coincidence, but rather to reveal the underlying structure and culture of the development industry itself.

There is also a political side to this question. This returns us to the earlier discussion of the different grounds on which child participation is advocated. If one starts from the situation in which these slum and street working children are living, does it really seem that children's participation is the most pressing issue? For the boys in Amra, at least, there is no shortage of opportunities to participate. They are constantly invited to do so: to front various kinds of politically inspired demonstrations; to join in petty business or petty crime; to participate in drug or gun running. Models of 'active youth' are all around them, in the form of the neighbourhood *maastans*, who represent a tantalising model of masculine empowerment. The question, therefore, becomes not whether young people participate, but in what, and on what and whose terms: how to foster participation *of the right kind*. This in turn directs attention to the implicit rules of what counts as participation, the structures within which it is governed, and the kind of world that different forms of participation imagine there to be.

Jason Hart (2007: 10) writes of the 'Peace Camps' which bring together Israeli and Palestinian young people in an attempt to reach across the divide of the Israel–Palestine conflict. For the Palestinians, he said, even describing the conflict in this neutral way is a denial of the real politics of oppression and colonisation that they experience. Within the peace camps, too, there is a denial of the everyday experience of politics that, for the Palestinians at least, keeps 'children's participation' in a 'virtual box'. This does not mean the camps are non-political, rather, the very denial of politics sustains a particular set of power relations. In a similar way the story of Amra suggests that child participation activities may lead to withdrawal from the dangers and complexities of trying to make tangible changes to poor children's lives, in order to produce symbolic goods of which the development industry is itself the primary consumer. These conjure a 'front-stage' of Bangladesh and development politics, characterised by rational policy and liberal democracy, which is very far from the lived reality of Amra members – or of anyone else in Bangladesh. The clear disjuncture between this picture and the violence and corruption that people experience on a daily basis raises the question: whose or what interests does this ideological construction serve?

Conclusion

This chapter poses a number of questions for the theory and practice of child participation. First, it contests any notion that children's agency can be understood as autonomous, untouched by the structure or culture through which it arises. Reflecting on violence suggests that the agency of children and others in promoting 'child participation' needs to be analysed in relation to the resources on which it draws, and the structures out of which it – and they – arise. It also means that we need to sit apart from approaches that set children off as essentially different from adults – especially when it comes to power differences among them, whether of age, class, gender, ethnicity, race, size or simple force of personality. Second, children, like adults, have the potential to organise among themselves a 'liberated zone', but they will not necessarily do so. The critical issue is not the exclusion of adults – in fact, children who have grown up in very difficult circumstances may need an adult presence to support their choice to act differently. Rather, the issue is the resources on which the children can draw. These include any adults who support them and the political commitments those adults have, as well as the social, political, economic and institutional contexts in which they are set. Third, children's participation is not just a challenge to power, but itself a means of its expression. This means that it is never politically neutral – it will challenge some power relations, while confirming others. While some at least of it is theatre, we need to look beyond the 'front-stage' to the 'back-stage' of realpolitik that this sustains. Finally, the chapter suggests that there is a limit to what can be achieved by an agency-centred model of participatory advocacy. If we are serious about learning from child participation we need to 'follow their feet' when marginalised children leave the air-conditioned office and design programmes that address the world they go and live within.

Notes

1. 'Big Brother'. This was Shyamol, who is otherwise referred to as 'the facilitator' in this paper.
2. This is a pseudonym, as are all the boys' names given here. Amra began as a boys' organisation but in the past 2 to 3 years it has opened up to involve girls also. As this occurred after the study on which this paper is based, we are unable to discuss the implications of this development.
3. This section is an abridged version of White's account of the event recorded in her evaluation of Amra, 2000–1.
4. See White and Choudhury (2007) for more description of the general practice of child participation in Bangladesh.
5. We are grateful to the University of Bath and the Shared Scholarship Scheme of DfID for funding this MSc study.
6. This involved interviews with 13 NGOs and 60 street and working children, see White (2002). We are grateful to ESCOR, the research-funding branch of the British Overseas Development Administration (now renamed the Department for International Development, DfID) for funding this.
7. We are grateful to the British Academy for funding this research.
8. These comprise the core and outer groups of child members, slightly better-off children who are classed as 'volunteers', 'beneficiary' members of street-based groups, and young men who were formerly in the core, who retain a link as graduated members.
9. We use the term 'street working' children to denote children who work in or around the street in irregular forms of (self-)employment. While few of these children are utterly homeless, many have experience of sleeping in the street on an occasional basis.
10. The Bengali permits either reading – it translates literally to 'having eaten beating he has got big'. However, the term 'eaten' (*kheye*) is used much more widely in Bengali than in English, to refer for example to being scolded, taking bribes etc., so not too much should be read into its use here.

References

Choudhury, S. A. (2003) 'Participation or mobilisation? Promoting the rights of the marginalised children in Bangladesh', unpublished MSc dissertation, Bath, UK: University of Bath.

Connell, R. W. (1987) *Gender and Power*, Cambridge: Polity Press.

Galtung, J. (1990) 'Cultural Violence', *Journal of Peace Research* 27(3): 291–305.

Goffman, E. (1990) [1959] *The Presentation of Self in Everyday Life*, Harmondwsorth: Penguin.

Hart, J. (2007) 'Empowerment or Frustration? Participatory programming with young Palestinians', *Children, Youth and Environments* 17(3): 1–23.

Khan, I. A. (2000) 'Struggle for survival: Networks and relationships in a Bangladesh slum', unpublished PhD thesis, Bath, UK: University of Bath.

Lee, N. (2001) *Childhood and Society: Growing up in an age of uncertainty*, Buckingham: Open University Press.

Lukes, S. (1974) *Power: A radical view*, Basingstoke: Macmillan.

Scheper-Hughes, N. (1992) *Death Without Weeping: The violence of everyday life in Brazil*, Berkeley/London: University of California Press.

White, S. C. (2002) 'From the politics of poverty to the politics of identity? Child rights and working children in Bangladesh', *Journal of International Development* 14(6): 725–35.

White, S. C. and Choudhury, S. A. (2007) 'The politics of child participation in international development: The dilemma of agency', *European Journal of Development Research* 19 (4), 529–50.

Part II

Learning about children's participation in practice

4 Children's participation in armed conflict and post-conflict peace building

Clare Feinstein, Annette Giertsen and Claire O'Kane

Introduction

Consideration of children in situations of conflict and post-conflict tends to focus on their protection and reflects a view that children are passive victims. However, ongoing research and evaluation conducted by Save the Children reveals the extent to which girls and boys are active participants in their own lives, while also influencing peers, families, school, communities and, in some contexts, political and military actors. This article explores the way in which children's participation is given meaning in situations of conflict and post-conflict peace building. In particular, it asks and explores how child-led organisations and children's capacities can be strengthened to enhance children's role as agents of peace, and how peace processes and peace agreements can become inclusive and responsive to children's perspectives.

Save the Children Norway undertook a global thematic evaluation on children's participation in armed conflict, post-conflict and peace building in Bosnia-Herzegovina, Guatemala, Nepal and Uganda to find answers to these questions. This chapter reflects on the process and some of the initial findings of this evaluation, which was undertaken over a two-year period[1] with the active involvement of children and young people who are part of existing children's associations, peace clubs and child clubs.

Save the Children Norway and the thematic evaluation

Save the Children Norway is an international non-governmental organisation working towards the realisation of children's rights. As a rights-based organisation Save the Children Norway understands and approaches children's participation as a need and a right, a working principle, a cross-cutting issue, a process, an objective, a political tool and a pedagogical approach (see Save the Children Norway 2005).

Save the Children Norway has introduced thematic evaluations as an organisational learning method to evaluate how it is working as an organisation, and with what results, in its different country programmes and in different thematic areas. In the case of a thematic evaluation on children's participation this relates to the need: to ensure that children's participation is part of all areas of Save the Children Norway's work; to improve quality in children's participation; to identify strengths and weaknesses, challenges and opportunities; and to document what has been achieved.

The decision to focus the global evaluation on children's participation in the specific area of armed conflict, post-conflict and peace building was based on children and young people's clear messages for peace and education, and their need for more support for their own participation and peace initiatives, articulated during an earlier global evaluation on children affected by armed conflict, displacement or disaster, undertaken in 2005 (Brown 2005).

Save the Children Norway country programmes which were affected by conflict or post-conflict and which support children's groups, participation or peace initiatives were encouraged to take part in the thematic evaluation. Country teams in Bosnia-Herzegovina, Guatemala, Nepal and Uganda committed themselves to the process.

Engaging children as active agents in the thematic evaluation process

A commitment to participatory research and evaluation with and by children, young people and adults provides an approach to participation which brings together reflection, learning and action to build upon their lived experience. Girls and boys from different ages and backgrounds have been actively involved as peer researchers, advisers, documenters, peace agents and advocates. They have gathered and analysed information on children's experiences of armed conflict, living in and through post-conflict situations, their understanding of peace building, and their role as agents of peace. Giving value to children's own views, perspectives, insights and their ability to problem-solve, to dialogue and negotiate with adults to strengthen their own initiatives and organisations has been integral to the way in which the thematic evaluation has been carried out.

Formative dialogue research (FDR) has been used as a methodological framework and a tool during the thematic evaluation, complemented by the use of a wide range of participatory tools,[2] as well as strong adherence to ethical guidelines.[3] The framework, tools and guidelines are all designed to ensure the active involvement of girls and boys of different ages, backgrounds and abilities at all levels and stages of the evaluation. This has included identification of key research issues based on children's priorities, support to children to shape their meaningful and safe contributions to the evaluation, and support to children's advocacy and media initiatives.

Key elements of FDR include dialogue to better explore and understand different perspectives, as well as the sharing of information and different perspectives to address challenges or to modify and improve projects – so that projects, and in this case children's own initiatives, can be strengthened *during* the research and evaluation process (see Baklien 2004). Key aspects of the participatory process, the methodological and ethical framework have been described and analysed elsewhere (Save the Children Norway 2008). This short contribution therefore focuses primarily on practical experiences and reflections on children's participation, including an identification of factors which either hinder or enable children's participation in peace building.

Building upon the FDR approach, this contribution also highlights significant efforts being undertaken by children and young people during the thematic evaluation process to strengthen their peace-building initiatives. Examples of child-led advocacy, media and documentation initiatives clearly illustrate children's strong wishes to be taken more seriously as social and political actors – and as agents of peace. They also illustrate the need to better address the root causes of conflict – including violence, poverty, discrimination, inequality, exclusion, corruption and violations of human rights – to ensure peace and reconstruction processes which promote equitable, participatory and protective environments for all citizens, including children.

Children's participation in conflict, post-conflict and peace building

Meaningful participation and space to come together with their peers, to share their experiences and express their views, can give children strength and increase their life skills and self-confidence – especially in situations characterised by conflict or insecurity. Support for child clubs, groups or initiatives has therefore been integral to Save the Children Norway's strategy to support meaningful children's participation. Children's active participation in this evaluation, through their clubs, groups and associations, has also been important in helping them to make sense of and come to terms with the situations they have confronted.

> I stayed alone, with no parents. I used to think about the past. It was difficult to forget what happened to me in the bush. I felt alone. No one wanted to stay with me, to share with me. I then joined an association and began to find peace within myself. My family came back to me. I have friends and I have learned from others. These days I am fine. I know what to do at the right time and right place.
>
> (Former abducted child, Northern Uganda)[4]

Children's participation in conflict, post-conflict and peace building takes different forms. In their respective child clubs, groups and associations girls and boys are participating actively to ensure their own protection and to contribute to peace building through:

- organising children's meetings, how to live, to relate to each other and to respect each other, and to better protect themselves;
- preparing poems, songs, dance, drama, debates, (wall) magazines and radio programmes to sensitise peers, family, school and community members on child rights and peace;
- promoting conflict transformation, dialogue and supporting peer advice, peer support, peer education and peer counselling;
- encouraging all girls and boys to go to school and to study (including children who were formerly associated with armed forces, and children with disabilities);
- raising their voice to tackle discrimination, abuse, violence and corruption within school and community settings;

- promoting children's participation in school governance, local governance and policy and practice developments to address issues which affect them;
- taking specific action according to the particular sociocultural, political context of their country and immediate environment.

Children's contributions to peace building

Children's main activities towards peace building have largely focused on raising awareness of peace, promoting the social values needed for peace, strengthening (and in some cases rebuilding) social relationships, and in some contexts demonstrating peaceful ways of resolving conflicts with families, schools and communities. To some extent children are also rebuilding social structures and contributing to the creation of safer environments and a stronger civil society, by organising

---

Box 4.1 Country-specific examples of children's participation

1 **Nepal** has been characterised by both conflict and post-conflict during the thematic evaluation process, as the conflict between the government and the Maoists has entered a new phase and a constitutional election process has taken place. Throughout this period, children have played an active role, especially through their Child Clubs:

- promoting understanding and respect for 'Children as Zones of Peace' and 'Schools as Zones of Peace' – including negotiations with Maoist and government army officials not to interrupt children's lives or education;
- advocating for peace through the organisation of peace campaigns, rallies and workshops at local, district and national levels;
- raising their voice against violations of children's rights, including early marriage, discrimination, abuse and violence;
- engaging in the constitutional election process through the development of a twelve-point Declaration by children's representatives from across the country which has been presented to concerned political parties and agencies.

2 In **Northern Uganda** a formal peace-talk process has been under way in Juba throughout the duration of the thematic evaluation, which has contributed to hopes of peace and security, resulting in some resettlement of children and adults from camps of internally displaced people. However, levels of insecurity continue as a peace agreement had not yet been reached. Children have been participating actively in school-based peace clubs, and out-of-school associations:

- promoting unity at community level through cultural dance and drumming;
- praying for peace and reconciliation;
- initiating community activities to build cooperation and solidarity among children and adults, to raise awareness of HIV/AIDS, and to support reintegration of formerly abducted children back into their communities;
- engaging in consultations on Agenda 3 of the peace talks on accountability and reconciliation and influencing the preparations of the peace agreement.

3 In **Bosnia-Herzegovina** living in a post-conflict scenario children have been:
   - undertaking public advocacy through highlighting the importance of creating safe and protective environments for children. They have designed 'risk maps' of areas in their localities showing where and why they feel unsafe, and have developed action plans to make these places safe and protective for children, which they have presented to the local authorities, including the mayor, for action;
   - organising a children's delegation to meet with the prime minister to advocate for the provision of quality education where no child is discriminated against;
   - organising round-table discussions on issues relating to children's rights and peace building – for example, young people in Srebrenica were concerned about the effect of the 1995 massacre. Young people from the region, together with internally displaced and returnee children, initiated and organised a round-table conference to discuss issues of importance for children living in the town and invited community leaders, local stakeholders and religious leaders to talk together with them;
   - advocating for their involvement in developing the school curriculum.

4 In **Guatemala**, which has also been characterised by a post-conflict scenario, girls and boys have been active:
   - working to maintain the historical memory of the internal armed conflict and highlighting the importance of including the study of the history of the conflict – its reasons and its impact – as part of the school curriculum;
   - working as 'mental health promoters' to promote better mental health among peers, especially those affected by the civil war, such as orphans;
   - sharing their ideas with representatives of the Human Rights Ombudsman's Office;
   - undertaking public advocacy through radio programmes, the painting of wall murals and the development of articles for a magazine to promote their messages about conflict and peace and the need for justice.

Box 4.2 Uganda: case illustration

Children involved in the thematic evaluation in Northern Uganda have been persistent in advocating for inclusion of children's voices and children's representation in the formal peace talks, and played a catalytic role in ensuring the inclusion of girls and boys in civil society consultations on Agenda 3 of the peace talks on reconciliation and accountability. On reading a draft report of children's views on reconciliation and accountability (Concerned Parents' Association 2007), the government delegation extended its own formal consultation process by a day to directly meet with children's representatives from four districts in Northern Uganda and listen to their views. The ensuing agreement on reconciliation and accountability clearly reflects a commitment to children's participation.

children's clubs and networks, groups and organisations; and by influencing school, community, local and national governance planning through dialogue between children and adults, which, in turn, contributes to monitoring and better implementation of children's rights. However, children are also advocating for increased space in political processes affecting them, including formal peace-talk, reconciliation and reconstruction processes, so that they may more meaningfully contribute to efforts to identify, address and monitor the structural factors which inhibit peace and the fulfilment of children's rights.[5]

Factors which hinder and enable children's participation in peace building

'Intolerance, violence, mistrust, adult attitudes, lack of support from the authorities, the lack of a culture of peace' are all factors which inhibit children's participation in peace building according to children and young people in Guatemala.

(National Reflection Workshop, November 2007)

Consideration of factors which hinder or enable children's participation in peace building further reinforces the importance of efforts by adults – parents, teachers, community elders, NGO workers, government officials and UN agencies and procedures – to recognise and more positively engage with girls and boys as social and political actors.

Children and young people have also emphasised the need to recognise and address discrimination and subtle power relations that exist among them – among girls and boys of different ages, abilities and ethnic, class, caste, religious or income groups – so that more inclusive, democratic forms of participation and organisation can be fostered.

Social and traditional values continue to be the main stumbling block for children's participation – both generally and in peace building. The proverb 'children should be seen and not heard' remains prevalent in diverse sociocultural contexts. Children's capabilities are generally undermined by adults, and it is not considered important to take their views into consideration in decision-making processes. Negative social attitudes towards particular groups of children, including children with disabilities, girls, ethnic/minority groups, and children associated with the armed forces, may further undermine opportunities for certain children to participate. In most contexts the school environment also continues to reinforce power relations, traditional learning and disciplinary methods which are antagonistic to participatory ways of engaging children.

As a result of the prevailing attitudes and behaviour towards children, practices and policies (at different levels – school, community, district, nation) which promote and support children's participation are generally the exception rather than the norm. In most contexts children have been excluded from formal peace-building processes and child rights have been marginalised in the development and monitoring of peace agreements and peace accords.

It is therefore not surprising that many girls and boys lack confidence in speaking out or playing an active role in trying to transform violence into peace. Children's fears of reprisal, abuse, abduction or other violations of children's rights are further amplified in situations which have been characterised by insecurity or conflict. As highlighted by one girl in Nepal: 'Before, Child Club members felt afraid to talk with Maoist community leaders, but now we can freely mingle with them, since there is less fear of abduction now peace negotiations are under way.'[6]

Inequality and discrimination among children is also a barrier to children's participation, as younger children, in some contexts girls, children from lower caste, class or income groups, children with disabilities, children from minority ethnic groups, or non-school-going children may participate less as older, male, more educated children tend to dominate. This domination may be reinforced by adults, especially teachers, who often select the more vocal, confident children to represent their peers.

Despite these negative aspects, there are positive examples of social change through which children are gaining increased space to organise themselves, to undertake child-rights and peace-building activities and to participate in decision-making processes affecting them. Such space, however, needs to be further explored and expanded.

From children's perspectives, key enabling factors for children's participation – both in general and for their participation in peace building – include:

- sensitisation of key adults in their lives – parents, teachers, community, religious and political leaders – to recognise the importance of listening to children's views and to support children's participation in peace building;
- support for girls and boys to regularly come together in their own clubs, groups or associations to express their views, to analyse and plan action on issues affecting them;
- capacity building of children on children's rights, life skills, non-discrimination and inclusion, peace building and conflict resolution, organisational development, media and advocacy;
- practical support from NGOs or local community in terms of material and financial support, for example for transport and costs of organising action initiatives;
- access to child-friendly information on national policy and practice issues affecting them, including peace-agreement, peace-talk, constitutional or election processes;
- the establishment and strengthening of partnerships between child clubs or associations and schools, such as school management committees, other civil society groups, for example women's groups, youth groups, village child protection committees, and government bodies such as the district child welfare board in Nepal, or the Uganda Parliamentary Forum for Children;
- the development of inclusive governance structures and political processes, including peace talks, constitutional and election processes which include children's representatives;
- increased efforts by government, rebel groups, the UN, INGOs, NGOs, civil society groups and other actors to respect, protect and fulfil children's rights.

Examples of child-led advocacy, media and documentation initiatives

Creative examples of how children are using documentation for advocacy work and how this is providing inspiration to, and guidance for, children involved in peace-building work include: the development and publication of 'Children's Peace Albums' in Northern Uganda, which bring together children's poetry, drawings and stories on conflict and peace; publication of poetry and stories in newspapers in Nepal; children's involvement in community and district-based radio programmes in Guatemala, Uganda and Nepal to share key messages and stories; and the development of a children's newsletter which has been presented by children's representatives to the prime minister of Bosnia-Herzegovina.

Children and young people involved in the thematic evaluation in each country have also been supported to draft a memorandum outlining the key issues of importance to them so as to enhance their participation in peace building, and which they are bringing to the attention of key duty bearers in their communities and at national level.[7] While each country focuses on specific issues that are of particular relevance to their context, they have also identified issues in common across countries, such as greater support and priority to children's rights, the importance of listening to children and taking into account what they say, and the importance of promoting peace building.

Box 4.3 Priority issues identified by children and young people in their memorandums

Nepal: The importance of child clubs developing and implementing rules, regulations and action plans; ensuring inclusive and active participation; building the capacity of all child club members; ending all forms of social discrimination; promoting peace building.

Bosnia-Herzegovina: Lack of knowledge about child rights; child participation in the curriculum; peace building; promotion of child initiatives and skills; peer violence.

Uganda: Ignoring children's views; negligence of child rights; corruption; the International Criminal Court (and arrest warrants as a barrier to securing the peace agreement); land disputes.

Guatemala: Absence of taking children's opinions into account; considering children to be incapable; importance of including the real history of the war in the school curriculum; learning the causes of the internal armed conflict; promoting respect for cultural differences; concerns about insecurity and increased violence due to maras (gangs).

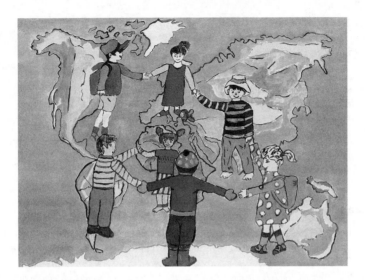

Figure 4.1   'Children as agents of peace', drawing by a 14-year-old girl from Bosnia-Herzegovina

Concluding comments

This chapter has looked at children's participation in armed conflict and post-conflict peace building. Through the documentation, analysis and advocacy of their experiences of, and contributions to, peace building, it is clear that the issue is no longer *whether* they should be part of peace processes, but *how* to ensure that their voices are heard in consistent and substantive ways in peace agreements and decision-making processes related to the building of peace in their communities and countries. Through the thematic evaluation, children and young people have demonstrated how they are deeply affected by armed conflict and by the continuing aggressiveness and violence which surrounds them. However, they have also shown the valuable contributions they have made and can make to peace and reconciliation processes and their feeling of responsibility for the future of their countries. As summed up by children in Bosnia-Herzegovina, they want to be 'the generation that is capable of thinking about the possibilities for change'.[8] As adults, we need to make sure that we are ready to continue to support this generation with the necessary child-friendly structures and processes that will make their participation in decisions affecting them meaningful, sustainable and inclusive.

Acknowledgements

We would like to acknowledge the creativity, dedication and hard work of the children and young people, and supporting adults, who have been actively engaged in the thematic evaluation in Bosnia-Herzegovina, Guatemala, Nepal and Uganda.

Notes

1. October 2006–October 2008.
2. See Kit of Tools on www.reddbarna.no/chp/www.reddbarna.no/default.asp?V_ITEM _ID=19028.
3. Which are underpinned by application of practice standards in children's participation and adherence to organisational child protection policies.
4. See Save the Children Norway (2006).
5. See also O'Kane, Feinstein and Giertsen (2009).
6. Expressed during National Reflection workshop in Nepal December 2007 – see Save the Children Norway Nepal, 2008.
7. See   www.reddbarna.no/chp/www.reddbarna.no/default.asp?V_ITEM_ID=11749 for the full text of the Children's Memorandum from each country.
8. National Reflection Workshop, Bosnia-Herzegovina, January 2008.

References

Baklien, Bergljot (2004) 'Formative dialogue research', English version of article published in the *Journal of Sosiologi idag* 4, 2004, available at: www.reddbarna.no/default. asp?V_ITEM_ID=11025

Brown, M. (2005) *Global Evaluation: Children affected by armed conflict, displacement or disaster (CACD)*, Oslo: Save the Children Norway.

Concerned Parents' Association (2007) *Accountability and Reconciliation, Perspectives from Children and the Youth in Northern and Eastern Uganda*, Uganda: CPA in association with Transcultural Psychosocial Organisation, Save the Children and UNICEF.

O'Kane, C., Feinstein, C. and Giertsen, A. (2009) 'Children and young people in post-conflict peace-building', in D. Nosworthy (ed.) *Seen, but not Heard! Placing children and youth on the security agenda*, Geneva: Centre for the Democratic Control of Armed Forces (DCAF).

Save the Children Norway (2005) *Save the Children Norway's Framework for Increasing Quality Work in Child Participation*, Oslo: Save the Children.

Save the Children Norway (2006) 'Thematic evaluation of children's participation in armed conflict, post conflict and peace-building', International Start-up Workshop, November 2006, Uganda, report by Clare Feinstein, Claire O'Kane and Annette Giertsen.

Save the Children Norway Nepal (2008) 'National Reflection Workshop Report: Thematic Evaluation on Children's Participation in Armed Conflict, Post Conflict and Peace Building', National Reflection Workshop, 3–7 December 2007, Pokhara, Nepal.

5 The participation of children living in the poorest and most difficult situations

Patricia Ray

Introduction

Under the influence of the Convention on the Rights of the Child, the promotion of children's participation has become a key component of the approach of many child-focused development organisations. At the same time, the child rights principle of non-discrimination has led to an increasing focus on groups of children whose rights are most violated and who are living in very poor and difficult situations. From this work, the participation of children in decisions that affect their lives emerges not only as a right but as a key strategy in enabling them to transform their relationships with adults, exercise their other rights and become active citizens.

Traditionally, most organisations have worked with children in difficult situations on a group-by-group basis according to the different categories of 'Children in Especially Difficult Circumstances', such as street and working children and children with disabilities. The best practices and lessons learned in working with specific groups of children are important. However, engaging with children on a group-by-group basis tends to focus attention on certain groups at the expense of others and fails to recognise the many and varied ways in which children can be marginalised by their societies (Feeny and Boyden 2003). Children in the poorest and most difficult situations are still largely excluded from 'mainstream' child-centred community development activities. There is a need for a more integrated approach that identifies common principles for working with children and communities to identify, understand and assist children in difficult situations to improve their quality of life. This chapter seeks to contribute by identifying common lessons learned in facilitating the participation of these children.

The chapter looks at who the children in the poorest and most difficult situations are, examines the barriers that they experience to their participation and draws out some of the common lessons learned in facilitating the participation of these children. The chapter draws largely from a global review that was conducted for Plan International on its work with children in the poorest and most difficult situations (Ray and Carter 2007) as well as other studies and materials produced by Plan and its partners. The review involved a study of the literature and visits to eight countries to meet with children, their communities and representatives from the organisations that work with them. The countries were Egypt, Uganda, Senegal, Sierra Leone, Nepal, India, Vietnam and Guatemala and were chosen in order to provide a range of examples of the kind of work that Plan does with children in difficult situations.

Who are children in the poorest and most difficult situations?

Over the years, many different terms have been used to describe those children whose rights are most violated and who are most at risk within their societies, the most commonly used being 'Children in Especially Difficult Circumstances', which was coined by UNICEF in the 1980s. However, many documents simply list different groups of children and few clear definitions are to be found. In reality, the children who are most at risk vary by location and over time and need to be identified within each country and local context.

Children in the poorest and most difficult situations are those whose quality of life and ability to fulfil their potential is most affected by the violation of their rights, caused by one or more of the following forms of marginalisation:

- extreme poverty
- violence, abuse, neglect and exploitation
- discrimination and social exclusion
- catastrophic events, such as conflict and disaster.

What most clearly distinguishes these children is that they lack adequate care and support and live their lives outside the mainstream of society. The term 'children in the poorest and most difficult situations' has been adopted in this article because it is understood and accepted by children and because it expresses the important link between extreme poverty and other situations of risk.

Many children's groups are very sympathetic to the situation of children who are worse off than themselves, and can play a key role in identifying and promoting the inclusion of children in difficult situations within their societies (see Box 5.1).

The participation of children in the poorest and most difficult situations

Children living in the poorest and most difficult situations experience great difficulties in making contributions to community development processes, but do exercise varying degrees of agency over their own situation. For them, participation is concerned principally with the struggle to access basic human rights at an individual or group level. Children are affected in their ability to participate by the relationships of power that adults exercise over them. For children in the poorest and most difficult situations, these barriers are magnified and complicated by disadvantage, discrimination and the extreme violation of their other rights. The following discussion illustrates what participation means for children in the context of the four main causes of marginalisation identified above.

Children who live in extreme poverty have great difficulties in meeting their very basic needs for food, clothing, shelter and personal hygiene. This in turn

Box 5.1 'Who are the children with the most difficult lives in your community?'

Members of a children's group in a poor urban area of Delhi conducted a consultation with their peers on the question 'Who are the children with the most difficult lives in your community?' Here are their responses:

- Those involved in child labour
- Children who work on the railways are abused physically and sexually
- Those whose parents suffer from alcoholism
- Children who are exploited mentally and physically, particularly girl children who are abused at home
- Those who are very poor
- Girl children, orphans
- Children involved in sexual exploitation
- Children who are trafficked
- Children who are denied education
- Those who drop out from school and then get involved in substance abuse.

brings fear, shame, lack of self-esteem and stigmatisation by others, making it very difficult for children to participate in the life of their communities or to benefit from public services. In these situations participation is characterised by children's own actions and decisions as they develop methods for coping. Their options are often very limited and may involve them in activities such as street migration and prostitution, which put them at even greater risk. We found that finding enough food to eat was the main preoccupation of very poor child-headed households in Uganda. Older children from these families drop out of school to work and find food. Boys frequently migrate to the cities for work, while some girls have sex for money and many marry very young.

Children who are subject to violence, abuse, neglect and exploitation are also restricted in their ability to participate. The UN Study on Violence Against Children has shown that violence and abuse are very common in homes, schools and communities, particularly against already marginalised groups, such as girl children in some societies. A group of children from an urban community in Delhi commented very perceptively on the harm that abuse does and how it inhibits children from actively participating in their own development. They said:

It is difficult for children, particularly girl children who are exploited mentally and physically, to speak out and develop. They lack self-esteem and start to hate themselves.

Discrimination and social exclusion set children apart from the mainstream of society and severely limit their opportunities and their agency. Patterns of discrimination vary between different cultures and traditions, but children with disabilities face discrimination worldwide. In Egypt, the birth of a child with a disability is viewed as something shameful, and such children are frequently neglected and excluded from playing with other children or participating in the life of their families and communities. The mother of a child with disabilities told us:

> We had a problem in our minds. Before [the programme] we did not give our children with disabilities enough to eat, take them to the health centre when they were sick or let them play with the other children.

Children are disproportionately affected by catastrophic events, such as natural disasters or conflict, in terms of loss of life, injury, loss of parents, loss of development opportunities and vulnerability to protection violations. Yet children's and young people's situations, and in turn their participation in humanitarian relief and rehabilitation efforts, are consistently ignored. In a study of children's participation in disaster response and recovery following the Asian tsunami, Plan found that government and relief organisation officials felt that there were more important things to do than to try to engage with children, even though children were willing and able to help (Plan International 2005a). Among children affected by conflict and disaster, children from marginalised groups, such as those from ethnic minorities, are at an even greater disadvantage. Following the tsunami, children in Thailand reported that no effort was made to include children from marginalised groups in the participatory activities for children that were implemented in the camps.

These examples illustrate how the participation of children in the poorest and most difficult situations is characterised by a struggle to survive and engage in everyday activities. This lack of fulfilment of the basic rights of the most marginalised children is often neglected in child-centred community development programmes, which unintentionally reproduce existing patterns of exclusion and discrimination. To this extent, these children experience two levels of exclusion by being denied basic rights and by being denied opportunities to participate in responses to their situations.

Lessons learned in promoting the participation of children in the poorest and most difficult situations

Children's participation is a key strategy in assisting children in the poorest and most difficult situations to realise their rights. However, efforts to support their participation need to take account of the fact that society has failed in its duty of care towards them. Strategies need to be put in place to ensure that they do not come to further harm, and that are sensitive to the particular situation, context and experience not only of each group of children but, in many cases, of each child. Some of the lessons learned by Plan and its partners in promoting the participation of children in the poorest and most difficult situations are summarised below.

Targeted and community-wide approaches

Promotion of the participation of children in the poorest and most difficult situations may be targeted to particular groups or may be part of community-wide approaches. Although ultimately the aim is for all children to be included and

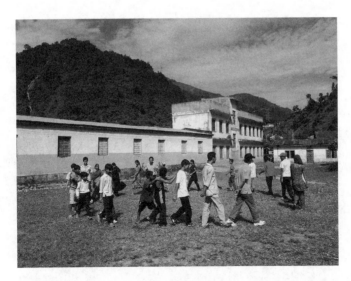

Plate 5.1 Which children are absent from the circle? These children and young people
are members of a school-based children's club in Nepal who were 'warming
up' for a discussion with visiting researchers. Sitting on the wall watching them
was a group of children who were not members of the club because they were
not in school. Enquiry revealed that all of them were children from *dalit* families
(discriminated castes). No out-of-school clubs had been set up, thus reinforcing
existing patterns of exclusion. Copyright: Patricia Ray

to benefit equally from their societies, targeted approaches are often necessary
in order for children to have time and space to address their particular issues
together with children in the same situation. This is especially true for children
who have been separated from their families and communities, such as street children and some working children.

Many child domestic workers, for example, are very isolated. They work long
hours and often are not allowed out of their employer's house. If they complain,
they may be dealt with very harshly. As a result, they become withdrawn and
cope by internalising their problems. Children and Women in Social Service and
Human Rights (CWISH), a national NGO, works with child domestic workers in
Kathmandu, Nepal. It invites children to attend a day centre and participate in
non-formal education classes. Initially the children are very fearful and withdrawn.
Careful approaches that build their confidence and skills are necessary. With time,
the children make friends and begin to support each other. They told us:

> Through coming here we have regained our happiness and now we can build
> up a vision of the future. We now know how to make friends and how to deal
> with other people like our employers and people on the street.

Community-wide approaches may be adopted to promote the participation and
social inclusion of children in difficult situations who have not separated from their

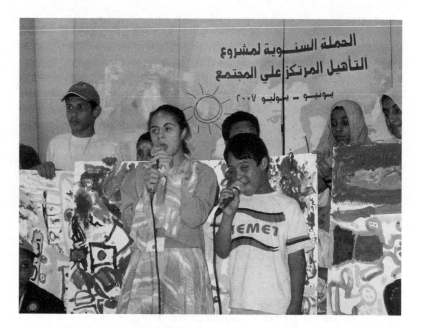

Plate 5.2   Children with and without disabilities participating in a conference to promote
access to services for children with disabilities in Egypt. Copyright: Patricia Ray

families and communities. Existing children's groups can play an important role
in these programmes. The Child Focused Community Rehabilitation Programme
implemented by Plan and its partners in Egypt involved children's groups in the
awareness-raising and social mobilisation component of the programme and
members became actively involved in working with children with disabilities.
Children with and without disabilities now participate together in cultural, sporting
and social activities and in advocating for improved attitudes and behaviours towards
children with disabilities and for improved services. As one girl put it:

> In the beginning we feared disabled children, now we have come to love them like
> brothers and sisters. They have their rights and we want to help them get them.

Individual approaches

Many children in the poorest and most difficult situations experience complex
problems. Their participation in the decisions that are made about their futures is
crucial if lasting solutions to improving their quality of life are to be found.

Plan in Uganda found that the participation of children from very poor
child-headed households in vocational training schemes was not sustained (Plan
International 2005b). One girl who had been provided with a sewing machine
only used it to put her cloths on top of it. Asked why, she said:

I find it more important to stay home and grow and prepare food for my brothers and sisters than to continue going for lessons in tailoring.

Plan Uganda realised that programmes of assistance needed to be based on a deeper understanding of the children's view of their particular family situation and on their existing coping strategies, which would have become apparent if these children had been involved in the design of programmes. It also realised that this would be better facilitated by community members than by the staff of an external organisation. Plan has now trained volunteer counsellors to visit child-headed households on a regular basis, to build trust, gain an in-depth understanding of the situation of each household and provide them with support and advice. This generates confidence in the children to participate in decisions made about the assistance that is provided for them and also strengthens the commitment of the community to supporting children from these households.

Peer and role-model approaches

As children grow, the importance of their peers and older children in guiding their behaviour and forming their values increases. This is the basis for the use of peer and role-model approaches to behavioural change. Separated children lack care and support from their families. They therefore form particularly strong peer groupings and are often distrustful of adults (see Box 5.2 for examples of how peer approaches can be used to make contact with children).

The testimonies of young people who have survived difficult situations are important in motivating others to take action to prevent risks. Following a series of landslides that have engulfed villages and caused serious loss of life on the island

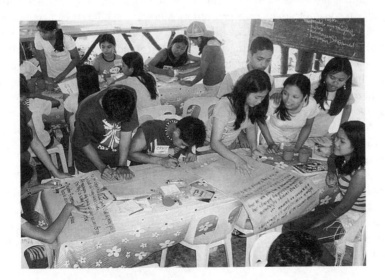

Plate 5.3 Young people engaged in participatory risk mapping in Southern Leyte, Philippines. Copyright: Patricia Ray

Box 5.2 Peer and role-model approaches

It took three years for Community Action Centre Nepal – an organisation in Nepal that works with girls who are commercial sex workers – to establish meaningful contact with them. Their outreach with the girls is conducted largely through peer support and education. Similarly, street children who have participated in their programmes are trained as peer educators by Childhood Enhancement through Training and Action (CHETNA), a partner of Plan India in Delhi. They identify and make contact with newly arrived street children and introduce them to the services that CHETNA provides.

of Southern Leyte, in the Philippines, Plan is promoting a child-centred approach to disaster risk reduction. Children and young people who experienced the landslides at first hand are very motivated to be involved and lead the process of risk mapping and the implementation of activities to reduce the risk of further disasters. As one of them said:

> Being a student survivor, I have my responsibility to get involved with this. We lost our loved ones and we have to honour and treasure the memories.
>
> (Plan International et al. 2008)

Participation in protection

Children in the poorest and most difficult situations are frequently surrounded by adults who exhibit deep-seated negative attitudes and behaviours towards them. They cannot always be 'rescued' from their situation, and their participation in activities to promote their own protection is crucial. Children can be taught to protect themselves through discussion of the potential risks that they face, how to deal with them and how to access help from the police and service providers. Children are able to protect themselves more easily when they look out for each other. In Delhi, CHETNA (Childhood Enhancement through Training and Action) forms children into groups that support each other, report violations and lobby for the rights of street children.

Children can be assisted in identifying those people in their environment who pose a threat to them, and supported in developing responses to reduce the threat that they pose (White 2002). Many organisations have found that, in most cases, positive dialogue and involvement with those who pose a threat is the best way forward. For example, Plan works with Concern in Nepal to establish clubs for children who work in hazardous forms of child labour. The challenges that the children face include violence within the family, often triggered by alcohol, violence in the work place and discrimination at school. Together they engage their employers and parents in dialogue to see how their situation at work and at home can be improved. One girl said:

> There has been a change in the whole family. My parents used to drink and then quarrel, but after I spoke to them about it they have stopped.

communities heavily affected by HIV/AIDS, others were from urban areas with high rates of abuse and crime. The Children's Institute worked with a partner non-governmental organisation (NGO) in each province. These organisations selected the children after explaining the project and seeking their consent, and that of their guardians, to participate in the project. Three of the four partner NGOs each provided an adult caregiver to accompany and support the three children selected to participate in the project. The fourth group did not have an adult caregiver, which was a shortcoming.

There was a detailed and continuous consent procedure (Mniki and Rosa 2007). The project and its objectives were explained in detail before it started, and children were given the choice of opting in or out of any of the activities. It was also important to ensure that the children did not expect immediate results from the law reform. The project team explained that developing and implementing legislation can take years, so that the children knew that they could change the law but that the law would take effect in the future, making a difference not to them but to younger members of their families and communities.

Preparatory phase

Discussing abuse and traumatic experiences

The Children's Institute organised three workshops with the children and their caregivers prior to the first public hearings in parliament. The first workshop concentrated on building legislative literacy, i.e. explaining children's rights and the law-making process, and starting discussions about children's experiences and appropriate service responses. The project team was concerned that, while discussing the children's life experiences would yield rich advocacy material, it would inevitably stir up difficult feelings. A psychologist joined the team to help deal with catharsis and prevent secondary trauma. He used a narrative therapy methodology, whereby children produced personal 'Hero Books' to gain mastery over specific problems and challenges. The children were encouraged to see their problems as having a political dimension, and that participation in the law-making process is one way of gaining control over these challenges. They came to realise that the fact that legislation does not provide the right services to protect children from abuse, or prevent them from having to look after cattle, is part of the problem; therefore part of the solution was to mobilise in the political arena.

Making the text accessible

The consolidated Children's Bill was written in complex legal language and contained over 300 clauses that covered a range of different services. To make it accessible, the team drafted an illustrated resource pack containing a child-friendly version of the Bill (Proudlock et al. 2004). The pack was designed after the first workshop, during which children identified the challenges facing them, and it focused on the chapters and clauses corresponding to the issues raised, namely children's rights, parental responsibilities and rights, prevention and protection services. It also contained activities designed to enable children to learn about, and develop opinions on, what was lacking in the Bill and what clauses they were satisfied with. At the second workshop children used the resource pack to develop submissions for presentation at the parliamentary hearings, as well as action plans for an advocacy campaign in their own neighbourhoods, which they called 'Children are the Future, Give them their Rights'.

The national process[2]

National Assembly public hearings

In August 2004, 30 children's sector organisations, including children's groups, presented submissions on the Children's Bill to the National Assembly. In preparation, the Dikwankwetla went on a tour of parliament, and met with the chair of the Parliamentary Portfolio Committee on Social Development. They also used one of the committee rooms to create a mock parliament, with members of the team challenging the children and asking them questions so they could practise using the microphones and gain confidence.

At the hearings, the Dikwankwetla described the challenges facing them and children in their communities:

> I've got six other siblings, four of which are HIV positive. I am taking care of my four siblings with my old grandmother and that doesn't mean my mother is not alive. She is very alive but the problem is that she doesn't stay at home with us and take care of us. She is always away and when she comes home she comes drunk and she abuses us emotionally. This affects me mentally. I cannot cope well with my school and I don't have enough time to rest.

One child spoke of the rape of a close relative by another family member. The stories clearly illustrated the lack of service delivery and support for children, and how that lack of support violated their rights. Once they had described the challenges, they called on the members of parliament (MPs) and government officials to fulfil their rights, for example:

• the right to be looked after and have a home
• the right to equal opportunities and to development.

After two of the children spoke, the chair of the Portfolio Committee said: 'Thank you, we have now heard from the nation', but the project staff had to tell the chair that the submission was not finished. (Project staff interpreted this as a dismissive act, but during the evaluation the children and caregivers mentioned this comment as a highlight.) The session ended with questions and comments from the MPs. They were cynical about the high standard of the presentation; one even asked whether the children had been told what to say. However, as children answered the questions their replies dispelled any doubts. At the end of the session some of the MPs spoke to them individually, and some of the children showed the MPs copies of their 'Hero Books' during these conversations.

Media exposure

The Dikwankwetla children were told that both the public and the media would attend. They chose to give their own first names and where they came from. During the hearings one child spoke of the rape of a close relative by another family member. An article on the children's submission was published in a newspaper the following day, which included the child's submission, the content of the story and the disclosure of the child's home province, which made her identifiable. The article was not published where the child lives, but about a year after the hearings the article was copied and printed in a textbook that was used in the child's school. This caused distress to the child and her family. The local NGO intervened by providing counselling and support to the child and her family.

NCOP public hearings

The deliberations took much longer than anticipated and, although information on the debate was passed to the caregivers, the children were not regrouped to lobby or respond. In June 2005, when the National Assembly passed the Bill, the matters of virginity testing, circumcision and access to contraception caused a furore in the media. The public outcry was such that the Select Committee on Social Services in the National Council of Provinces (NCOP) decided to hold more hearings to consult on the controversial topics. The clauses under debate did not correspond to the issues raised by the children during the Dikwankwetla workshops, therefore the project coordinator did not involve the group. If the principles of participation had been fully applied, this decision should have been made by the children. When the groups met with the project staff in preparation for the provincial hearings they expressed strong opinions on these matters.

Reflection and evaluation

Parliament passed the Children's Bill in December 2005. Dikwankwetla held a further workshop to evaluate progress and plan for advocacy around the second Bill. During the workshop certain weaknesses of the campaign came to light. Needing to follow the parliamentary timetable but also school holidays meant that there were gaps either between the workshops or between the time the workshop was held and when the public hearings took place.

> We feel that we were neglected by the CI in that we were not contacted or informed about the progress of the Bill and our work.

Advocacy is a process that relies on constant communication. The financial and logistical challenges meant that communication with the children was principally through the workshops. In between there was little in the way of progress updates or engagement that would have enabled them to follow the debates and lobby decision makers. The children drafted new advocacy plans which included teleconferencing as a means of filling the extended gaps between parliamentary sessions, and asked for their own budgets for provincial meetings and campaigns. This helped with the groups that had a local caregiver, but the children from one province did not have an adult caregiver to coordinate activities and hold the group together.

The provincial process

Provincial hearings on the Children's Amendment Bill were held in rural community halls, and in some cases large numbers of the general public came to observe the proceedings; hence the children chose to travel to areas where they would not be known. The submissions gave a description of the challenges they faced and their suggestions for changes to the Bill:

> I suffered a lot when both my parents died, I had to live with my relatives. They said they will take care of me and bring me up, because I was still very young, but they failed to keep their promise. I had to wake up in the morning and go to the field before I go to school. I sometimes had to sleep outside the house. I had to be absent at school because I had to stay home, it was very hard so we [I and my siblings] decided to move out and stay alone because we couldn't take all the abuse. We decided to become orphans at our own home which is child-headed household, it's very hard because we need parental care.
>
> You should change the Bill and you should add to the list of who should report abuse, you should add principals of schools, foster-parents and LoveLife staff.[3]

Another child spoke of the rape of her sister and praised the local service providers for the support her family received after the event, and she called for stronger prevention services to stop abuse. One MP responded with shock and outrage, promising to personally give protection to her and her family.

The levels of commitment to public participation varied greatly. In the province of KwaZulu-Natal (KZN) the legislature organised educational workshops to maximise involvement. In contrast, in Limpopo the MPs refused to allow members of the public to speak. One of the children described what happened:

> At first we were not allowed by the parliamentary administrator to present because the Committee didn't know about us. Lucy [CI staff member] insisted that we be allowed to present. Someone from the DoSD [Department of Social Development] who knew about Dikwankwetla informed the Chairperson and we were allowed to present. ... The Chairperson was the only parliamentarian in the Committee, the others were councillors. The MP has now been appointed MEC [Member of the Executive Council] for Transport. We are worried that our submissions may not make it to Parliament.

All of the recommendations made by the Western Cape and KZN groups were included in the provincial mandates. As the children had feared, none of the recommendations made in Limpopo was included in the detailed mandate. The NCOP accepted all of the changes proposed by the provinces, and passed the Bill on 29 May 2007. Some of these changes were extremely controversial (e.g. a ban on corporal punishment in the home), so the National Assembly took the unusual decision to hold a series of community consultations in rural communities. The Children's Institute complained about the hearings in Limpopo and this was taken into consideration by the consultation planning team. Limpopo and North West were on the itinerary; therefore the children from these provinces got a second chance to address the decision makers.

At the community consultations in Limpopo, two of the children asked for the camera to be turned off while they presented. The Committee agreed to make an exception when the first child asked, but an official raised a concern that this would result in the lack of a public record; therefore, when the second child asked for the camera to be turned off, the Committee declined. It did, however, offer to meet with the child separately after the close of the official hearing. This shows that there are options available to parliamentarians and that they can be flexible; however, the participation of children is not planned for and therefore measures are ad hoc.

Evaluation by participants

In December 2006 the Children's Institute conducted a four-day project evaluation with the Dikwankwetla. Their evaluation of the parliamentary hearings is summarised in Table 6.1.

Adult evaluation

Interviews were conducted with the adults who participated in the hearings, including MPs. When asked about which submissions stood out, the majority of respondents replied that the children's submissions made a great impact on the MPs because they were 'different' and 'came from the heart'. Many commented on how the children's submissions complemented the adult submissions: 'they spoke for themselves and they sort of emphasised everything that the experts were saying. How it impacts on them.'

Impact on the Children's Act

There were public hearings in eighty locations over the course of four years, and hundreds of written submissions. It is virtually impossible to isolate the impact of any individual or group on the final legislation. However, the MPs incorporated some of the changes raised by the Dikwankwetla, for example they changed the definition of child-headed households to include children living alone whose parents are still alive. Furthermore, to ensure that children are not overburdened by taking on full adult responsibilities, MPs insisted that the eldest child must be at least 16 and be assisted and supported by a 'supervising adult'.

Table 6.1 Children's evaluation of parliamentary hearings

Positive experiences	Negative experiences
• Our submissions made a difference and were heard by parliamentarians because Dikwankwetla was mentioned in magazines, articles on the internet and quoted by parliamentarians.[a] • Our submissions were appreciated because a few parliamentarians came up and thanked us. • Our submissions influenced the passing of the Children's Bill. • We felt very important to be in parliament. • It was a process of personal growth. • We were nervous but it was an experience of a lifetime. • We managed to make our submissions even though the committee was made up of only adults with no youth representatives. • The first objective of the project was to convey the message to the members of parliament. That goal was reached. • There is a positive impact because [the Children's Bill] is now an Act and we were part of it. • The MPs were influenced by children because they responded well.	• Not all the correct people heard us or agreed with what we were saying. • Some of the things we said ended up in the wrong space, like articles in the media. • It was difficult to get time for submission to the local public hearing. • It is difficult to get hold of parliamentarians to invite them to visit our project. • Some of the parliamentarians thought the CI told us what to say in our speeches. • Even after the workshops with the CI, we were still nervous to speak in parliament.

Source: Mūkoma 2007.

Note

a The Minister for Social Development, Dr Zola Skweyiya, quoted Dikwankwetla in his keynote address at the South African launch of UNICEF's the 'State of the world's children report 2006' in Cape Town, 6 February 2006.

Implications for children's participation in the legislative arena

What value is there in children participating in the law reform process?

The Dikwankwetla project was unique in South Africa because it attempted to facilitate the sustained involvement of one group of children during a four-year legislative process. Their participation brought many benefits, e.g. the children developed a thorough understanding of democratic processes, the institutions of government and children's rights, which they in turn shared with others in their home communities. Given the right support materials and a safe space, the children were able to understand the complex legislation and to relate it to their own experiences in a positive and empowering way. The gap between the different stages of the process also enabled the children to consult with their peers, and to inspire other children to join the campaign.

The children brought something unique to the process, and their experiences highlighted the challenges children face as well as the gaps in services to support and protect them. Although the MPs did not recall the children's submissions specifically, the concerns raised by the children were repeatedly raised by the MPs during the many months of deliberation.

The children's presentations moved the adult activists who attended the hearings, and during the course of the law reform process an increasing number of children were consulted or helped to participate. That the final Act contains some of the measures that were recommended by the children is testament to the fact that children are capable of participating meaningfully in the process.

Do the benefits outweigh the risks?

When the Dikwankwetla project was established the team knew that the children would be exposed to risk, but that risk was managed for the most part; and when one child's story was published there was support for the child and family in their own community. This incident highlights the need for support long after the event and raises questions about whether these kinds of disclosure should take place in a public space. There is value to children sharing their experiences of abuse with decision makers who are writing child protection legislation. However, it is important that disclosure does not have negative repercussions for the child. When a child gives evidence of abuse in court cases special protective measures are taken, e.g. CCTV and intermediaries are used, and the media are not permitted to disclose the name of the child in any news coverage. It would certainly be possible for parliament to offer such protection to children. Reporting guidelines could be issued; alternatively, hearings could be held in a separate room, or on a different day from the other submissions. Parliament needs to plan for the participation of children and give consideration to how it can create a safe space where children can give evidence of their own experiences, and at the very least to train MPs on how to interact with children. Ultimately, the children evaluated the project very positively and described a number of benefits that outweighed the risks.

However, to enable children to participate, such a project needs extra support. Facilitating the active participation of these twelve children cost approximately $125,000 per year over a four-year period. This funding was sourced by the Children's Institute from donors. Even with this support, the law reform process remained daunting and complex.

Conclusion

Facilitating children's participation raises ethical concerns. On the one hand, there is the duty to realise children's right to participate. On the other, such participation could compromise children's right to protection. The success of the Dikwankwetla project indicates the potential of children to fulfil their citizenship by participating in a country's legislative processes. However, law reform is a complex process and children, like adults, need expert guidance to understand and make the most of the opportunities available.

Challenges identified through this project included the need for more resources, especially for sustained advocacy and lobbying. Such a process has to involve a continuous cycle of action and reflection in attempting to balance the rights to participation and protection. This calls for increased understanding among all stakeholders of the delicacy of this balance – including MPs, who need to be trained on children's rights and how to dialogue with children. Some serious consideration needs to be given to how the executive and parliament can adapt their processes to enable children to participate in settings which are child friendly.

Notes

1. At the time of writing the exchange rate was R8 / USD1.
2. The national parliament has two chambers: the National Assembly, and the National Council of Provinces.
3. LoveLife is an HIV prevention programme targeted at young people.

References

Giese, S., Meintjes, H. and Motsieloa, M. (2003) 'Project proposal: Facilitating children's participation in the debates and decision-making processes that inform the final provisions of the Children's Bill', Cape Town: Children's Institute, University of Cape Town, April .

Marera, D. (2008) 'Analysis of General Household Survey 2006', in P. Proudlock, M. Dutschke, L. Jamieson, J. Monson and C. Smith (eds) *South African Child Gauge 2007/ 2008*, Cape Town: Children's Institute, University of Cape Town.

Mniki, N. and Rosa, S. (2007) 'Heroes in action: A case study of child advocates in South Africa', *Children, Youth and Environments* 17(3): 179–97.

Mūkoma, W. (2007) *Dikwankwetla Children in Action Project Evaluation Workshop Report*, Cape Town: Children's Institute, University of Cape Town.

Proudlock, P., Nicholson, J. and Dyason, B. (2004) *The Children's Bill Resource Pack*, Cape Town: Children's Institute, University of Cape Town.

Skelton, Ann (2008) 'Transforming the youth and child justice system', available at www. anc.org.za/ancdocs/pubs/umrabulo/umrabulo14/childjustice.html, accessed 11 July 2008.

Commentary 1

Participation in contexts of social change

Fran Farrar, Talha Ghannam, Jake Manning and Ellie Munro

Equality and rights

Throughout the examples, the underlying principle that participation is a human rights issue is evident, and as such supports the strong links between equality, the rights of children and young people and participation as a means of fulfilling those rights. More specifically, in South Africa the issue is the struggle for equal access to support, services and protection; in the post-conflict examples it is about equal access to education, reliable information, an end to social stigma and the 'freedom' to be a child; in Plan UK's work it is about equality of access for all children, regardless of disability, poverty, social stigma etc. The underlying theme of the child/young person as an equal citizen is of paramount importance as the foundation for participatory practice.

Considering participation as a right (Article 12, UNCRC), how might we best balance this with other rights at issue within a conflict situation (e.g. the right to live safely)?

The hierarchy of need

Participation is a fundamental building block of a coherent and caring society. However, it is recognised that in conflict situations practical issues of food, shelter and safety may be the primary ones for attention. We must therefore consider carefully the point at which the participation of those involved in conflict is best addressed. The examples give specific insight into the significant risk attached to participation for some in a conflict or post-conflict situation, and the adult management of processes needs to have careful consideration of children and young people most at risk, whilst balancing this with their right to participate.

- In order for children and young people to participate, processes and structures must be in place to safeguard them.
- Is it always necessary to rectify the problems of immediate, physical and emotional need first, or can participation be part of the solution?
- How can participation help to alleviate child poverty?

Individual and community engagement

In order to achieve embedded participation, both individual and community-focused participation are needed. While an individual may be empowered to participate, it is also necessary to promote the integration of social and cultural considerations in order to bring about genuine change. Taking these contributions as exemplars in their field, it is evident that a coherent and bespoke approach to each situation is necessary – there is no one approach that can be universally identified as best practice. One might consider that a collective, community approach is of greater influence, for example when campaigning to bring about a significant community change. However, the individual child or young person must also be able to identify positive change in their own lived life in order for us to be able to say that a process has been successful. The two approaches must come together in order to fulfil the rights of all while not overlooking the rights of the individual.

All the chapters mention the benefits of participation for confidence, self-esteem and improved well-being. Participation as a form of intervention works on several levels to improve the lived lives of children and young people. The examples illustrate the importance of supporting children and young people to gain the confidence to participate, in particular, in challenging situations where trust has been eroded. The chapters on peace building and the work of Plan also mention the crucial role of participation as a 'strengthener' and 'rebuilder' of social relationships.

- How might the rights of the individual be best addressed in a community approach?
- When resources are limited, should we concentrate first on the individual or the community?
- How can we educate societies in the power of participation for social relationships, and will this help to win hearts and minds?

Grassroots vs government-led

In order to bring about genuine change in the lived lives of children and young people there must be a committed approach from both senior decision makers (governmental) and individuals and communities. The South African example suggests that there are considerable risks of children and young people becoming disillusioned with progress if the two do not actively work together closely. In order for participation to be embedded, there must be 'buy-in' from the top, supported by activism at the grassroots level. In order to bring about organisational change, those with prescribed power need to acknowledge, accept and act upon the right of those at the grassroots to participate as individuals and as communities. The hierarchy of power is needed in order to provide opportunities to participate in some cases, and this can be supported by legislative and strategic change at the top to provide opportunity at the individual and community level.

There are examples of powerful individuals supporting change, but to ensure the sustainability of children and young people's participation, a unified governmental approach needs ultimately to be agreed, by means of policy on participation. This policy needs further to be monitored and evaluated to ensure that change is brought about.

Whatever the starting point, it is important to map current practice across all levels of engagement and then to plan how improved participation might best be achieved through dialogue within the hierarchy. It is evident that children and young people have the capability to engage with adults at all levels, particularly when supported and informed. In order for participation to improve, a joint approach, with open dialogue, is necessary.

- How might grassroots practitioners best approach governments in order to bring about change?

Informal and formal approaches

While it is recognised that formal approaches may well be needed in order to approach governments and senior decision makers, an informal approach may work best with individuals and groups. It is also recognised that in a conflict situation informal approaches may be necessary, in order to facilitate a more immediate change.

Participation methodologies might be adopted on an informal basis but, in order to sustain the participation of children and young people, a formal approach will be necessary in the longer term.

- In conflict situations, might a grassroots informal approach lack the necessary urgency to bring about a quick enough change?

What's changed?

Unless the children and young people involved can recognise the positive changes resulting from their participation, then the activities and processes have done little to support the lived lives of the individuals and communities. It is imperative that all participation practice is able to identify what has changed as a result of the activity. The examples of participation practice focus very much on activities, and it is hoped that the longer-term evaluation of these will include the voice of children and young people and their accounts of what's changed as a result of their own actions.

- How might we best identify and share the changes brought about by the participation of children and young people?

Universality of barriers to participation

Practice sharing is an important part of successful participation practice and the examples bring both insight and a reality from inspirational children and young people. Participation in conflict and post-conflict situations illustrates the resilience and adaptability of children and young people in extreme situations and is a reminder that the children's rights agenda needs to be upheld across all countries and situations.

The negative perceptions of adults and their expectation of what children and young people can achieve remain a significant barrier to the participation of children and young people universally. It is important for us all to recognise that UNCRC is an international convention for all children and young people and is of particular significance to those most at risk, as illustrated here. In the face of negative perceptions that continue to be supported internationally by the media, as the examples show, positive portrayals of children and young people may help to improve and support participation and bring about direct change.

- How do we, as a relatively stable society in the UK, use the sharply focused learning around effective participation in challenging situations?
- What can we learn from participation in conflict situations that applies to children and young people in situations of violence in other societies (domestic violence etc.)?
- How might we ensure that the media take responsibility for their portrayal of children and young people?

Summary

There is an infinite number of practice approaches to the participation of children and young people, and a variety of activities and processes is necessary in order to change the hearts and minds both of adults and of children and young people. Through a focus on the children's rights agenda and the sharing of good practice, a basis can be developed for positive participatory practice. The lessons we can learn from the experiences of those in the particular situations described in these chapters strengthen and enhance our universal understanding of participation as a right, not a privilege.

The authors

Fran is a Development Officer for the National Youth Agency in England. She has been working in participatory youth work for the past decade, working with national and local statutory and third-sector organisations to help develop improved services for young people, and help promote their voice and influence to bring about positive change in their lives.

Talha is a Young Trainer in the Participation Team at the National Youth Agency in England. He has been working to promote youth engagement since the age of 13. In 2006, Talha was elected as Member of the UK Youth Parliament. He is currently studying for a degree and sits on a government advisory group on issues affecting young Muslims around the UK.

Jake works as a Development Officer for Participation Works at the National Youth Agency. He has worked extensively with a diverse range of children, young people, practitioners and managers in many local, national, statutory and non-statutory organisations to support the development and embedding of participation.

Ellie is a participation consultant with the National Youth Agency and has been working to promote children and young people's rights since she was 14. This has included helping a range of organisations to map and plan for participation, delivering training sessions around the country and developing resources for practitioners.

7   Younger children's individual participation in 'all matters affecting the child'

Priscilla Alderson

Studies of children's participation frequently look at their shared activities in groups when children comment or make decisions about adult-led policies and services (as other chapters in this book illustrate). However, people may demonstrate and exercise their competence more fully in their individual personal life and relationships, where they are agents and contributors rather than service users or members of formal groups.

Individual child–adult participation can also offer greater scope for sustained, original, deep conversations than groups can, as differences between research interviews and focus groups usually show. Transcripts of 4-year-old girls' conversations vividly reveal how much more rich and complicated their talk is with their mothers in private, everyday life at home, than in the more formal public space of pre-school services (Tizard and Hughes 1984). As agents, young children may alter relationships, decisions and the working of social assumptions or constraints (Mayall 2002: 21). The Convention on the Rights of the Child (UN 1989) speaks of the rights of 'all members of the human family', and understanding of children's conscious awareness obliges adults to value their views and participation and their present life now, besides their potential and future. This chapter therefore concentrates on individual two-way participation.

From the start, children appear to be intensely concerned with the quality of relationships and trust. I will give an example later of premature babies' responses to certain adults. I do not want to over-individualise participation; collective political engagement is vital. And yet strong groups recognise and respect every individual member, and this chapter considers the personal beginnings that can lay foundations for later political engagement, as well as showing that participation and rights involve personal agency and relationships set in families and communities.

In terms of Article 12 of the CRC, when does a child become 'capable of forming his or her own views', and so of having 'the right to express those views freely in all matters affecting the child'? At what stage do adults give 'due weight' to children's views 'in accordance with the age and maturity of the child'? The CRC allows for national laws which 'are more conducive to the realization of the rights of the child' (Article 41). Case law in England and Wales arguably goes beyond Article 12 in allowing 'competent' children to be sole decision makers, without a stated lower age bar (Gillick 1985).[1]

'All matters affecting the child' may include the continuing complexities of everyday life, frequent informal choice making, formal decision making (more rare, but a usual topic in participation literature) and the innumerable concealed prior 'decisions' now set in habits and routines, customs and structures, which adults tend to assume but children often question or have to learn, such as how to stand in line at school (Waksler 1991).

This chapter aims to show how children's participation is broader and more varied, and begins at a younger age, than is usually acknowledged. The first section reviews early informal participation at home. A second aim is to suggest that what passes for formal 'participation' when groups of children are consulted is more often concerned with provision and protection than with genuine participation, and so the second part of the chapter reviews these competing emphases in the context of public services.

Early participation at home

Participation begins in the less-observed private world of the family. This section provides a few examples of children's early and often underestimated participation. Widespread violence, abuse and neglect at home warn against taking idealised views of the family. However, children generally report having more respect and choice, free time and space at home, away from the demands of formal care and education. Mayall (2002; 2007) reviews how parents tend to respect their very young children as individual persons, competent interactors and interesting, supportive and amusing companions. Parent–child relationships are complex intellectually and morally, and can involve the personal respect that children most value. Mayall considers this is because of the wide range of shared activities, experiences and responsibilities, shared events and relationships, shared social and cultural worlds, including television, which they discuss, narrate and interpret together. Parents and siblings have time to listen to young children and to understand and encourage their earliest communication. Very young children can take part in family dramas as actor, victim and observer, and can understand different viewpoints (Dunn 2004). Family life mainly inhabits the present, which can connect to Kantian respect for children as ends in themselves, in contrast to instrumental, future-orientated child-professional relationships, when children may be the means towards the ends of the school, service or government. In many homes, the aims, topics, methods, processes, values and outcomes of participation within child–parent and sibling relationships are framed around respect for children's agency.

Although many majority-world parents may be stricter and *talk* less about autonomy, they may *allow* much more autonomous activity (Katz 2004; Penn 2004). Children aged 5 years may have far more freedom over their time, space, friendships and activities when herding goats all day, than wealthy minority-world children are allowed. Child workers who contribute in cash or kind to their family can have higher status than wholly dependent richer children. Poverty may force parents to respect their child's independence and autonomy, as when mothers in Peru agree that their young children will earn and learn more by working their own business than by helping with their mother's business (Invernizzi 2008).

Research reports tend to analyse brief extracts from transcripts, which can misleadingly imply that young children cannot engage in the kind of sustained talk shown in the next example. When aged 40 months, Robbie told me this story in the park (quoted with permission).

> There was a Baby and the Baby said, 'I don't want to go to school.' And the Mummy said, 'You've got to go.' And the Mummy took the Baby to school … and the Baby do reading … But the Baby said, 'I want to go to London.' And they went to London and the Baby runned away home and the Mummy said, 'Don't run away,' and took him home. And the Mummy cooked the dinner, and the Baby said, 'I want pasta,' and the Baby wouldn't eat dinner [more details] and then the Mummy came to get the Baby and put him in a bin and the Baby cried, 'Waah, waah', and then the Baby died.

Robbie went on with a story about a little boy who

> weared all these clothes in bed … and ate all his porridge up in bed [gobble noises] and he ate everything – all the windows, the glass, and then all people's hair, and then the sky, and then his house, and he was this BIG [shows with finger and thumb] yum, yum, yum, yum, the things went down into his body and into his tummy and then kerching and kerching, waah, waah, and then he died and dropped dead. He was sick from his eating. Then the doctor made him better again.

The boy ate more surreal items, including birds, his own eyes and mouth, and the book in which I was recording the story. Robbie illustrated a range of participation *activities* – conversing, communicating, story-telling, entertaining, imagining, playing with plausible and implausible ideas, making connections, meanings and sense, mixing his own experiences with fantasy and notions from films and stories. There is also participation within his deeply loving parent–child *relationships* of care and conflict, freedom and control, adventure, danger and protection, rule making and breaking, power and resistance, and continuous health care.

In neonatal units, where the private family world combines with public health services, we observed premature babies react with excitement to their parents' voices, in preference to other adults' voices. Parents and staff noted how babies appeared to prefer and relax with and 'trust' some adults and to be wary and tense with other adults (Alderson et al. 2005). Als (1999) writes of premature babies' 'autonomy'; influenced by her work, a few neonatal units have 'baby-led' policies, with low lighting and noise, and attention to 'reading' each baby's 'language'.

Babies take part in 'cultural life and the arts' when they are first wrapped or clothed, hear a lullaby and their family language, and smell food cooking. Breastfeeding depends on the baby's expressed 'views' about setting the pace and timing and the 'demand' that builds up the supply. By proxy, babies enjoy their parents' rights to freedom of association and peaceful assembly, to information, thought, conscience and religion, and they suffer if these rights are denied through family poverty or persecution. Young children soon learn when they are cold enough to need a coat, and tend to assert their autonomy and dignity through strenuous resistance to being strapped into a pushchair without warning or negotiation. At 2 years, Robbie refused to use his bike brakes, until his parents showed him exactly how and why they worked.

Many child patients have long-term conditions, with repeated health care treatments, so they make chains of countless informal decisions, based on their former experiences and growing understanding. Children with serious conditions, such as diabetes, learn early responsibility. At 3 years, Maisie warned her mother when she was feeling hypo (shaky from low blood sugar). At 4 years, Ruby could be trusted not to eat chocolates when her friend did and no adults were nearby, and by 5 she could test her blood sugar level and decide how much cake she could eat at a birthday party (Alderson et al. 2006).

Participation rights in formal services and welfare: provision and protection

Disappointingly, participation projects rarely lead to real change and action (Willow et al. 2004). This section reviews how, and possibly why, children's formal 'participation' is mainly about adults protecting and providing for them rather than working for change.

For example, staff and researchers in education, play, community, youth and childcare services might say to children: 'I am going to consult you as a group so that the expert adults can know how to provide better services or policies for you. You will learn about cooperating, listening, speaking, sharing, collecting and discussing different views and choices, and about democracy, citizenship and social inclusion. You will gain new skills, self-esteem and consideration for others.' The main aims are to teach children, to improve their trust, compliance and involvement, and to provide better services. However, adults are primarily accountable to systems that manage, evaluate and fund the services, not to the children. The aims, topics, methods, processes, values and outcomes, child–adult relationships and 'participation' itself are all framed around provision and the smooth running of cost-effective services, which discourages the disruption and change that may follow genuine consultation. Fielding (2008) criticises the aims of 'effectiveness'-based policies and considers that they displace person-centred participation. When participation primarily means 'sharing', children are encouraged to share rather than challenge group consensus and decisions.

In child protection, the literature implies that social workers will say, or think: 'I will listen to the child as part of supportive, semi-therapeutic, expert practice, to learn about the child's problems and ways I can help. I must balance my decisions about the child's best interests with those of other family members and within available resources. I will give information and support in order to help the child to trust me and accept my decision as effortlessly as possible. This may mean avoiding painful areas where I may not be able to help, to save the child (and myself) from unnecessary distress and false hopes. I may need to hold back some information and overemphasise certain hopes or dangers to persuade the child and parents to comply. Child development research proves that it is not worthwhile to discuss much with children aged under 8 years' (paraphrased from Winter 2006; 2009).

Here, the main aims include protecting the child's safety and welfare. The social worker is ultimately accountable not to the child, but to line managers, the courts and the public, while balancing costly over-intrusion into family life against the risk of failing to prevent fatal injury to the child. The aims, topics, methods, processes, values and outcomes, child–adult relationships and 'participation' itself are framed around protection of the child, the practitioner and society. Growing tiers of management and inspection allow less autonomy to professionals and thereby restrict the children they work with even more.

The above can all be valuable activities, in which children take part at various levels. However, the examples, like cut flowers in a vase, are detached from the roots of 'participation', its origins, meaning and purpose, context and grounding, so that the participation literature mainly describes the equivalent of the varieties of flowers, vases, arrangements and settings, but not the root and growth of participation.

The background to participation: autonomy and freedom rights

UNCRC participation rights originated in adults' autonomy rights, exemplified in the European Convention on Human Rights but reaching back to Locke and Paine: freedom of information and expression, thought, conscience and religion, association and peaceful assembly; rights to life and survival, to privacy and family life, to a legal identity, to cultural life and the arts, and due legal process; freedom from discrimination, violence, torture, cruel or degrading treatment, exploitation, and arbitrary punishment, arrest, detention or interference. The whole UNCRC is imbued with respect for the child's person, worth and dignity, and concerned with the social, economic and political means of promoting these within a 'free society'.

There is not space here to respond to the main objections to children having autonomy rights (Guggenheim 2005). Such objections echo centuries of debate when powerful groups resisted the assertion of their rights by commoners, ethnic minorities, women and others. Autonomy rights are essential defences against violent oppression, inequality, injustice and abuse of power. These politics may seem far too extreme to apply to child–adult relationships. It may appear obvious that adults are children's best and most loving providers and protectors; and yet each year countless young children suffer and die through violations of their human rights (UNICEF 2008). Besides love and care, conflict, power and risk are central to human relationships, as even very young children know.

Paradox is at the heart of autonomy rights, which break down and also build up barriers: the individual is freely integrated into society and community but also distinct from it, with strong non-interference rights over person, property and privacy. The common thread is the belief that each person is best placed to make informed personal decisions without interference, in public civic life and also in private life, although many people want to share their decision making with others.

Pure Kantian autonomy rights are not advanced here as totally realisable or desirable. All rights are qualified by respect for others and for common interests, while relationships involve interdependence and intimacy. Yet if the term 'participation' implies only community, harmony and unity, it sidelines the vital counterpart of autonomy that is necessary when interests conflict. It is the ultimate defence of privacy, and of the crucial freedom to choose whether, when and how to participate. Autonomy rights enshrine equal respect for the worth and dignity of every person, for her unique and essential knowledge about her own best interests, and for defence of her inviolable physical and mental integrity against assault.

Participation rights and autonomy in formal services and welfare: medical decisions

One type of child participation uniquely illustrates autonomy: medical and surgical decision making. Unlike the professionals discussed earlier, doctors in effect say to the child and/or parents: 'This is the intervention I recommend to treat this problem. Treatment involves these hoped-for benefits, these methods and processes, risks and discomforts, and these alternatives. I must warn you of all the potential difficulties, and not put any pressure on you, so that you can give your informed, voluntary, autonomous consent or refusal'.

The aims, topics, methods, processes, values and outcomes, child–adult relationships and 'participation' itself are all organised around the patient's and/or parents' autonomy, qualified by concern for the child's 'best interests'. Why and how is this approach so different from the two earlier examples? The emphasis is on truth about risk, caution about benefit, respect for physical integrity, deference to the patient's and/or parents' decision, and concern with direct intended outcomes, but not with ulterior learning and benefits for the child. Trust is based on honesty, not on protective paternalism. The medical decisions also affect not groups with mixed interests but one *individual* child most directly (and potentially dangerously), whereas groups can have conflicting interests. The universal value of respect for each child's bodily integrity is shown, for example, by the grief and horror felt by families when children are injured or killed during armed conflict.

Frequently, the child knows most about the bodily problems, the needs and benefits of treatment, the risks and costs. A study of 120 experienced children aged 8 to 15 years having repeated major surgery found that 13 of them were the 'main decision-makers', in the view of the child and parents (Alderson 1993: 164) and some surgeons respected children's preferences from around 8 years. With non-emergency surgery, practitioners have time to recognise and enhance children's informed decision making. If children were reluctant to have surgery, there were usually great efforts to inform and involve them, sort out misunderstandings, negotiate, and avoid imposing a decision on a fearful, resisting child.

Practical medico-legal concerns have developed most of the research, law and guidance on children's competence and consent. Child patients share the status and long history of adult patients, including the trials about Nazi medical experiments, which produced the definitive statement on autonomous voluntary consent: 'Free power of choice, without the intervention of any element of force, fraud, deceit, duress, overreaching, or any ulterior form of constraint or coercion' and sufficient information to be able to make 'an understanding and enlightened decision' (*Nuremberg* 1947). Human rights gradually emerged through resistance to oppression; patients' autonomy rights developed in reaction to scandals about abusive research and treatment (Beauchamp and Childress 2001; Alderson and Morrow 2004: 25–34).

Unlike the other professionals above, health care practitioners cannot simply overrule the family if there is disagreement. Also uniquely, health care professionals are ultimately accountable to the courts and the public, not for making a correct decision themselves, but for ensuring that they enabled the patient/parent to make an informed voluntary decision. The doctor cannot claim that the child or parents were all incompetent to decide, whereas teachers and social workers may validate their decisions by presenting parents as incompetent; the doctor, however, who acted without consent would be tried for negligence or assault. Consent transfers responsibility for risk from the doctor to the patient, and doctors have gradually accepted that codes of ethics and consent protect not only patients, but also doctors, researchers and high standards of treatment and research. Doctors accept that they can do immense harm as well as good, whereas other professionals tend not to acknowledge this – another possible reason why they favour managing 'participation' over respecting autonomy.

Learning from children about rights: some conclusions

Human rights are not simply abstract theories. As even babies show, rights inhere in inalienable, practical, embodied human experiences and relationships, freely expressed through bodies, and often denied by confining or punishing bodies. The child who is, and is in, the body concerned may have unique and essential knowledge about human rights and participation generally (Alderson 2008).

The director of a children's rights centre involving disadvantaged 'school rejects' thought that they had such deep, broad, generic understanding of rights 'Because they know what it means when your rights are denied'. Children's active participation covers innumerable experiences, activities and relationships, the 'all matters' in Article 12. It ranges far beyond formal, adult-led consultations, from explicit choices and decisions into challenges to the innumerable concealed and assumed prior 'decisions' now set into routines, structures and interests that affect children, as mentioned earlier. Hence the importance of respect for everyone's integral autonomy rights, when even premature babies' 'views' can inform policies in neonatal units to promote their health and welfare.

Fielding (2008: 59) warns against the dominant, instrumental, impersonal market model of education and participation, divorced from personal relationships, meaning, narrative, community and history, and he speaks of its 'deep dishonesty'. Fielding's 'person-centred' learning communities and services enable children to take part at higher levels of agency, beyond manipulation and tokenism (Hart 1992). Often unintentionally, however, participation projects with children may promise respect, listening and future changes, which cannot be achieved. To guard against this, adults need to be wary about the aims and sponsorship, the political and economic context of each project. Is it possible to achieve real participation within short-term relationships and working contracts? Might the consulting adults be used and abused as much as the children during a pretence of participation within rigid hierarchical contexts? How often is the hidden agenda during consultation a determination to improve the children but not the service?

These few examples illustrate young children's early capacities to form and express views freely, with the higher level of Gillick competence to weigh choices and make formal decisions, which is being increasingly recognised and respected in young children. Obviously the youngest children cannot form and express complex, legally valid decisions, but I suggest that this competence does not involve a Piagetian step up to a new and different stage of life, but exists on a continuum from birth, while young children gradually acquire the language to analyse, reason and express complex experiences and decisions.

Note

1. Gillick *v* Wisbech and W. Norfolk AHA [1985], 3All ER.

References

Alderson, P. (1993) *Children's Consent to Surgery*, Buckingham: Open University Press.
Alderson, P. (2008) *Young Children's Rights: Revised second edition*, London: Jessica Kingsley/ Save the Children.
Alderson, P. and Morrow, V. (2004) *Ethics, Social Research and Consulting with Children and Young People*, Barkingside: Barnardo's.
Alderson, P., Hawthorne, J. and Killen, M. (2005) 'The participation rights of premature babies', *International Journal of Children's Rights* 13: 31–50.
Alderson, P., Sutcliffe, K. and Curtis, K. (2006) 'Children's consent to medical treatment', *Hastings Center Report*, 36(6): 25–34.
Als, H. (1999) 'Reading the premature infant', in E. Goldson (ed.) *Developmental Interventions in the Neonatal Intensive Care Nursery*, New York: Oxford University Press, pp. 18–85.
Beauchamp, T. and Childress, J. (2001) *Principles of Biomedical Ethics*, New York: Oxford University Press.
Dunn, J. (2004) *Children's Friendships*, Malden, MA: Blackwell.
Fielding, M. (2008) 'Personalisation, education and the market', *Soundings* 38: 56–69.
Guggenheim, M. (2005) *What's Wrong With Children's Rights?* Cambridge, MA: Harvard University Press.
Hart, R. (1992) *Children's Participation: From tokenism to citizenship*, Paris: UNICEF.
Invernizzi, A. (2008) 'Everyday lives of working children and notions of citizenship', in A. Invernizzi and J. Williams (eds) *Children and Citizenship*, London: Sage.
Katz, C. (2004) *Growing Up Global*, Minneapolis, MN: University of Minnesota Press.
Lyon, C. (2006) 'Toothless tigers and dogs' breakfasts', *Representing Children* 18(2): 111–26.
Mayall, B. (2002) *Towards a Sociology for Childhood*, Buckingham: Open University Press.
Mayall, B. (2007) 'Children's lives outside school', *Primary Review Research Survey 8/1*, Cambridge: University of Cambridge Faculty of Education.
Nuremberg Code (1947) ohsr.od.nih.gov/guidelines/nuremberg.html, accessed 23 June 2004.
Penn, H. (2004) *Unequal Childhoods*, London: Routledge Falmer.
Tizard, B. and Hughes, M. (1984) *Young Children Learning*, London: Faber.

UN (1989) *Convention on the Rights of the Child*, New York: UNICEF.

UNICEF (2008) *State of the World's Children*, New York: UNICEF.

Waksler, F. (1991) *Studying the Social Worlds of Children*, London: Falmer.

Willow, C., Marchant, R., Kirby, P. and Neale B. (2004) *Young Children's Citizenship: Ideas into practice*, York: Joseph Rowntree Foundation.

Winter, K. (2006) 'The participation rights of looked after children in their health care', *International Journal of Children's Rights*, 14(1): 77–95.

Winter, K. (2009) 'The participation of young children in the 'looked-after' children decision-making process', unpublished PhD thesis, London: University of London.

8 Disabled children and participation in the UK

Reality or rhetoric?

Kate Martin and Anita Franklin

> If you make decisions without us, it makes us upset.
> Don't put us down, don't tell us how we feel.[1]

Introduction

In England, disabled children and young people are frequently denied their right to participate in decision-making arenas, despite a plethora of government policy and guidance encouraging their full involvement. There is evidence to suggest that despite an overall increase in the participation of children and young people, disabled children are much less likely than their peers to be engaged in decisions about their own lives, particularly those with complex needs or communication impairments (Sinclair and Franklin 2000; Sinclair 2004; Department of Health/ Department for Education and Skills 2004; Cavet and Sloper 2004; Franklin and Sloper 2007; 2008). In addition, despite a growing body of literature examining the context, and the impact on children and young people, of participation, there is little reference to disabled children's place within this. This chapter will start to address this gap.

Disabled children and the rhetoric of participation

> Don't want adults to make decisions for me – I want to make decisions for myself.

Since the late 1990s the UK government has included within policy developments a commitment to increasing the involvement of children in decision-making processes concerning their own care and service development. These include the government's responsibilities to fulfil the requirements of the Children Acts 1989 and 2004, the UN Convention on the Rights of the Child (CRC) 1989, the Human Rights Act 1998 and the Convention on the Rights of Persons with Disabilities 2006, all of which embody the participation of disabled children and young people.

A central theme of the National Service Framework for Children, Young People and Maternity Services in England (Department of Health/Department for Education and Skills 2004) stresses the need to consult and involve children. This framework sets standards aimed at raising the quality of health and social care services for children. Standard 8 for disabled children and those with complex health needs states:

> Professionals should ensure that disabled children, especially children with high communication needs, are not excluded from decision-making processes. In particular, professionals should consider the needs of children who rely on communication equipment or who use non-verbal communication such as sign language.
>
> (Department of Health/Department for Education and Skills 2004: 29)

Thus, disabled children and young people are afforded the same participation rights as all children, yet a review of the literature concluded that the participation of disabled children needs further development, with little available evidence of good practice (Cavet and Sloper 2004). Franklin and Sloper (2007) report on the fragile nature of disabled children's participation in social care, wherein participation is dependent on the skills and capacity of a few people, and often confined to limited, short-term funded projects, with the result that the participation of disabled children and young people is still not embedded in practice. Those who are engaged are usually the more able, articulate disabled children, those with complex needs or communication impairments being less likely to be engaged in decisions and issues which affect them, meaning that their needs, wishes and opinions remain invisible and unheard. So what are the barriers preventing participation from becoming a reality?

Dilemmas and barriers to disabled children's participation

> Don't guess what we can or can't do. Listen to me.

Franklin and Sloper (2008) report on some of the practical barriers to disabled children's participation. In this chapter we explore some of the main theoretical debates concerning participation and disability and start to draw them together in order to stimulate further consideration of this issue. These include an examination of how disabled children's rights to participate and be seen as competent social actors are affected by a combination of three factors: conflicts and dilemmas within current policy; social constructions of disabled children; and power as a barrier to participation.

> If you listen to us you can help us get a positive outcome – it helps us.

Conflicts and dilemmas within current child policy

One of the key issues impacting on children's participation *per se*, and in particular the participation of disabled children, is the inherent conflicts and dilemmas
posed by current child policy, namely *Every Child Matters* (ECM) (DfES 2003), the
Children Act 2004 (which gave ECM legislative force), the model of social investment inherent within them and the way children are constructed within this. Such
policies are focused upon improving outcomes for children, which have been
defined as *being healthy; staying safe; enjoying and achieving; making a positive contribution;*
and *achieving economic well-being*, arguably on the basis that investment in children
in the present will improve their outcomes in the future and thus reduce social
exclusion.

However, such a model of social investment, as Williams suggests, regards children as citizen-workers of the future (2004). This focus on children for who they
will be in the future (and what they will contribute to the economy) has many
implications for children's participation in the present; not least, as Lister (2003)
argues, the focus is on the processes of becoming an adult, rather than on the
quality of children's lives, equality and rights in the present. Evidence of this disre-
gard for participation in decision making can be seen in many ways, including, for
example, children's participation only being referred to as a passing expectation
within ECM; in the weaknesses of the powers accorded to the newly created post
of the Children's Commissioner in the Children Act 2004 (Hudson 2005); and in
the government's failure to place Article 12 of the UNCRC high on the agenda
(Committee on the Rights of the Child 2002), thus calling into question the levels
of importance being placed on all children's participation, but with a particular
impact on disabled children, due to the additional barriers to participation they
experience. Specific policy regarding disabled children provides further evidence.
For example, £5 million was made available to fund parent/carer participation
as part of a comprehensive spending review of services for disabled children, but
none was forthcoming to support disabled children themselves to participate,
although the importance of their participation was highlighted throughout the
review (HM Treasury/Department for Education and Skills 2007). Although the
policy developments noted above have implications for all children, the current
model of social investment poses a number of additional issues for disabled children and young people.

The value placed on disabled children as children

It has been argued that the social investment model fails to adequately address the
needs of specific groups of children, particularly those such as disabled children,
who may not be regarded as worthy of such social investment in the present, as
they are not deemed to be 'opportunities for promoting a market friendly society'
(Lister 2006). In addition, the strong focus on educational attainment within ECM
overshadows that of participation, thus highlighting the lack of commitment to
children's views and opinions in the present in favour of ensuring that they achieve
academically. This potentially has a disproportionately higher impact on children

and young people with learning difficulties who may not follow the standard course of development, but who will nevertheless achieve in other ways (Williams 2004).

Not only does the current policy context place limited importance on participation in favour of educational attainment, it could be argued that it is based on prejudicial assumptions that disabled children and young people will not be workers of the future, when indeed many will be, thus perpetuating low expectations for disabled children. If value is being placed on children primarily for their potential future economic contribution, what implications does this hold for the value placed on those disabled children who will not be part of the future workforce, and more broadly for the value we place on children for being children?

The model of social investment can also be regarded as a desire to control the future through children by imposing outcomes which have been 'defined by adults and legitimated in relation to the needs of adults and the state of adulthood' (Moss and Petrie 2005: 91) rather than the needs of children, their opportunities for self-realisation and the 'better lives children will lead as children' in the present (Prout 2000). Wyness and Buchanan (2004) see this in terms of a conflict between children's participation and pressures to protect children and regulate their development. This promotes the perception of children as 'becomings' rather than 'beings' (Prout 2005) and an image of children being incomplete, passive and incompetent, rather than active agents able to participate in decisions and issues that affect them (Thomas and O'Kane 1999; Willow 2002).

Disabled children's competence to participate

As argued above, an image of children being incomplete and passive reinforces the underlying tension within participation of children's perceived competence to participate. Thus children's participation hinges on adults' perceptions of their 'ability' to participate, and is subject to the inherent power imbalance that exists between adults and children. Wyness and Buchanan (2004) argue that the 'child's status as an incompetent is measured against a model of competent adult', rather than approaches that recognise children's rights to participate and that are adapted accordingly to ensure that this is realised. The construction of children as 'becomings' draws us away from the need to respect children's rights in the present and recognise their rights to participation. Although this would potentially apply to all children, for disabled children and young people this issue is twofold – disabled children experience discrimination and oppression on the grounds not only of being children, but also of being disabled.

Social constructions of disabled children

Compared to their non-disabled peers, disabled children and young people experience multiple discrimination, low expectations and social exclusion (Russell 2003). Further to this, as Davis et al. (2005) argue, 'policy decisions rarely take account of disabled children's opinions because professional practices and vested interests of service providers are promoted before those of children', meaning that disabled children's 'needs' are often primarily defined by non-disabled adults' perceptions of what they 'need' (ibid.). Hence, policy is often shaped by non-disabled adult assumptions, prejudices or stereotypes about disabled children and young people. Policies and structures that are developed for all children and young people often fail to take into account the needs and opinions of disabled children and young people, rendering them inaccessible and not inclusive. For example, mainstream participation structures tend to be exclusive of disabled children and young people, often utilising inaccessible participation methods.

Regarding children as 'becomings' has an even more profound impact on disabled children's realisation of their right to participate, in that not only do they have this perception to contend with, but in addition, historical medical notions individualised disability and equated it to suffering, dependency, passivity and vulnerability (Davis et al. 2005), rather than addressing the societal and structural causes of disability, such as prejudice and discriminatory processes and practices. This view has led to disabled people having a poor self-image and low expectations (Davis et al. 2005), with few visible positive role models to aspire to. This is compounded by the fact that disabled children are constructed in policy as vulnerable (Priestley 2000) and often have to pronounce 'difference' to get the support to be 'included' (Davis et al. 2005). Disabled children and young people, particularly those who use methods other than speech to communicate, continue to be defined by what they cannot do, rather than what they can do (Rabiee et al. 2005), again impacting upon their right to be regarded as competent social actors. This construction of disabled children as vulnerable, and the discourse this creates, impacts upon professionals' attitudes towards disabled children and is often reflected in the power adults exert over children.

Don't judge a book by its cover – we can all make choices.

Power as a barrier to participation

Power therefore can present a significant barrier to meaningful participation. Issues of power, including both adult–child relations and the structural power of organisations (Cockburn 2005) and their impact on participation do not receive adequate attention, particularly where 'state authorities play a significant role in their lives' (Badham 2004). This can impact disproportionately on disabled children and young people, as many will be subject to increased surveillance in their lives, leading to increased adult control (Priestley 2000). This can create additional barriers to participation for disabled children and young people, who may often have to rely on the discretion of adults to facilitate and support them to access the opportunities to participate. For example, disabled children who use alternative methods of communication often have to rely on a small number of people trained or experienced in that method to interpret/facilitate all their communication.

On a demonstrable level, these issues can be witnessed in the attitudes of some adults. Concerns over the capabilities of children with cognitive impairments and complex needs to understand the concepts of decision making, and whether participation could be achieved in a meaningful way with these children, were raised in study by Franklin and Sloper (2007; 2008). This study highlighted among some practitioners a notion of 'ideal participation', based on the main-stream participation agenda in the UK whereby participation activity was not embracing or recognising methods of participation which are more accessible to some disabled young people. For example, an over-reliance on the notion that good practice should include young people attending bureaucratic, adult-focused review meetings of their care appeared to create a hierarchy of 'ideal partici-pation' which could create barriers for disabled children and young people. To illustrate: when a child with learning difficulties had given their views on 'what they like' and 'what they don't like' about a short break service through symbols and non-verbal methods of communication, this was viewed as limited and its validity was questioned, as it was felt the child could not categorically state that they wanted to attend the service.

A way forward

Time – help us make decisions by giving your time and talking to us.

For participation to be a reality for disabled children a number of areas need addressing. First, approaches to participation must be viewed flexibly, using methods that are accessible and suitable for the child in question (Kirby et al. 2003; Rabiee et al. 2005). For disabled children with cognitive impairments, participation may be at a level of choosing between two objects or options, but this should be seen as a valid means of participation and afforded equal status and priority with other levels of participation. Competence also relies on the ability of practitioners to gain informed consent (Alderson 2007). The question needs to be not whether a child can participate, but how. Furthermore, adults need to be reflective about the inherent power imbalance that exists, and ensure that disabled children, regardless of age or perceived 'ability', are regarded as competent social actors and ensure that methods to support children's participation are adapted and responsive to meet the needs of individual children, rather than expecting children to fit in with adult structures or notions of 'ideal participation'. For this to happen, adults need to 'examine assumptions about children, increase recognition of diversity and attune to children's own perspective' (Davis and Hill 2006).

Got to make choices for ourselves. Something we have to learn when we become adults.

Second, there needs to be a fundamental shift in attitude, which starts with the recognition that it is the basic human right of all children to be involved in deci-sions about matters that affect them and to have their views, however they are expressed, valued and accorded equal importance. When asked how it feels when adults listen, young people at the Council for Disabled Children workshops stated: 'I feel happy and don't feel sad' and 'It makes me feel normal, good'. This suggests that the act of involvement in a meaningful way is as important as the outcome of that involvement. While this is also pertinent for all young people (Percy-Smith

2008), it is especially important for disabled children, who may experience being, or at least feeling, socially excluded.

A third issue for participation to become a reality for disabled children is to embrace a rights-based approach. In addition to empowering disabled children, more regard needs to be paid to the rights of disabled children. The creation of a rights-based perspective would provide a basis for recognising the barriers disabled children face and provide a solid basis from which the participation of disabled children and young people can evolve into more than just rhetoric. As one young disabled woman put it, with a passion that cannot be conveyed through the written word:

> Listen to me, no one else, listen to me. It's my body. Listen to me; it's my life, listen to me.

> (Martin 2008)

Notes

1   All quotations are from disabled young people attending workshops on participation facilitated by the Council for Disabled Children (CDC). These workshops resulted in the creation of a poster entitled Top Tips for Participation. This poster can be downloaded from the website: www.ncb.org.uk/cdc

References

Alderson, P. (2007) 'Competent children? Minors' consent to health care treatment and research', *Social Science and Medicine*, 65: 2272–83.

Badham, B. (2004) 'Participation – for a change: Disabled young people lead the way', *Children & Society*, 18: 143–54.

Cavet, J. and Sloper, P. (2004) 'Participation of disabled children in individual decisions about their lives and in public decisions about service development', *Children & Society* 18(4): 278–90.

Cockburn, T. (2005) 'Children's participation in social policy: Inclusion, chimera or authenticity?', *Social Policy and Society*, 4 (2): 109–19.

Committee on the Rights of the Child (2002) *Concluding Observations of the Committee on the Rights of the Child: United Kingdom of Great Britain and Northern Ireland*, 4 October, Geneva: United Nations.

Davis, J., Watson, N., Corker, M. and Shakespeare, T. (2005) 'Reconstructing disability, childhood and social policy in the UK', in H. Hendrick (ed.), *Child Welfare and Social Policy: An essential reader* (pp. 323–37), Bristol: The Policy Press.

Davis, J. M. and Hill, M. (2006) 'Introduction', in E. K. M. Tisdall, J. M. Davis, M. Hill and A. Prout (eds) *Children, Young People and Social Exclusion: Participation for what?* (pp. 256), Bristol: The Policy Press.

Department for Education and Skills (2003) *Every Child Matters*, London: The Stationery Office.

Department of Health/Department for Education and Skills (2004) *National Service Framework for Children, Young People and Maternity Services: Disabled Children and Young People and those with Complex Health Needs*, London: Department of Health.

Franklin, A. and Sloper, P. (2007) *Participation of Disabled Children and Young People in Decision-Making relating to Social Care*, York: Social Policy Research Unit, University of York.

Franklin, A. and Sloper, P. (2008) 'Supporting the participation of disabled children and young people in decision-making', *Children & Society*, 23(1): 3–15.

HM Treasury and Department for Education and Skills (2007) *Aiming High for Disabled Children: Better support for families*, London: Her Majesty's Treasury and Department for Education and Skills.

Hudson, B. (2005) 'User outcomes and children's services reform: Ambiguity and conflict in the policy implementation process', *Social Policy and Society*, 5 (2): 227–36.

Kirby, P., Lanyon, C., Cronin, K., Sinclair, R. (2003) *Building a Culture of Participation: Involving children and young people in policy, service planning, delivery and evaluation – research report*, London: Department for Education and Skills.

Lister, R. (2003) 'Investing in the citizen workers of the future: Transformations in citizenship and the state under New Labour', *Social Policy and Administration*, 37 (5): 427–43.

Lister, R. (2006) 'Children (but not women) first: New Labour, child welfare and gender', *Critical Social Policy*, 26 (2): 315–35.

Martin, K. (2008) *Top Tips for Participation: What disabled young people want*, London: Council for Disabled Children.

Moss, P. and Petrie, P. (2005) 'Children – Who do they think they are?', in, Hendrick, H (ed.) *Child Welfare and Social Policy*, Bristol: The Policy Press.

Percy-Smith, B. (2008) *Evaluating the Development of Young People's Participation in Two Children's Trusts*, Evaluation Report, Year 2. Leicester: National Youth Agency.

Priestley, M. (2000) 'Adults only: Disability, social policy and the life course', *Journal of Social Policy*, 29 (3): 421–39.

Prout, A. (2000) 'Children's participation: control and self-realisation in British late modernity', *Children & Society*, 14: 304–15.

Prout, A. (2005) *The Future of Childhood: Towards the interdisciplinary study of children*. Oxon: RoutledgeFalmer.

Rabiee, P., Sloper, P. and Beresford, B. (2005) 'Doing research with children and young people who do not use speech for communication', *Children & Society*, 19: 385–96.

Russell, P. (2003) ' "Access and achievement or social exclusion?" Are the government's policies working for disabled children and their families', *Children & Society*. 17: 215–25.

Sinclair R. (2004) 'Participation in practice: making it meaningful, effective and sustainable', *Children & Society*, 18: 106–18.

Sinclair, R. and Franklin, A. (2000) *Young People's Participation, Quality Protects Research Briefing, No.3*, London: Department of Health.

Thomas, N. and O'Kane, C. (1999) 'Experiences of decision-making in middle childhood: The example of children "looked after" by local authorities', *Childhood* 6(3): 369–87.

United Nations (1989) *Convention on the Rights of the Child*, Geneva: United Nations.

United Nations (2006) *Convention on the Rights of Persons with Disabilities*, New York: United Nations.

Williams, F. (2004) 'What matters is who works: why every child matters to New Labour. Commentary on the DfES Green Paper *Every Child Matters*', *Critical Social Policy*, 24 (3): 406–27.

Willow, C. (2002) *Participation in Practice: Children and young people as partners in change*, London: The Children Society.

Wyness, M. and Buchanan, L. H. (2004) 'Childhood, politics and ambiguity: Towards an agenda for children's political inclusion', *Sociology*, 38 (1): 81–99.

9 Participation among young people with mental health issues

Redefining the boundaries

Ann Dadich

Introduction

This chapter extends extant literature on youth participation in two ways. First, it argues that current understandings of youth participation, particularly those espoused by government policy, need to be broadened. Although participation is often used to refer to involvement in mainstream decision making and change processes, this paper argues that non-conventional forms of *social* participation can offer meaningful alternatives for enhancing the participation of excluded groups such as young people with mental health problems. Second, the chapter suggests that broadening current understandings of youth participation should not be done without careful consideration of possible implications – especially for young people. The paper draws on research into the experiences of young people with mental health issues in self-help support groups (SHSGs) in New South Wales, Australia.

To explain these two key arguments, the chapter begins by explicating the concept of youth participation. It then illustrates the way in which young people, especially those with mental health issues, are often excluded from mainstream society. The chapter then examines how SHSGs have provided opportunities to young people with mental health issues for participation and engagement in mainstream society. While the findings suggest that current understandings of youth participation need to be revisited, the chapter concludes with a discussion of possible ramifications that deserve careful consideration.

Youth participation – does rhetoric equal reality?

Youth participation permeates much official rhetoric (ALP 2007; UN Human Rights 1989). Although variously defined, the current and preceding Australian federal governments have interpreted youth participation in terms of involvement in *education*, *employment* and *election* processes (Wyn 2007); yet, the accent is heavily on economic participation. However, rhetoric does not necessarily reflect reality, and policy alone does not guarantee youth participation (Davis and Watson 2001). In fact, socio-political structures typically disengage young people, especially those with mental health issues, from important processes, like the management of their own mental health.

Political science literature affirms the exclusion many young people experience from mainstream society (Bellamy 2002). Conventional social systems use a range of processes to disengage (and maintain the disengagement of) these individuals. Many are excluded from accessing information and from particular decision-making processes (Bessant et al. 1998) by the very strategies that are meant to close the divide. Social alienation leads to cynicism, fatalistic attitudes and a sense of hopelessness about their own state of affairs (Eckersley 1999). This is particularly the case for young people who are part of minority groups (Stanton-Salazar 1997), like those with mental health issues.

Young people with mental illness largely remain on society's fringe (Fuller et al. 1998). Mental illness and emotional problems seriously impact on the various domains of a young person's life, such as their ability to continue educational pursuits, initiate employment and form strong support networks with family or peers (Daniel and Cornwall 1993), with the result that they remain on the periphery of societal structures and institutions. Although people with mental health issues have long experienced disengagement and social exclusion, one vehicle that has helped them to (re-)engage with and participate in mainstream society is the SHSG (Nash 1999).

Self-help support groups

The SHSG can be defined as:

> a non-profit support group run by and for people who join together on the basis of common experience to help one another. It is not professionally run, although professionals are frequently found in supportive ancillary roles.
>
> (Madara 1999: 171)

There are a number of benefits associated with SHSGs, particularly those that meet around mental health issues. At an individual level, these include behavioural, cognitive and spiritual transformation (Kyrouz et al. 2003). At a social level, SHSGs are said to offer an *environmental antidote* (Davidson et al. 1999) to the social isolation often experienced by those with mental illness (Noordsy et al. 1996).

As 'pockets of alternative, collective power' (Orford 1992: 235), SHSGs have the capacity to lobby and initiate effective change (Deegan 1992). Some have proven successful in challenging laws and other socio-political practices. Riessman and Carroll (1995) for instance, recall the crucial role of Mothers Against Drunk Driving (MADD) and the Association for Retarded Citizens (ARC), which, although they began as SHSGs, evolved into powerful advocacy constituents.

These groups have a valuable place in bringing the concerns of disenfranchised populations to the fore. Examining women's involvement in SHSGs, Scoffy (1991, cited in Clark, 1995) found that the groups empowered women to take responsibility in their own lives. The groups offered opportunities to explore personal issues in a supportive milieu with other women and, within these contexts, to find strength in unity. Similarly for young people with mental health difficulties, SHSGs offer possibilities for counter-narratives to social constructions held by community services characterised by dependence and without the ability to act and make informed choices (Clark 1995).

Meaningful participation among young people with mental health issues

The study on which this paper draws involved young people who had experienced a range of mental health issues, including a diagnosable mental illness, substance use issues, alcoholism, drug addiction, issues related to sexual identity, or emotional health issues; and had participated in an SHSG. For these young people, in spite of the extensive therapeutic benefits associated with these groups (see Dadich 2005), there was no explicit mention of socio-political activity that attempted to further group cause. However, closer analysis revealed the significance of socio-political activity at an intra-group level. Despite no explicit mention of advocacy efforts beyond the group context, approximately two-fifths of the young people spoke of supporting or advocating on behalf of individual group participants. These individuals suggested that opportunities to give *and* receive assistance were helpful, enhancing psychological well-being and enabling young people to become more than passive recipients of support:

> It's taking the focus off myself and really trying to help others, and by doing that … I feel like *I am healing*.

Over three-quarters of the young people valued the learning opportunities and reciprocal support afforded by the groups, particularly when these involved the sharing of personal narratives:

> It's been good just having that contact with positive people, like the people who have got the clean time[1] up who are able to give you that kind of peer-based support, advice, and information about recovery.

Sharing personal narratives was believed to be beneficial in improving the situation of young people, regardless of whether the young person *listened* to the stories of others, or *shared* their own story. By listening to the stories of fellow group participants, the young people could compare their situation with others, learn of successful coping strategies and gain hope through others' victories:

> When you hear of someone doing well and … they give you a bit of hope … you'd come out you know, uplifted and feeling positive.

Others suggested that by sharing *their own* story, they developed articulation skills and greater self-confidence. This, it might be argued, might be the foundation for greater engagement with socio-political activity in the future. Sharing their own story also reminded the young people of the journey they had travelled and the progress they had made thus far:

> I'm not so fearful, not paranoid, whatever, so I'm not sort of scared to reach out.

Through opportunities to partake in supportive efforts, a number of young people spoke of a transformed sense of self – not only for the recipient, who was often stigmatised by their mental health issue, but also for the young person who had conventionally been the *recipient* of mental health care. As *beneficiaries* of support, the young people were cradled by the collective care of people with whom they could identify; and despite their concerns with personal shortcomings, their worth was validated:

> They weren't judgemental when I told them what I'd been doing the last couple of years. They were, 'That's okay, just keep coming back'.

As *providers* of such support, the young people often experienced an altered understanding of their abilities and of their valuable role within the group:

> being able to help other people too ... you just like to feel you can contribute something.

The SHSGs were thus an important way for many young people to challenge and change social constructions they had of themselves and reframe their self-identity, giving rise to different self-understandings:

> You see like the women who come in and they're struggling and ... their husbands or their boyfriends are beating them up and they have no idea like, they don't know up from down or what the hell's going on, but they still have ... sobriety and just the way they hold themselves, the dignity that they have, and the grace that you can only get from being ... humiliated beyond belief, that's the only way you can get that kind of grace, and they have it and it's in their eyes, and it's the way they hold themselves, in the way they treat one another ... it's so what I want to be like ... I want to be like those women ... they're just the hardest workers, like the most incredible women I have ever come across.

Rather than being seen as young people with a debilitating mental health issue who lack the ability to engage socio-politically in changing their situations, through SHSGs young people were able to actively engage in collectively reflecting on and transforming their own marginalisation.

> I sort of lost faith in my brain capacity because ... of the illness, and I'd attempted study so many times and had failed ... now ... there's something that you can aspire to, even when you have a mental illness you know, you can still have a career and, and I'm involved in the consumer movement now, so ... [I'm] not just at home doing nothing ... all the time and isolated from the community and, and sort of 'a nobody' sort of thing; you know that, that you can do things and contribute to, to society.

Transforming self-identity and social constructions are key components in participatory learning and action, particularly among disenfranchised communities (Linton 1998). By uniting and recognising afflictions as assets, personal strengths can be harnessed and channelled into effective socio-political change (Rappaport 1993).

As Adamsen and Rasmussen (2001) note, 'self-help groups ... contribute positively to the self-reflexive process of participants and to a strengthening of their self-perception, which is a prerequisite for social interaction with others on equal terms' (p. 915). It is through such empowerment that individuals are able to critically analyse the social and political environment and execute choice (Zimmerman 1985).

Several young people also recognised it as an opportunity to challenge stereotypical views about SHSGs, particularly among service providers. Some professionals regard SHSGs as mere examples of the *blind leading the blind*. Group participants are thought to be provided with false or misleading information from peers who lack academic credentials (Galanter 1990). In the hope of defying these sentiments, a number of young people chose to participate in the study knowing that the findings would be disseminated through academe. These individuals were keen to promote the potential value of SHSGs as arenas for social participation and to assert the place of these groups in a gestalt of support systems. As such, these young people were engaged in socio-political efforts that aimed to raise the profile of SHSGs to service providers – many of whom are potential gatekeepers to community-based support networks (Woff et al. 1996) – and reconstruct views of SHSG participants as active participants in improving their situations.

These findings suggest that, while young people with mental health issues are often disengaged from important social processes, they are not always inactive agents; indeed, their participation may simply take a different form. The findings extend, as well as challenge, current understandings of youth participation within government discourses by suggesting that marginalised young people are participating in social and/or political endeavours, but not in conventional ways. The evidence suggests that participation is more than being a student, an employee or a voter, or partaking in a community activity or informing health services. It is about challenging the status quo by contesting and transforming self-identity and the dependency implicit in prevailing models of mental health care responses.

These broader understandings of youth participation are more inclusive, acknowledging a greater sense of plurality. However, there are possible ramifications if social policy is to reflect this broader view of participation, particularly for young people.

Implications

To develop social policy that supports wider interpretations of youth participation, a number of key questions need to be considered. Without such deliberation, social policy might in fact thwart participation and, in so doing, fall short of fulfilling its role in facilitating community well-being (Dean 2006).

While not exhaustive, the following questions provide a useful starting point.

1   *How is it possible to develop a social policy that has the flexibility needed to encompass the diverse and changing nature of participation among young people?*

Not only does this require the development of a coherent and an inclusive policy, but it also requires ongoing opportunities to test the strength of the policy and amend it accordingly, so that it reflects the realities of participation among young people. Through this process, inadequacies in the current discourse might also become apparent.

2   *How will a broader understanding of youth participation affect the exchange of dialogue between policy makers, researchers, theoreticians, practitioners and, ultimately, young people?*

Changing the way in which key concepts are understood can stymie effective communication between stakeholders. While this can be problematic at a global level when international discussions are held, it can also hinder communication at a national or state level.

3   *Will broadening the concept of youth participation diminish experiences with, and consequences of, social exclusion?*

If government rhetoric is to encompass more diverse instances of youth participation, it then follows that more young people might be regarded as socially active, and thus *not* disenfranchised. Consequently, this might minimise the prevalence of disengagement among young people, particularly from conventional social systems (like education, employment and community services); it might also under-value the consequences of disengagement for young people. The more that young people are seen to be *participating*, the more comfortable our consciences will be.

Within the current political climate of neoliberalism (Béland 2007), this point warrants particular consideration. Under the guise of economic rationalism, neoliberalism supports a range of practices, including the reduction of public expenditure for social services such as health and education, as well as redefining *public and community good* as the *promotion of individual needs* and *individual responsibility* (Martinez and Garcia 1997). Consequently, those who are in most need of support become less likely to receive it (Hamilton and Maddison 2007) – this includes young people with mental health issues. For this reason, there is a need to exercise caution when broadening social policy, as it might in fact shadow experiences of disadvantage.

4   *Will broadening the concept of youth participation provide policy makers with the opportunity to falsely claim greater political clout?*

Following from the previous question, if more young people are regarded as socially active, it is possible that the government bodies that broaden current policy will claim ownership of positive change. More specifically, they might allege that it was they that encouraged participation among young people, particularly those who were (and perhaps remain) disenfranchised.

Evidently, these issues will not be overcome easily, as the questions posed do not have clear or definitive answers. However, as McNeish (1999) has stated, 'A good starting point ... is to make sure they are asked' (p. 202). Confronting these (and other) challenges is a useful reminder that the concept of participation is not necessarily without costs and consequences. Such an acknowledgement will help to ensure that future interpretations of participation will not be undertaken uncritically.

Conclusion

Although important for personal, social and political reasons, youth participation is variously understood and is not easily achieved, despite support from official rhetoric. However, as this chapter has demonstrated, this may partly be because youth participation reveals itself in non-conventional ways. Young people with mental health issues who have participated in SHSGs suggested that these community support systems can be an important channel for meaningful participation.

Although it is tempting to modify social policy to ensure that it facilitates community well-being, it is equally important to be cognisant of possible ramifications associated with policy change. Otherwise there is risk that young people will be further marginalised from opportunities to participate in their communities. Such awareness requires bona fide commitment to young people, regardless of whether their views concord with the adult-defined frameworks that dominate research and policy development with respect to young people.

Acknowledgements

The author would like to thank Nathan Frick and Sarah Alliston, members of HY NRG (the **headspace** Youth National Reference Group), for providing constructive feedback that informed the development of the chapter. Note: **headspace** is Australia's National Youth Mental Health Foundation.

Note

1 Abstinence from drugs and alcohol for an extended period.

References

Adamsen, L. and Rasmussen, J. M. (2001) 'Sociological perspectives on self-help groups: Reflections on conceptualisation and social processes', *Journal of Advanced Nursing* 35: 909–17.

ALP (Australian Labor Party) (2007) *National Platform and Constitution*, Canberra, ACT: ALP (Australian Labor Party).

Béland, D. (2007) 'Neo-liberalism and social policy: The politics of ownership', *Policy Studies* 28: 91–107.

Bellamy, C. (2002) *The State of the World's Children 2003*, Geneva, Switzerland: UNICEF (United Nations Children's Fund).

Bessant, J., Sercombe, H. and Watts, R. (1998) *Youth Studies: An Australian perspective*, Melbourne, VIC: Addison Wesley Longman.

Clark, C. (1995) *Drug Self Help Groups – Education for professionals: National drug strategy national education grant project: Stage 1 report*, Brunswick, VIC: SHASU Inc. (Self Help And Substance Use).

Dadich, A. (2005) 'The role of self-help support groups in fostering independence in young people', in J. Gaffey, A. Possamai-Inesedy and K. Richards (eds) *The Chameleon and the Quilt: A cross-disciplinary exploration in the social sciences*, Sydney, NSW: University of Western Sydney.

Daniel, A. and Cornwall, J. (1993) *A Lost Generation?* Canberra: Australian Youth Foundation (AYF).

Davidson, L., Chinman, M., Kloos, B., Weingarten, R., Stayner, D. and Kraemer Tebes, J. (1999) 'Peer support among individuals with severe mental illness: A review of the evidence', *Clinical Psychology: Science and Practice* 6: 165–87.

Davis, J. and Watson, N. (2001) 'Countering stereotypes of disability: Disabled children and resistance', in M. Corker and T. Shakespeare (eds) *Disability and Postmodernity*, London: Continuum.

Dean, H. (2006) *Social Policy*, Cambridge: Polity Press.

Deegan, P. E. (1992) 'The independent living movement and people with psychiatric disabilities: Taking back control over our own lives', *Psychosocial Rehabilitation Journal* 15: 3–19.

Eckersley, R. (1999) 'What the !#&* have values got to do with anything! Young people, youth culture and well-being', *Social Alternatives* 18: 29–32.

Fuller, A., Mcgraw, K. and Goodyear, M. (1998) *The Mind of Youth – Initial findings from the resiliency report*, VIC: Department of Education.

Galanter, M. (1990) 'Cults and zealous self-help movements: A psychiatric perspective', *American Journal of Psychiatry* 147: 543–51.

Hamilton, C. and Maddison, S. (eds) (2007) *Silencing Dissent: How the Australian government is controlling public opinion and stifling debate*, Crows Nest, NSW: Allen & Unwin.

Kyrouz, E. M., Humphreys, K. and Loomis, C. (2003) 'A review of the effectiveness of self-help mutual aid groups', in B. J. White and E. J. Madara (eds), *American Self-Help Group Clearinghouse self-help group sourcebook* (7th edn), Cedar Knolls, NJ: American Self-Help Clearinghouse, pp. 71–86.

Linton, S. (1998) *Claiming Disability: Knowledge and identity*, New York: New York University Press.

Madara, E. J. (1999) 'Self-help groups: Options for support, education, and advocacy', in P. G. O'Brien, W. Z. Kennedy and K. A. Ballard (eds) *Psychiatric Nursing: An integration of theory and practice*, New York: McGraw-Hill.

Martinez, E. and Garcia, A. (1997) 'What is "neo-liberalism"? A brief definition for activists', www.corpwatch.org/article.php?id=376, accessed 28 May 2007.

McNeish, D. (1999) 'Promoting participation for children and young people: Some key questions for health and social welfare organisations', *Journal of Social Work Practice* 13: 191–203.

Nash, S. (1999) *Self Help in Australia: The self help movement in Australia in the 1990s*, Carlton, VIC: COSHG (Collective Of Self Help Groups).

Noordsy, D. L., Schwab, B., Fox, L. and Drake, R. E. (1996) 'The role of self-help programmes in the rehabilitation of persons with severe mental illness and substance use disorders', *Community Mental Health Journal* 32: 71–81.

Orford, J. (1992) *Community Psychology: Theory and practice*, Chichester: John Wiley & Sons.

Rappaport, J. (1993) 'Narrative studies, personal stories, and identity transformation in the mutual help context', *Journal of Applied Behavioral Science* 29: 239–56.

Riessman, F. and Carroll, D. (1995) *Redefining Self-help Policy and Practice*, San Francisco: Jossey-Bass Publishers.

Stanton-Salazar, R. D. (1997) 'A social capital framework for understanding the socialisation of racial minority children and youths', *Harvard Educational Review* 67: 1–40.

UN (United Nations) Human Rights (1989) *Convention on the Rights of the Child*, Geneva: Office of the High Commissioner for Human Rights.

Woff, I., Toumbourou, J., Herlihy, E., Hamilton, M. and Wales, S. (1996) 'Service providers perceptions of substance use self-help groups, *Substance Use and Misuse* 31: 1241–58.

Wyn, J. (2007) 'Generation and class: Young people's new, diverse patterns of life and their implications for recognising participation in civic society', *International Journal of Children's Rights* 15: 165–79.

Zimmerman, M. (1985) *Empowerment, Perceived Control, and Citizen Participation*, Illinois: University of Illinois, Psychology Department.

10 Advocacy for children in family group conferences

Reflections on personal and public decision making

Perpetua Kirby and Sophie Laws

Introduction

How can children best be helped to have their views heard when decisions are made that are of personal importance to them? This chapter draws on research into the representation of children's views within family group conferences (FGCs), a particular type of family-led decision-making forum. We reflect on the findings of our in-depth case study research, and identify links to issues for participatory practice where children are involved in public-sphere decision making.

Within FGCs extended family and friends come together, with professional support, to discuss and decide future action for the care of their children. Typical questions for such a meeting might be, for example, what support can be offered by the extended family where parents are absent or where the child has challenging behaviour. These meetings are frequently held in a context where the state is highly likely to intervene, or may have already intervened, through legal action, due to concern about the adequacy of current parental care.

Children are now more often actively involved in FGCs (Ryan 2004) and may be supported by a family member or friend (family supporter), or increasingly by professional advocates. Professional advocates meet with the child before the conference, attend the conference and may spend some time in the private family stage of the meeting – which is not normally attended by professionals. They may also meet with the children after the conference.

We were commissioned by the Brighton and Hove Children's Fund Partnership and Brighton and Hove Daybreak FGC Project to examine support for children within FGCs. The research explored who is best placed, and how, to support children to think about and express their views to adults about major personal decisions. It was a comparative study examining how family supporters and professional advocates, respectively, supported children's participation within FGCs (Laws and Kirby 2007).

The research addresses a neglected area of children's involvement in important decisions *together with their families*. Children are starting to be engaged in intergenerational dialogue within some public settings, and within families they make daily decisions together with adults. Rarely, however, are both children and their families supported by professionals to make important decisions. The Royal College of Paediatrics and Child Health has been developing training in how to communicate with children and parents in clinical settings, recognising the complexity of three-way communication between doctors, parents and child (see www.rcpch.ac.uk). However, this type of work is in its infancy and its complexities are becoming clearer. The review by the Northern Ireland Commissioner for Children and Young People (2006) of participation in care planning processes found that in about one-third of cases birth parents were seen as an obstacle to children's participation.

The FGC model developed as a result of a perceived over-involvement of the state within the family, with a belief that families can make good decisions regarding the care of their children if supported through an FGC process. It originated in New Zealand, specifically trying to adapt official decision making to fit indigenous cultural practices involving the extended family. The growing involvement of children within FGCs has caused a tension: on the one hand, the state and professional intervention is perceived as disempowering for families, and yet there is an increasing tendency to involve professional advocates to help children represent their views within FGCs. The FGC is an exceptional situation for children's participation, which happens occasionally and with relatively few children, but it points up some of the issues in involving children in important decisions about their lives.

About the research

The research was primarily a qualitative and participatory study, in which we interviewed children aged 4 to 14 years and adults from ten families in the south of England who had attended an FGC, plus the advocates or family supporters, conference coordinators and other attending professionals. We talked to six families with independent advocacy support for the children, one in which the young person refused an advocate, and three families who used family supporters. The project staff were courageous in their openness to sharing and learning from their innovative work within this research process.

Children's influence

Children clearly have an important contribution to make in difficult decisions about their care. In our study the majority had some say, in that their issues were included in the FGC plan. Mostly they influenced small decisions, but in a few cases, including with young children, they influenced key decisions.

Hearing children's own words has a powerful impact, as adults learn both through listening and through observation in the meetings (see also Dalrymple 2002; Pennell and Burford 2000). Separated parents, for example, were struck by how much children wanted to see them. Some other family members discovered that children wanted to see them less. Even when what they wanted was not possible or appropriate – for example, for parents to remarry – expressing it sent a strong message about how children felt.

While children's direct personal contact with adults can be extremely powerful, there is also a role for professionals to consolidate the views of children and to represent these. One of the key factors that helped children to influence decisions within the FGCs was having adequate preparation and representation. At the conference they were more likely to get their views into the plan and acted upon if they had a professional advocate rather than a family supporter.

Children's participation in FGCs

Enthusiasm for children's participation within meetings needs to be balanced with consideration about children's motivation for attending and how they experience the meetings (see also Holland and O'Neill 2006; Bell and Wilson 2006). There was an ethos in the projects we studied which encouraged and enthused about children's attendance at the FGCs. Children were told it was a meeting for them, were asked what food they would like and looked forward to it as a fun family social occasion. Some of these children were motivated to attend more because it was a chance to see loved and often absent family members, rather than because they wanted to take part in a meeting, or necessarily appreciated the seriousness of it.

In reality, FGCs are difficult adult meetings, so even where children were helped to express some views, their participation was generally limited. The majority went 'in and out' of the meeting, and while some said what they felt, often their views were read out and communicated by the advocate or family supporter. The youngest children tended not to be invited to FGCs, their views being represented instead by advocates.

In this type of context there is potential harm for some children, by witnessing very difficult discussions and family conflict about their lives in front of many people (including other young people), or by fearing particular adults and possible repercussions from taking part. It is not always clear in advance what the risk of harm may be. For example, in one case the child's extended family all said in front of her that they were not able to look after her. We were told of another example, not in our research, where a mother had cut her wrists in the meeting. Fortunately it had been decided only the day before to exclude the child. Not surprisingly, in our research most children found the meetings boring and unpleasant. Some developed strategies to withdraw. And yet they mostly chose to attend, including subsequent review meetings, rather than be excluded. This reflects the picture found by Thomas and O'Kane in relation to attendance at LAC (looked-after children) review meetings (1999a; 1999b; Thomas 2000a).

> Annoying … because there was lots of speaking. So I just ran off after an hour or so, and went under the table.
>
> (Child)

> At the first bit I spoke lots … and then the second I didn't really, because every time I go to the meeting we always go in this hallway and like skid and that.
>
> (Child)

> So she went with a lot of power because the coordinator had spoken to her before. 'The meeting's about you, I'm going to get your favourite cakes, tell

me what you want me to get you, it's all about you.' So when we got there
and things were discussed over her head – because that's how things happen,
don't they? … she sat there and she really wanted someone to play with and
to go off.

(Foster carer)

Involving children in planning any meeting may help to build their commitment,
but care should be taken not to raise false expectations. FGCs are held because
there are real difficulties within the family, which exist whether children attend the
conference or not. Of course, children will be aware of and witness many of these
difficulties already. The challenge, however, is to involve them in ways that do not
replicate existing damaging situations or expose them to further harm.

Having a family supporter or advocate should allow children to present their
views without necessarily attending all or any of the formal meetings. The research
concluded by recommending a separate room with crèche/youth workers, food
and age-appropriate resources for all children attending, enabling adults to talk
alone at times while ensuring that children are not exposed to harm and can avoid
long, difficult discussions.

Children may not necessarily come up with solutions to their personal situation and sometimes it may only be possible or appropriate for them to tell us a
bit about how they experience their lives or what they want – by allowing space
for children to offer their own information rather than simply answering adult
questions – and for this to help inform adult decisions. There were several cases
in the research where the advocate or family supporter was unable to find out the
children's views on matters relevant to the FGC. They allowed these troubled
children largely to lead the interaction. In some cases this meant the FGC questions were not addressed, as this would have involved the child being persuaded
to do something unwanted. While what they tell us may be irrelevant to the adult
decisions being made, it is important to ask, as we cannot know in advance what
children will tell us, or how useful it will be.

Helping children to fully appreciate their real level of influence, and for adults
themselves to be clear, is a challenge in all contexts. Particular difficulties were
found in two cases where children were thought to exert considerable power
within their families and not to be given adequate 'boundaries'. In these cases, the
strong emphasis on the child's having a sense of control and importance within the
FGC was felt by some respondents to be unhelpful.

Engaging children

Children benefit from, and want, support to engage in difficult personal decisions.
Jane Dalrymple (2002) found that a large majority of children accept professional
advocates when these are offered. Providing adequate support requires skill and takes
time. We found that effective support for children included significant preparation
before the meeting, support during, plus a debriefing afterwards. Advocates' role
included assisting children in understanding the questions being discussed and considering their views, supporting them to express those views, plus increasing the focus

of the FGC on the children and helping to ensure that their voice was distinct from that of their carers. Advocates spent a lot of time before the FGC, meeting two to four times, including spending several hours playing, and carefully and skilfully raised difficult issues to discuss. This helped to build relationships, providing an engaging and safe way to explore feelings. For example, a 4-year-old child made known through play with trains his wish to be close to his father as well as to his mother.

Family supporters can also support children well, but we found that this varied widely between individuals, whereas professional advocates provided consistently high levels of support to the children. It can be a difficult role for family supporters to understand and undertake, and they have competing loyalties within the meeting. The challenge is to adequately brief and support them, without imposing too much on those who are volunteering their time.

Children attending FGCs have frequently experienced contact with many professionals, and some continuity of adult relationships may be of great value to them. It was notable that in our sample the advocates had not ceased their relationship with most of the children after the FGCs, although they were officially expected to do so. At the very least they had left the door open to further contact. Other research has found the absence of relationship with children based upon 'shared knowledge, communication and understanding' to be a barrier to their participation in care planning (NICCYP, 2006: 24), and the need for social workers in particular to have more time for understanding 'the viewpoint of a marginalised young person is a time consuming business' (McLeod 2007: 8). It is questionable whether advocacy that invests less time with children could achieve the kind of results that were found in our research. Other research (Dalrymple 2002) reported that young people need an optimum of two to three meetings for an effective advocacy relationship to develop.

Deciding which children to involve

Children's participation in FGCs internationally varies widely, but it seems that usually those under 10 years are excluded from meetings (Nixon et al. 2005; Thomas 2000b), and there are disagreements about whether children should attend or be given responsibility for agreeing the plan (Rasmussen 2003). In our research we found that even some very young children, while not attending the meetings, made active use of their professional advocates, appearing to understand that this was a way they could tell their families their views. Although they could not meaningfully consent to their participation in such a complex process, they had views about their life situation which some chose to share. It is important to assess each young child so as to decide whether they are able to understand the advocacy role and use it to share their thoughts and feelings. The difficulty is deciding who should assess their competency and how.

Supporting families within meetings

Families need support to involve their children in these kinds of meetings. Family groups are often large, they may include parents plus others with legal responsibility, and there are frequently conflicting sides of the family present, so it is not often clear who is 'in charge' of children during FGC meetings. It is important therefore to offer help to identify who will be responsible for supporting attending children (for example, if they become upset, disruptive or want to leave).

Families benefit from hearing their children's views and being supported to focus on these, but we found the insistence that children attend the meeting inhibited family discussion about their care. Families need support to decide whether and when a child should be excluded from all or parts of a meeting, and given 'permission' to do so when they want to talk freely.

Children do not have to be physically present, at least not for all of the meeting, in order to be effectively represented. Children's participation should not be confused with attendance. Hearing their views at first hand is powerful, but more important perhaps, particularly where there may be potentially harmful consequences from children's attendance, is the quality of their advocacy and checks to ensure that families address children's wishes. Even where advocates support children, it is important to actively encourage all adults to ensure that children are genuinely heard. Supporting understanding of children's motivations and concerns for attending (as well as helping children understand the reality of the meetings) can help families to decide how to involve them. For example, a primary desire to meet up socially with family members could be addressed separately through a designated lunch slot which the child attends.

Good advocacy support may also have wider benefits for family relationships. There were some examples in our research where participants said that the advocates had helped to change how a family listened to its own children, while in other families there was no clear impact. Some felt that adults now listened more and had learned new ways of engaging with children through observing the advocate (e.g. sitting on the floor with the child).

Relevance for public-sphere decision making

This research, while focused on a specific context of personal decision making, has resonance for participatory practice where children are involved in public-sphere decision making. Primarily, the importance of preparation and representation within the context of FGCs is pertinent for thinking about how to improve children's involvement in public decision making, as one of the greatest challenges here is trying to ensure that consulted children influence outcomes. Often too much emphasis is put on collecting their views and not enough on planning and managing the process by which those views are represented and fed into adult decision-making processes, with inadequate clarity about who has designated responsibility and accountability for ensuring that this happens.

FGCs raise specific concerns about how much children should participate, but other settings similarly struggle with how much to allow children to set the agenda, and how much adults should stipulate discussion topics and outputs. Within public consultations children (and adults) can be asked for solutions to service or policy issues about which they know little. Some might be better equipped simply to share their own related experiences, which can be used to inform change.

The question of which children should participate in making difficult decisions is relevant for public decisions too. It may not always be appropriate to include all children or even a diverse mix, depending on the purpose and context. For example, in an ongoing consultative group which requires long-term commitment and engagement in fairly complex policy discussions, there is an argument that selection might best focus on the personal characteristics of individuals who are able to provide consistency, develop a good understanding and provide relevant feedback (i.e. ability and proven motivation). When diversity is stressed as important – or when all or most children are expected to participate – then greater flexibility is needed to allow the project to meet their needs, more variety in how they can choose to participate, plus realistic expectations of what can be achieved.

The importance of giving children sufficient time when preparing for FGCs has relevance for all contexts. Many one-off or occasional consultations are constrained by limited timeframes and resources. Workers struggle with knowing how much to accommodate and support those who find it difficult to engage, when there is a pressure for outputs. Younger children or those with support needs, in particular, may need more time.

The advocates used fun in their preparation meetings, although not in the FGCs. Fun activities are used within many consultation contexts to help engage children in what might otherwise be difficult or boring discussions for some. Sometimes payment is offered, although this raises questions about how much a participant can then be expected to 'work' (i.e. participate). In some settings 'fun' might become a form of coercion, rather than true engagement and relationship building. When doing the one-off interviews for this research we spent some time playing and aimed to be *interesting* to the children (bringing along things they personally liked) as well as being *interested*, in the hope that this would encourage them to engage and be open. It was not always clear how much children, particularly the younger ones, clearly understood the purpose of our visits, despite our attempts to explain (for example, by showing photographs of their advocates). At times we felt uncomfortable that our use of fun might be a form of distraction that persuaded children to take part when they did not want to, although we tried to be mindful of when children did not want to participate (and terminated one interview within a few minutes). A researcher on another project had told us that she often distracted children with fun activities when they appeared to be disengaging in research interviews, and then carried on, rather than offering them the option of leaving, because of the pressure to ensure good sample sizes within a limited time.

Conclusion

It is clear that children can benefit from good advocacy support within FGCs to ensure that they can express their views and to help them to influence decisions. Adult family members also value some time without children present when discussing difficult issues about children's lives. More sharing of learning between professionals who engage children and families in different types of decisions is essential to take this work forward and to help ensure that the views of children are understood and heard, without placing children under unnecessary pressure.

There are many strands of learning in common between experiences of children's participation in public and private spheres. The importance of preparation, and the need for attention to practical arrangements that make children comfortable to take part, and giving them choices as to how to do so, are all frequently noted. But where decisions are being made about a child's own life, of course the consequences of *not* taking an active part in decision making are much more apparent and potentially serious for the individual. There is no option to get views instead from another child who is easier to engage, for example. There is more work to be done to bridge the gap between the commitment in law and policy for meaningful participation by children and young people in decisions concerning them, and the complex realities entailed in putting this into practice.

References

Bell, M. and Wilson, K. (2006) 'Children's views of family group conferences', *British Journal of Social Work* 36(2–6): 671–81.

Dalrymple, J. (2002) 'Family group conferences and youth advocacy: The participation of children and young people in family decision making', *European Journal of Social Work* 5(3): 287–99.

Holland, S. and O'Neill, S. (2006) ' "We had to be there to make sure it was what we wanted": Enabling children's participation in family decision-making through the family group conference', *Childhood* 13(1): 91–112.

Laws, S. and Kirby, P. (2007) *Under the Table or at the Table? Advocacy for children in Family Group Conferences*, Brighton, UK: Brighton and Hove Children's Fund Partnership and the Brighton and Hove Daybreak FGC Project. Full report and summary available.

McLeod, A. (2007) 'Whose agenda? Issues or power and relationship when listening to looked after young people', *Child and Family Social Work*, 12: 278–86.

NICCYP (2006) *Review of Children and Young People's Participation in the Care Planning Process*, Belfast: NICCYP.

Nixon, P., Burford, G. and Quinn, A. with Edelbaum, J. A. (2005) *Survey of International Practices: Policy and research on family group conferencing and related practices*, May 2005, www.frg.org.uk (accessed 24 January 2008).

Pennell, J. and Burford, G. (2000) 'Family group decision-making and family violence', in G. Burford and J. Hudson (eds) *Family Group Conferencing: New directions in community-centred child and family practice*, New York: Aldine de Gruyter.

Rasmussen, B. (2003) 'Vulnerability and energy: The study of the Danish experiment with family group conferencing', *Protecting Children*, 18 (1–2): 124–6.

Ryan, M. (2004) *Harnessing Family and Community Support*, Totnes: Research in Practice (Champions for Children, no. 2).

Thomas, N. (2000a) *Children, Family and the State: Decision-making and child participation*, Houndmills: Macmillan (paperback edition 2002, Bristol: The Policy Press).

Thomas, N. (2000b) 'Putting the family in the driving seat: The development of family group conferences in England and Wales', *Social Work and Social Sciences Review* 8(2): 101–15.

Thomas, N. and O'Kane, C. (1999a) 'Children's participation in reviews and planning meetings when they are "looked after" in middle childhood', *Child and Family Social Work* 4(3): 221–30.

Thomas, N. and O'Kane, C. (1999b) 'Children's experiences of decision making in middle childhood', *Childhood* 6(3): 369–88.

Commentary 2

Reflections on the participation of particular groups

Anita Mathew, Alessandro Martelli, Rita Bertozzi and Nicola De Luigi

What emerge from the chapters by Kirby and Laws; Alderson; Martin and Franklin; and Dadich are three key issues which reflect the challenges of participation for particular groups. First is the way in which adult interpretations of the dual concerns of protection and participation influence the social context in which children and young people seek to participate. Second, the chapters reveal the extent to which discrimination and exclusion, and social constructions of childhood, disability and the competence of children and young people can be detrimental to the participation of particular groups of children. Third, the chapters bring out the significance of the seldom referred-to Article 5 of the UNCRC, relating to the evolving capacity of children to participate, in turn raising the important issue of the role of adults in providing enabling environments for children to participate and to make participation inclusive, relevant and effective.

The issues raised in the four chapters around the mode and extent to which children and young people have opportunities to participate is closely related to one of the main arguments faced within debates about youth and participation in the last two decades: the problematic balance between protection and participation. This can be interpreted as a dichotomy between a paternalistic approach to children's participation (nurturance orientation) and an approach characterised by the promotion of autonomy (self-determination orientation). The authors stand in opposition to the current social construction of childhood, characterised by a liberal-market orientation; an attention to educational attainment; a semantics of control; an idea of children as 'becoming', as an effect of an adult-based definition; and a prevalence of provision and protection. The perspectives in the four chapters aim to 'redefine the boundaries', contesting policy rhetoric and professional practices by promoting an alternative social and cultural orientation towards children; giving attention to real participation; developing a semantics of self-realisation; an idea of children as 'beings'; a direct involvement of disabled children as active and competent agents; a redefinition of methods; and fostering reflexivity within organisations and social services. This debate is also present in Italy, where children and youth have recently received greater attention, particularly with the Law for the Promotion of Rights and Opportunities for Childhood and Adolescence (L. 285/1997) and through experimental services and initiatives. In contrast to the 'service-orientated' ethos of participation in the four chapters, in Italy (typical of southern European countries) the family is still central, with the result that there is a lack of nursery schools and an extended dependence by young people on the family (the 'long' family of young adults). This provides a contrasting context for children's participation, as it does in other parts of the world where family and community provide the primary social context for children.

A further key question arising from these chapters is the relation between the socio-political dimension of participation and other dimensions, such as education and economic and civil participation. Discourses developed within the four chapters seem to leave 'behind the scenes' the socio-economic context of the lives of disabled young people and, more, the social and individual capital they and their families can appropriate (family status; social attitudes, solidarity; technologies, services, territorial/urbanistic aspects and barriers; etc.). What is the relationship between individual and collective means of participation? And how can we make sense of participation, when it varies in relation to the kind of exclusion young people experience? In the case of mental health disability we may promote a form of direct participation, while in the case of conflicting families the emphasis seems to be on providing mediation, support and protection.

In the Indian context, although the child is central even in the relationship between parents, patriarchal values mean that women and children are subservient in family decision making, where 'arranged' marriages remain the norm and joint families, especially in the rural areas, are still prevalent. Given these circumstances, the prospect of the participating child is dependent on the status of the child. However, the example of family group conferences could provide a useful context for children's participation in resolving family conflict, even in contexts where cultural norms may appear restrictive. For example, Raju is 13 years old and lives in a government remand home. He relates:

> My parents don't know when and why I ran away, my father drinks and beats my mother as we have no money to live. My mother wants me around to help her and my other brothers and sisters. My father beats us all and my mother is now very sick. I have to stay away and work and want to send money back to them, but I don't and can't live there while my father is alive. I still love my family but I hate the way my father treats us.

Raju did participate, but decisions were being taken by others. The child, as per the rules of the home, had to be sent back home. The parents would be traced by the police and the child, even if opposed to returning, would be forced to make a decision without having a solution to the very cause of his running away in the first place. A family group conference would be most useful because a trained counsellor could work with the family, with the cooperation of the child, to solve the underlying problem and provide a way of ensuring protection through participation.

With regard to Alderson's chapter, reference to age in defining the capacities of children opens up a controversial field within which the relation between children and adults is a balancing act between protection and participation (as agency). Alderson states: 'children's participation is much broader and more varied, and begins at a much younger age, than is usually acknowledged, researched or reported'. However, the effects of broadening the definition to include 'informal' participation involving experiences, activities and relationships risk enlarging the concept to the extent that 'all is participation'. One could also argue that, notwithstanding the value of broader concepts of participation suggested in these chapters, they still appear to be 'adult based'. A key question concerns how children themselves would define the concept of participation in 'all matters affecting' them, according to their own terms of reference.

Participation takes on a whole new dimension when we work with disadvantaged children and young people. Adults have to take important steps to make sure that it is the present that matters for children – the here and now. The four chapters make it clear that inclusivity and non-discrimination, along with the best interests of the child and a change in the educational system, are key factors in transforming rhetoric into reality in enabling the participation of children. The chapters suggest that there is a need to challenge and change existing social constructs of childhood and particular groups – such as young people with disabilities or mental health issues. These discriminatory views centre on the idea that children, and these children in particular, are not to be seen as beings of the present, but more as only 'becomings' of the future, as yet without competence to participate and whose lives must be controlled by adults, often without ever consulting them on matters that affect their lives. To counteract notions of the adult knowing best, participation by the child is central to ensuring the best interests of the child.

Focusing on participation within families as opposed to organisations and wider society refocuses attention on individual rather than collective participation. As Alderson highlights, meaningful participation by younger children involves individual interaction and must entail affording children the role of being active agents rather than passive receivers, based on a presumption of lack of competence to make choices or decisions. The ethos of the UNCRC, which is now being gradually incorporated into legislation in many countries, is that children are to be protected not only as vulnerable, but because they have to be regarded as 'growing citizens' with their own citizenship rights. However, the notion of autonomy and the realisation of children as full citizens – in terms of playing an effective role (participating) in their community – is more difficult to achieve.

The chapter by Dadich about mental health service users' self-help support groups raises interesting questions about what constitutes meaningful and 'effective' forms of participation. The example of the self-help support groups reveals an approach to participation that is presented as an appropriate form of participation for this group, in essence seeking to maximise social capital within the group. Yet, in terms of 'linking' social capital there may be a risk of creating a sort of 'locked identity', a 'bounded' citizenship that allows young people to be recognised only within, and as members of, a specific group or community. How does this situation fit with ideas of universal human rights and the creation and maintenance of an 'open code' of inclusion?

Martin and Franklin, exploring the gaps between the rhetoric and reality of participation for disabled children, point out that social services allow only a fragile form of participation. How can – if they can – social policies and services promote stronger participation? Are timing, time and methods of social services suitable to young people's attitudes and agency? This raises questions about the role of the professional when children participate – an issue not mentioned in the chapters. Adults who work within an ethos of protecting or providing for children are more likely to play a more significant role. Yet the experiences related in Dadich's chapter suggest that there is considerable scope for children and young people themselves to play an increasingly active role as peer operators in providing peer support as a means of reforming approaches to participation at the interface of rhetoric and reality. However, there still remains a role for adults. Reflections on the four chapters suggest a key role for adults as providing 'an enabling environment' first and foremost, and ways in which this can be achieved. The chapters provide important insights into practical experiences of involving children and the importance of recognising different levels of participation according to children's evolving competencies and individual differences, as opposed to normative concepts of children's ability to participate.

The authors

Anita Mathew is a human rights activist and trainer. For the past decade she has worked in Goa with child and women's rights NGOs and with mental health issues. Raju's story speaks for all the children in many government remand homes in India who have no voice, nor have an enabling environment to participate.

Alessandro Martelli is Professor of Sociology at the Faculty of Political Science 'R. Ruffilli', University of Bologna (Italy). His professional interests largely concern young people in relation to active citizenship and social change; and transformations of welfare systems.

Rita Bertozzi is Assistant Professor of Sociology of Cultural Processes at the College of Education of the University of Modena and Reggio Emilia (Italy). Her main work concerns migrant children and families, child-centred research approaches and the construction of identity of the adolescent in multicultural contexts.

Nicola De Luigi is an Assistant Professor of Sociology at the Faculty of Political Science 'R. Ruffilli', University of Bologna. His research focuses mainly on social ex/inclusion and the relationship between youth, education and the job sector in different social contexts.

11 Questioning understandings of children's participation

Applying a cross-cultural lens

Jan Mason and Natalie Bolzan
(with Qing Ju, Chen Chen, Xia Zhao, Usha Nayar,
Anil Kumar, Swarna Wijetunge, Nittaya J Kotchabhakdi,
Nithivadee Noochaiya and Dalapat Yossatorn)

Introduction

Over the past few decades there has been an increasing emphasis on children's participation. This has been described as part of the two related global social trends of 'democratisation' and individualisation (Fairclough 1992; Prout 2000 citing Beck 1992). These trends, as Prout (2000) has pointed out, have facilitated the contemporary understanding of children as 'persons in their own right' (p. 308), as having agency and the right to have their voices heard. The UN Convention on the Rights of the Child (UNCRC) is generally seen as contributing to the global impetus on child participation and as the benchmark for a change in adult–child relations (e.g. John 1996).

In discussing different typologies for describing children's participation, Thomas (2007) has identified two distinct strands, which can coexist but are also, in essence, contradictory. The first of these typologies, as is the case with Hart's (1992) oft-cited development of Arnstein's (1969) ladder for social planning, articulates different levels at which children can be enabled to exercise power in decision making. These levels range from tokenism in the inclusion of children, to shared power between children and adults. Shared power is typically conceptualised in these typologies as a 'high point' for participation, but different levels of participation are considered as appropriate to different activities and situations (Thomas 2007). The second strand, as identified by Thomas (2007), conceptualises child partici-pation as necessitating adults giving away some of their power to children (e.g. Shier 2001; Mason and Urquhart 2001). Here, those developing the models place value on children having power to determine processes and outcomes (Thomas 2007). A UNICEF (2004) document defines 'authentic' participation by children as starting with children and young people themselves and demanding a change in adult thinking and behaviour, so that adults share with children in determining the way the world is defined.

The dominant understandings of child participation and their basic assump-tions, as represented in these typologies, are currently being challenged in some of the research literature. For example, Gallagher highlights assump-tions about power – implicit in these typologies – in which it is conceptualised as a commodity or capacity which powerful adults can transfer to powerless children (Gallagher 2008). His research challenges the adult concept in which attempts to empower children are seen as 'necessarily liberating' for children (p. 147), and makes a case for a reconceptualisation of relations of power in participatory research.

While there have been discussions on the conceptualisation of child participation in the context of initiatives to promote child participation globally, in 2004, when we commenced the project discussed in this chapter, there had been little research reported in the literature on the conceptualisation of child participation across cultures. This is despite the fact that an Editorial in *Childhood* (1997) had acknowledged the importance of 'different concerns and approaches coming out of different world regions' in contributing to more comprehensive knowledge about children's lives and the policies impacting on them (ibid.: 197). Where there has been documentation in the literature of child participation approaches in the Asia-Pacific region, it is 'often written by international agencies or their English-writing consultants', and therefore much of it 'reflects the experiences and priorities of the(se) agencies and individuals' (Theis 2007: 12).

In this chapter, we explore some of the ways in which participation is being understood and implemented in five countries in the Asia-Pacific region: Australia, China, India, Sri Lanka and Thailand, and discuss the significance of these cross-cultural perspectives on children's participation.

The cross-cultural project

This chapter draws on findings from a cross-cultural research project involving partners from the Asia-Pacific Regional Study Group of Childwatch International Research Network, all of whom had an interest in the topic of child participation. The partners were researchers from universities as well as other institutional settings, such as government-funded research centres. A collaborative approach was adopted, with all researchers responsible for implementing the project in their own countries while also engaging in learning across countries in response to findings at different stages of the research. Although this chapter has been written by the English-speaking members of the team, it is the product of written contributions, dialogue and feedback between all partners throughout the project. Cross-country research workshops were conducted in Bangkok, Mumbai, Sydney and Beijing between 2004 and 2006 to plan and discuss parallel studies exploring the concept and practice of the participatory principles of the UN Convention on the Rights of the Child, as implemented in our own countries, at the levels of family, community and society. Through reflexive cross-project dialogue it became evident that cultural context and traditions were pivotal in the undertaking of this research as well as in interpreting findings. For example, while all researchers shared a commitment to a concept of 'children's participation', we had different understandings among us of what we meant by the term 'child participation'. In some important respects these different understandings of participation paralleled the findings from the empirical studies of the way the concept is applied in different national contexts. The project involved research at family, community and policy levels to explore:

- the meanings being attributed to the concept of child participation;
- what was considered appropriate in terms of child participation;
- to what extent it was being implemented;
- what factors were supporting and/or limiting child participation in each of the countries.

Constructions of child participation across the study region

Initial discussions identified a lack of clarity across the group concerning the use of the term 'participation', reflected in much of the literature on participation in our own countries. While 'child participation' was used as a shorthand term to describe the pertinent UNCRC principles, the meanings of the term were rarely made explicit. Below we discuss the different interpretations of participation, based on discussion of empirical data throughout the project.

Child participation as a right

According to our overall findings, construction of child participation as a right for children to have their views heard was not being consistently or significantly operationalised in any of the Asia-Pacific region countries in which our study was situated. There was some recognition in all countries of this right in terms of rhetoric and changes in legislation; however, there was only limited evidence that the right is implemented in practice in children's interactions with adults. Findings from the one country with Western-liberalist value traditions, Australia, paralleled the findings reported on in the Australian non-governmental report to the UN on the implementation of the UNCRC in Australia (NCYLC 2005), which noted that while there had been some developments in relation to this right, there remained 'significant restrictions and tokenistic or manipulative processes in some important areas of children and young people's involvement in society' (p. 3). Discussion among project partners from Asian countries, where the value traditions were not Western liberalist, indicated that, where there was an emphasis on child participation as a right, it was often as a result of NGO influence. This is particularly the case in Sri Lanka. Tensions can arise in the implementation of the global agenda on child participation around financial and in-kind aid contribution when administered through multinational non-governmental organisations that have a rights base. Indeed, concern had been expressed among some adult respondents in all countries that a rights-based approach to child participation should be treated warily, in case it should contribute to instability in the social order.

Child participation as 'taking part in'

The dominant construction of the concept of child participation that emerged from our findings was of children 'taking part in' activities. In the preliminary stages of the research process all researchers appeared to share this understanding of child participation as 'taking part in'. However, as the discussions progressed it became apparent that there were differences. In the Australian data, this concept of 'taking part in' was about children participating as individuals in adult-organised activities. In data from Sri Lanka and Thailand, this was also likely to be the case, but in these countries the emphasis in the use of the term was on children participating *with others*, as a group. It became evident that the use of the English word 'participation' by us as a study group camouflaged semantic and associated conceptual subtleties, which implied fundamental differences in the meanings attributed to the phrase 'child participation' within the different countries in the study. This was exemplified with reference to the use of the term 'participation' in Sri Lanka.

In Sri Lanka, the Sinhala term for participation – '*sahabagithvaya*' – literally translated means 'to join in with others'; the group emphasis of this word tends to be contextual and communal in focus. It is often associated with concepts of obligation, important also in the other Asian countries. This connotation had resonances with the understandings of the dominant meaning of child participation in other majority-world countries in this study. The participants from Thailand, Sri Lanka, China and India considered that in their countries, where the ethos of collectivism has been dominant, responsibility to family and community has traditionally taken precedence over individual rights. For example, in Thailand, families, aware of the rapid ageing of their society, encourage their children to participate in caring for family members, while children's participation in agrarian pursuits has been understood as an economic imperative rather than as a right; when the harvest is due, all hands are required, children included. In the data from Sri Lanka the conceptualisation of child participation as a social obligation rather than an individual right, by both adults and children themselves, is associated, at the extreme, with examples of the way children's participation has occurred in the northern and eastern provinces, where continuous cycles of war and destruction have resulted in children taking on increased responsibilities. Further, the findings from Sri Lanka informed us that some children participated in war as child soldiers not because they had a right to choose to do so, but because they considered it an obligation to participate in this way.

Such implications of the use of the word 'participation' by the majority-world countries in this study contrasted with the use of the English word 'participation' by the Australian study group members, who perceived the idea of participation as 'taking part in' as having a more individualistic connotation. The Australian researchers referred to the liberalist ethos behind their 'Western' culture's focus on children as individuals who are in the process of *becoming* adults. This liberalism, as applied to the dominant understanding of child participation in the Australian study, was reflected in practices where children, but more usually young people, were encouraged by adults to take part in activities designed and structured by adults and frequently intended as training to enable the young people to acquire citizenship skills relevant to their futures as adults. This understanding of participation as investment in the future contrasts with majority-world conceptions of participation as making an active contribution in the present.

Interestingly, the children in the Australian study offered a challenge to this individualist perspective of participation in a way which, at surface level, seemed consistent with the more collectivist value systems of the majority-world countries, by defining participation in terms of 'obligation'. They were focusing on making contributions to their communities in the *present*, through working together with adults, by 'doing your share' in joining activities such as volunteering. They saw that participation was a responsibility they carried, rather than simply a right. In the context of the other findings of this research we can only raise the question as to whether the concept of 'obligation', like that of participation, means something different in societies where the emphasis is on deference to adults and collectivist or markedly patriarchal values, from what it means in contexts where more individualist values and an emphasis on democratic principles prevail.

Participation as involvement in decision making

A more minor construction of child participation across all countries was about children being involved in decision making. It is in this construction of child participation that sharing or transferring of power between adults and children has been understood as fundamental, and indeed potentially transformative of adult–child relations (e.g. Mason and Urquhart 2001). This construction did have some resonance across all countries, from both adults and children, but was not a strong theme. In Australia there was some rhetoric around the participation of children in decision making, but there frequently appeared to be a gap between rhetoric and practice.

In Australia, as indeed in China to a lesser degree, child participation in decision making appears to have been applied most to family interactions around clothes, family consumption and extra-curricular activities. It was around decision making in families that there was some evidence for tensions in child–adult relations around sharing power. The Australian children alluded most clearly to these tensions, indicating that where adults imposed restrictions on their decision making, they typically resisted or challenged these restrictions by taking matters into their own hands, with actions they considered appropriate.

In the data from Chinese children there were indications that some of them were challenging the rights asserted by their parents to decide on their friendships or emotional involvements. This challenge can be understood in terms of a cultural shift, with adult–child relations changing as the implementation of the one-child policy leads to an intensification of focus on 'only' children. In the other countries in our study, such as Sri Lanka and Thailand, where adult–child relations are still predicated on deference to elders, child participation around decision making continues to be constructed as occurring within a context of responsibility to family and community, rather than of individual rights. When children saw that they had a role in decision making in Sri Lanka, it was not in relation to themselves as individuals, but in relation to their contributions as participants in communal decision making.

Structural factors and cultural contexts as determinants of child participation

The way existing adult–child relations are structured and the contexts in which these relations are situated emerged from our analysis as being highly significant for how 'child participation' is constructed. Generation is recognised as a significant structural factor in determining adult–child relations (e.g. Alanen 2005). In our study generational structuring as signified by age was significant across all countries in determining which children could participate in what, with older children being more likely to be able to participate both in terms of 'taking part in' and in being involved in decision making. In Australia, for example, it seemed that those children most resembling adults, that is, older and more articulate younger people, had greater opportunities to participate.

Other structural factors were also significant in influencing child participation. Data from India indicated that its complex system of class, caste, religion, gender and location placed constraints on children's participation in decision making, while in China and Thailand location, gender, age and socio-economic factors were of greater significance, with different types of participation possible in urban and rural settings as a result of socio-economic status. Rural or more working-class children were generally likely to be required to, for example, participate in harvesting and farm work at times of increased demand, in line with the needs of the family or community.

Conclusion

Experiences from across these five countries located in the Asia-Pacific region reveals an ambiguity in the interpretation and implementation of participation – an ambiguity easily obscured by assumptions associated with cultural meanings of participation. This ambiguity is connected with the conceptual shifts involved in moving between understanding child participation as: putting into practice obligation as a community member (particularly evident in rural communities), asserting responsibility to educate young people for their futures as adults, or promoting child participation as a right of individuals in a democracy. While in each of the countries involved in this research there was a commitment to children being 'part of' activities, what they were able to be part of was culturally specific. Cultural contexts structure adult–child relations in different ways, so that it cannot be assumed that the meaning of 'participation' in a liberal democracy is the same as it is in a country with a hierarchical system of social relations, a predominantly communist country, or one racked by internal strife. In each of these countries the concept of citizenship structures relations in different ways, giving rise to a variety of ways in which participation is interpreted and enacted.

Acknowledgement of the existence of some marked differences in the way child participation and associated concepts tend to be understood is significant for the development of policies and practices, particularly those at the global level. Advocacy for children's 'empowerment' through the right to participate and in challenging existing adult–child relations may contribute to unintended negative repercussions, where it conceptually separates children as individuals from their communities. As White and Choudhury argue in Chapter 3 and elsewhere (2007), child participation is not just about facilitating children's agency, but also about paying attention to the structural factors of their environments.

Attention to the significance of differences between countries in, for example, responding to global mandates for child participation does not mean institutionalising these differences. Our findings also indicated that cultural systems are dynamic, not static. For example, the current tensions in the way some children and young people are now relating to adults in China and in some of the other Asian countries, where small numbers of children are defining participation as involvement in decision making, is an expression of very real changes currently occurring in the way childhood is being understood and reconceptualised in these countries. In some cases this is happening as a result of internal policy or practice changes, at other times through the interventions of NGOs, and sometimes through the actions of children themselves.

The complexity of issues associated with changes in adult–child relations, posed by promoting child participation across cultures, highlights the importance, as argued by Dallmayr (2002), of having critical dialogue around the potential consequences of introducing an individualistic approach to universalised human rights (in this instance, to child participation) through hegemonic top-down global policies. Citing An-Na'im (1992), Dallmayr notes the importance of this dialogue ideally coming 'from below' rather than 'from above' and including 'both intra-cultural' and 'cross-cultural sensibilities for justice and rightness'. The value and challenge posed by this form of dialogue were exemplified by the cross-cultural learning which resulted from sharing across all project partners, and the opportunities the study provided for various stakeholders, including children, to contribute through intra-cultural and bottom-up knowledge to this dialogue. The challenges for child participation advocates are to facilitate this process in a way that enables children's voices to be heard and at the same time avoids destabilising the very cultures which sustain and further the interests of the children who live their lives in these cultures. Our research has reminded us of the relevance of the argument of the Western liberal philosopher John Locke, that individual well-being cannot be separated from the well-being of communities (Weinberg 2007).

References

Alanen, L. (2005) 'Women's studies/childhood studies: Parallels, links and perspectives', in J. Mason and T. Fattore (eds) *Children Taken Seriously: In theory, policy and practice*, London: Jessica Kingsley.

An-Na'im, A. A. (ed.) (1992) *Introduction in Human Rights in Cross-Cultural Perspectives: A quest for consensus*, Philadelphia: University of Pennsylvania Press.

Arnstein, S. (1969) 'A ladder of citizen participation', *Journal of the American Institute of Planners* 35(4): 216–24.

Beck, U. (1992) *Risk Society: Towards a new modernity*, London: Sage.

Childhood (1997) Editorial: 'International child research: Promise and challenge', *Childhood* 4: 147.

Dallmayr, F. (2002) '"Asian values" and global human rights', *Philosophy East and West* 52(2): 173–89.

Fairclough, N. (1992) *Discourse and Social Change*, Cambridge: Polity Press.

Gallagher, M. (2008) '"Power is not an evil": Rethinking power in participatory methods', *Children's Geographies* 6: 137–50.

Hart, R. A. (1992) *Children's Participation: From tokenism to citizenship*, Florence: UNICEF International Child Development Centre.

John, M. (1996) 'Voicing: Research and practice with the "silenced"', in M. John (ed.) *The Child's Right to a Fair Hearing*, London: Jessica Kingsley Publishers.

Mason, J. and Urquart, R. (2001) 'Confronting the dilemmas of involving children as partners: A collaborative research project around decision making', *Children Australia* 26(4): 16–21.

NCYLC (The National Children's and Youth Law Centre) (2005) The Non-government Report on the Implementation of the United Nations Convention on the Rights of the Child in Australia, www.ncylc.org.au/croc/images/CROC_Report_for_Web.pdf (accessed 10 May 2009).

Prout, A. (2000) 'Children's participation: Control and self-realisation in British late modernity', *Children & Society* 14: 304–15.

Shier, H. (2001) 'Pathways to participation: Openings, opportunities and obligations', *Children & Society* 15: 107–17.

Theis, J. (2007) 'Performance, responsibility and political decision-making: Child and youth participation in Southeast Asia and the Pacific', *Children, Youth and Environments* 17(1): 1–13.

Thomas, N. (2007) 'Towards a theory of children's participation', *International Journal of Children's Rights* 15: 199–218.

UNICEF (2004) *The State of the World's Children*, Available as PDF at www.unicef.org/sowc.

Weinberg, M. (2007) 'The Human Rights Discourse: A Bahá'í Perspective', Bahá'í International Community, available at http://info.bahai.org/article-1-8-3-2.html, accessed 7 January 2008.

White, S. and Choudhury, S. (2007) 'The politics of child participation in international development: The dilemma of agency', *The European Journal of Development Research* 19(4): 529–50.

12 The construction of childhood and the socialisation of children in Ghana

Implications for the implementation of Article 12 of the CRC

Afua Twum-Danso

Introduction

In many ways the 1989 Convention on the Rights of the Child is a first in the history of the United Nations. Not only because it is the world's most widely and rapidly ratified international convention, but also because it was the first to articulate the civil and political rights to which children are entitled. These refer to the rights of children to: influence decisions made on their behalf, express their views on issues affecting them (Articles 12 and 13); freedom of thought, conscience and religion (Article 14); form associations (Article 15); and receive information (Article 17). Article 12, in particular, is a powerful assertion that children have the right to be actors in their own lives and not merely passive recipients of adult decision making (Lansdown 1995 in Percy-Smith 1998).

Despite the fact that almost all governments in the world have ratified the Convention, this particular article has faced seemingly insurmountable obstacles in societies around the world where children are seen as the property of their parents who must do as they are told and not question. Culture and its attendant values are central to the limited implementation of this article, due to the fact that they guide the way parents and other adults perceive and react to the principles on which Article 12 is based.

Hence, this chapter seeks to explore the context in which Article 12 is implemented within the family sphere in Ghana and the reasons behind its limited progress, as well as to explore opportunities that may facilitate its implementation within this social and cultural context. Data presented in this chapter were collected during 10 months of fieldwork in two local communities in Ghana (Nima and Ga Mashie) between May 2005 and March 2006 for my PhD research, which focused on local perceptions of the construction of childhood and the socialisation of children in order to understand the implications for the concept of children's rights and the implementation of the Convention within this social and cultural context. Focus group discussions were conducted with 291 children in the case study communities as well as in three private schools and with approximately 100 adults.

The implementation of Article 12 in Ghana: setting the context

Ghana was the first country to ratify the Convention on the Rights of the Child in February 1990, and not only did it do so with no reservations, but it also proceeded to incorporate the principles of Article 12 into the country's Children's Act. However, almost 10 years later, the government has acknowledged that this provision of the Act has proven the most problematic to enforce.

This is largely because, within the Ghanaian social and cultural context, consulting children is not seen as a right that children should have or an obligation that parents must meet. As a result, those children who do express their views or show signs of assertiveness are seen as social deviants, disrespectful, and are thus punished or insulted (as witches or devils). They are seen as bringing shame on their parents, as their behaviour shows that they have not been raised properly and thus are not aware of the role of key cultural values such as respect and obedience in regulating all interactions between adults and children in the Ghanaian social and cultural context. Conversely, children who are respectful therefore know how to behave in the company of adults and are not seen as assertive, which indicates that they have been trained properly by their parents.

Child participants in the study did not rate Article 12 highly among their list of rights. A number of them claimed that this article was not important, since children 'are not equal to adults' and hence 'do not know anything'. As one child put it: 'It is not everything that comes children's way that they should participate in' (focus group discussion [FGD] with Nima Basic I JSS pupils, October–December 2005). According to another child in Nima, it was not important for children to be involved in decision making or to express their views because 'some parents will spoil their children' (FGD with Nima Basic I primary pupils, 12 December 2005). This highlights the emphasis children themselves placed on the need for their parents to discipline them, as well as pointing to the social disapproval, even among children, of those children who are able to express their views, as it is thought they are spoilt and thus not trained properly in the values of society.

This attitude among children themselves was evident in the FGDs conducted with all groups of children during my fieldwork. Children did not feel that it was their role to speak, not even on issues that affect them. Many did not understand why I sought to obtain their views, and some informed me that I would be better off talking to their mothers, who they felt would be better positioned to engage in this discussion. Children themselves pointed to this attitude of their peers as a challenge. According to one participant:

> It is sometimes because of the children's own doing that they are not involved. The children wonder why they are being asked about this, they say they know nothing about it.
>
> (First FGD with out-of-school children organised at Freeman's Memorial Chapel, Bukom Square, Ga Mashie, 20 February 2006)

Even on the few occasions when children pointed to Article 12 as a right to which they are entitled, it was not seen as a high priority, because it was not 'necessary for dire survival' as compared to other rights such as those to education, shelter, health care and food, which are critical to survival and development (FGD with Christ the King pupils, 28 February 2006). There was a feeling among child participants that while children would not develop, or even survive, if they were not provided with food, shelter, education and medical attention, they could still develop into well-rounded, responsible citizens if they were not given the opportunity to express their views or participate in decision making during their childhood. Thus, there is a hierarchy of rights and needs which prioritises rights such as education, life, food, shelter and medical attention and parental care ahead of rights to express opinions and participate in decision making. As several children explained to me quite simply when prioritising their rights, 'if you do not express your opinions you will not die'.

One of the key reasons for the low priority allocated to the principles behind Article 12 is the belief expressed by almost all children in the study that they do not need to participate in decision making and express their opinions on issues affecting them, because parents will have their best interests at heart. However, contained in this belief is the assumption that all parents are looking out for the best interests of their children, which is at odds with the current literature on parent–child relations in Ghana, which shows that parents are retreating from the responsibilities of parenthood (see Oppong 2006). Therefore, there is a need to further explore this contradiction between children's insistence on parents having their best interests at heart and the reality within the country, which shows increasing numbers of parents abandoning their responsibilities.

The role of culture in understanding the limited implementation of Article 12

In order to understand this attitude towards Article 12 and the wider concept of children's participation in decision making, it is necessary to explore the impact of cultural beliefs and values on the way childhood is constructed and the implications for Article 12. Knowing your place in society is central to the maintenance of the Ghanaian social system, and every effort is made to ensure that each child is taught her place from a very early age. In fact, childhood is constructed and children are socialised in a manner that will ensure that they know their place in this societal structure and do not overstep the boundaries when interacting with their parents and other adults. Data collected highlighted four key components of the childhood-construction and child-rearing process which, while crucial to ensuring that children know their place in society, also restrict their ability to express their opinions, and thus limit the implementation of Article 12 in Ghana.

Childhood as a period of dependency

The first component of the childhood-construction and child-rearing process is dependency. This factor makes it possible for a 40-year-old who does not work and cannot take care of himself to be considered a child. As a dependant, such a person relies on his parents for all his needs and, to ensure that these needs are met, he must submit to their control and authority. In trying to explain this to me several children claimed that this was due to the perception in society that 'a child is fed by an adult; a child does not feed an adult'. This point was further elaborated by the elders at the Sempe Mantse Palace, who informed me that:

> Parents expect you to agree with their decisions, because you are a child, and like it or not, you do it ... because you do not feed yourself, you are fed.
>
> (FGD with elders at the Sempe Mantse We, 8 February 2006)

Thus, as a dependant who is fed, a child is restricted in his ability to express his views. In fact, I was told on several occasions that freedom of speech is a privilege for those who feed people, and which applies not only to parents but also to the elite who often look after entire families in addition to their own in return for their labour and loyalty.[1]

However, it is important to ask what this means for those children who work and whose families actually depend on the income they bring home. In discussions with children who hawk products after school, they informed me that, though they make money, they give it to their parents who then give them some for food or school fees. In this way, they do not have control over their earnings and their parents are still able to claim that they are feeding their children. Hence, the immediate transfer of earnings to parents/guardians reduces any autonomy or control to which a child may make claims as a result of engaging in an income-generating activity.

Childhood as a period of parental control and ownership

The second component of the child-rearing process, which closely relates to dependency, is parental control and ownership. Many children participating in the study informed me that, as a dependant or as someone who 'is fed by an adult', a child is 'under the control of his parents' and is ordered about. In a discussion with a group of women, they stressed the fact that a child is someone 'whose life is in the hands of her parents' (FGD with Women's Orientation Centre, Maamobi, 31 December 2005). Therefore, she has no say in decision making within the family and 'does not have the right to speak, but only to listen'. According to one participant in an FGD with a group of mature students from the University of Ghana, Legon, 'in this traditional context children are ordered about and once you are ordered about you have no say' (FGD with mature students, 8 November 2005). Parents may inform, and explain decisions to a child, but they will not necessarily involve her in decision making because they 'own' the child and will, it is believed, do their best for her. As one child participant explained to me:

> They do not consult me even in my choice of school. If they think it is something they must do they will not consult me because they think it is for my own good.
>
> (FGD with Christ the King JSS pupils, 28 February 2006)

However, it is important to note that even in cases where a child claims to accept the authority of his parents and other elders, he may still go ahead and do what he wants to do. While this was never stated explicitly during the data collection process, one observation I made was that while children always said 'yes' or 'no' to adults when asked to do something, they found ways of avoiding being sent on errands in the first place; for example, by pretending that they did not hear their name being called.

Childhood as never-ending

Even once a person achieves independence, marries and becomes a parent, he will always be perceived as a child by some. No matter how much one ages, there will always be people who are older and who will perceive that person as a child. Not only does this reflect the ways in which childhood can be seen as never-ending, but it also illustrates the corresponding eternal nature of parental/elder authority and control. According to the elders at the Sempe Mantse Palace:

> You can be 40/30, but you will still be a child in the eyes of the older people. As long as the older people are alive and you are sitting down with them you are a child. When the fishermen go fishing and they distribute the catch, they do not give any to the youngest – no matter how old he is.
>
> (FGD with elders at Sempe Mantse We, 8 February 2006)

Essentially, it is believed that in a group of adults the youngest is seen as a child, no matter what his actual age. Writing about West Africa more generally, Nsamenang posits that 'as long as one's parents are alive a child is always a child' and must come under 'some sphere of parental authority even vicariously' (1992: 151). Interestingly, children reproduce such practices among their own peer groups, as they tend to recreate the hierarchy of society in their own worlds, leading to teenagers treating younger children in the same way in which the age group ahead of themselves treats them.

Parental control and the perception that childhood is never-ending result in the marginalisation of a person within a group, due to the perception that he is a 'child', even though he may be married, own a house, have children and even be looking after his parents. As noted by some adult participants, 'a person in his 20s/30s can still be pushed aside by elder relatives even if they are married and have their own house' (FGD with media professionals, 14 September 2005). The key point to note here is that so long as he is with older people, he will always be a child, even if he has passed through all the necessary rituals to become an adult. As a result of this attitude, he will be treated as a child, which will impose limitations on his behaviour and freedom to speak his mind within these spheres, even though in other circles, such as with his own wife and children, he will be seen as the elder and thus possessing authority.[2] This notion of childhood as never-ending may lead some to conclude that age is an important criterion for defining someone's status in this society. However, what is actually being suggested here relates not so much to biological age, but more to the relativity of ages and the ideas surrounding gerontocracy and seniority.

Childhood as period of obedience and respect

In Ghanaian culture children are trained from a very early age that they must respect and obey all elders, be humble towards adults and take their advice. They are not expected to challenge adults, and certainly not expected to question what they are told to do. This has contributed to the perception among commentators that participatory rights are antipathetic to the fundamental values of community and family in Ghana, and in Africa more generally (see Temba and de Waal 2002: 219). Children must not consider themselves as superior to elders and must submit themselves to parental control (see Gyeke 1996). As a result of the strong emphasis placed on respect and obedience, virtually all the children who participated in this study put respect and obedience as the two most important duties they have in society:

- Children have to obey people in the community, not just parents.
- Children must be obedient and do what they are asked to do.
- Children must always listen to their parents' advice.
- Children have to respect mother and father.
- When sent, they [children] should go.

Thus, at the core of the very notion of what constitutes childhood are respect and obedience. This focus on respect and obedience means that children find it difficult to challenge, disagree with, question or correct adults if they are wrong. Pellow describes the implications of this emphasis on the need to respect adults succinctly: 'respect for one's elders, when carried to an extreme, rules out any chance of exercising one's free will' (1977: 56). It also affects the ability of children even to talk to adults if they have a problem. As one child participant explained, 'there are some of us who want adults to do something for us, but we cannot speak' (FGD with children organised by the Sempe Mantse Palace, 10 February 2006). Furthermore, the impact of respect and obedience on children's ability to express views also has implications for their development. According to one group of children, 'when children try to express their views adults say they do not respect. When they raise a good point they will reject it and this affects the children because when they go somewhere they cannot express their opinions' (FGD with Christ the King pupils, 28 February 2006). Obeng corroborates this point when she argues that, despite the importance of children to Ghanaian families, some cultural values such as respect and obedience destroy the initiative and creativity of the child, who is afraid to confront traditional norms and is thus unable to speak her mind easily (1998: 133).[3] As a result, large numbers of children not only struggle to formulate and articulate their views, but also find it difficult even to answer questions or simply to talk, unless it is in the company of their peers.

Opportunities for the implementation of Article 12 within the family

However, this does not mean that opportunities do not exist for children to participate in decision making. In some families, especially those that are nuclear, where biological parents head the household, there is evidence put forward by both adults and children to suggest that some parents do listen to and take on board the views of their children, especially on issues affecting them, such as their choice of school or trade, or whether they even want to continue to senior secondary school or enter a trade following the completion of compulsory schooling at the age of 15.

I was able to identify some general factors that would facilitate the ability of children to express their views within the family. One example is the parent–child relationship, which was identified as an important consideration if Article 12 is to be implemented. As one child participant summed up aptly, 'if you have a good relationship with your child, when there is an issue you can call your child and discuss it with him/her' (FGD with the Youth Wing of the Women's Orientation Centre, 4 February 2006). In both the case study communities, both children and adults believed that there is much more exchange of opinion between mothers and their children than between fathers and children. This was attributed to the relatively good relationship between mothers and children. Some children expressed their difficulty in talking to their fathers, who are seen as distant figures whose word is law. Thus, participants in adult FGDs informed me that if a child wants to express her view she will do so to her mother. In turn, mothers are more likely to ask their children for their opinions than are fathers. However, this will always be done in the privacy of their homes, as opposed to the public domain, because of the belief that in public children must, at the very least, show their submission to their mother's authority. This highlights the need to improve parent–child relations, which, according to several participants, may facilitate the implementation of Article 12.

Conclusion

This chapter has shown that, while many adults reject Article 12 and the principles behind it outright, on closer examination a middle ground can be identified, both in parental attitudes and in children's actual experiences of this Article in their families and communities. This indicates that opportunities do exist for children to express their views and participate in decision making in these spheres of their environment. However, due to the importance both adults and children within this social context place on cultural values such as respect and obedience, policy makers at both the international and the national levels need to explore how the cultural framework of a particular society can be used to engage communities in dialogue and explore the ways in which Article 12 can be implemented within the existing social and cultural context.

Notes

1. This is further supported by Vigh, who, in his study of youth in Guinea Bissau, documents the story of a young man who, although 26, continues to be totally dependent on his family. Therefore, although he often complained of his father's efforts to control him, he was aware that challenging his father's control would probably entail going to bed hungry; thus, he made himself eligible for meals by being subservient – doing what he was told, doing favours and running errands (2006: 39).
2. There are exceptions to the image depicted above, which is to be expected in this monetised and salaried age where money, more than land, plays a vital role in defining social

relationships. The socio-economic changes that have taken place in recent years have resulted in the creation of a new generation of educated young people who work and have access to better resources than their parents, particularly those remaining in the rural areas. Consequently, in some instances, this has transformed power relations in the family in favour of the youth and against the elders, who hitherto relied on their control of land for the power they wielded over their children. In this new relationship the younger members of a family who are well educated, have achieved success, gained financial stability and are now in a position to support the extended family and contribute significantly to the community may wield considerable power in these spheres (See Azu 1974; Therborn 2006).

3. Writing of the Tanzanian context, Esther Obdam claims that the school system, in particular, teaches children that they are not important, that their ideas and opinions do not matter. They are to do as they are told without question. When a child disagrees or fails to do what is expected of her she is punished, often beaten. Children grow up believing that they are not worth being listened to. They find it hard to formulate their thoughts and opinions because they are never asked for their views; they are told what to think. They are reluctant to speak up, out of fear of doing something 'wrong' and being punished for it. The school system forces children to learn through memorisation and does not give them the opportunity to think for themselves or to take part in decisions that affect them. Together with the harsh punishments for mistakes and any behaviour that is out of the ordinary, this crushes creativity and imagination (1998: 212).

References

Azu, D. G. (1974) *Ga Family and Social Change*, Leiden: Afrikastudiecentrum.

Gyeke, K. (1996) *African Cultural Values: An Introduction*, Accra: Sankofa Publishing Company.

Lansdown, G. (1995) *Taking Part: Children's Participation in decision making*, London: IPPR

Nsamenang, A. B. (1992) *Human Development in Cultural Context: A third world perspective*, Newbury Park: Sage Publications.

Obdam, E. (1998) 'Mambo Leo, Sauti ya Watoto: Child participation in Tanzania', in V. Johnson, E. Ivan-Smith, G. Gordon, P. Pridmore and P. Scott (eds) *Stepping Forward: Children and young people's participation in the development process*, London: Intermediate Technology Publications Ltd.

Obeng, C. (1998) 'Cultural relativity in Ghana: Perspectives and attitudes', in V. Johnson, E. Ivan-Smith, G. Gordon, P. Pridmore and P. Scott (eds) *Stepping Forward: Children and young people's participation in the development process*, London: Intermediate Technology Publications Ltd.

Oppong, C. (2006) 'Demographic innovation and nutritional catastrophe: Change, lack of change and difference in Ghanaian family systems', in G. Therborn (ed.) *African Families in a Global Context*, Uppsala: Nordiska Afrikainstitutet.

Pellow, D. (1977) *Women in Accra: Options for autonomy*, Michigan: Reference Publications Inc.

Percy-Smith, B. (1998) 'Children's participation in local decision-making: The challenge of local governance', in V. Johnson, E. Ivan-Smith, G. Gordon, P. Pridmore and P. Scott (eds) *Stepping Forward: Children and young people's participation in the development process*, London: Intermediate Technology Publications Ltd.

Temba, K. and de Waal, A. (2002) 'Implementing the Convention on the Rights of the Child', in A. de Waal and N. Argenti (eds) *Young Africa: Realising the rights of children and youth*, Trenton and Asmara: Africa World Press Inc.

Therborn, G. (2006) 'African families in a global context', in G. Therborn (ed.) *African Families in a Global Context*, Uppsala: Nordiska Afrikainstitutet.

Vigh, H. (2006) 'Social death and violent life chances', in C. Christiansen, M. Utas and H. E. Vigh (eds) *Navigating Youth, Generating Adulthood: Social becoming in an African context*, Uppsala: Nordiska Afrikainstitutet.

13 Youth participation in indigenous traditional communities

Yolanda Corona Caraveo, Carlos Pérez and Julián Hernández

This chapter discusses the meaning of youth participation in indigenous traditional communities in Mexico. It draws on the results of a series of in-depth interviews with young people who have taken part both in projects supported by civil associations and in projects developed from within the community. Its main purpose is to introduce some of the most frequent ways in which the young engage in collective activities, as well as the lessons and obstacles that this type of participation entails for them. All quotations in the chapter are from the interviews with young people.

In order to provide a context for the discussion on youth participation, we present the characteristics of the town where the research was carried out, as well as a recent account of what happens in these types of communities when they come in contact with the social and political processes characteristic of globalisation.

Setting: the town of Tepoztlán

Tepoztlán is a town located in the state of Morelos, less than 50 miles from Mexico City. It has a population of 17,000, who until the beginning of the twentieth century spoke mostly Nahuatl.

Because of its geographical position and its natural diversity, from pre-Hispanic times Tepoztlán has been involved in a wide variety of exchanges between various political and cultural groups and has been on the route between the basin of Mexico and the peoples of the Pacific coast. As a result, the town's inhabitants have developed a great ability to assimilate external influences while preserving their own cultural identity, a process that Bartolomé (2006) has called 'strategic adaptability'.

Despite the influence of modernisation processes and a series of economic, political and social changes that have had a strong impact on this community, its population retains a cultural logic of its own, related to the preservation of a collective organisation, a view of the world closely related to nature and a community life that guides and strengthens its social relationships.

Because certain customs and traditions have regulated the ways in which this town engages in local political life, its inhabitants have taken on a complex identity. Although they are Mexican citizens, they also see themselves in relation to other referents specifically related to their home town. They are fully fledged citizens, with full rights and responsibilities before the state and the nation, but above all they belong to their home town and are representatives of its culture and therefore respond zealously to their roles and duties toward their community.

Bearing in mind that the notion of citizenship is built historically, the current situation calls for its redefinition. For although the notions of civil, political and social citizenship seem to point towards an integration process, the facts point in the opposite direction. Local identities and movements for the defence of native cultures have re-emerged, demonstrating the presence of ethnic minorities or culturally diverse communities that, according to Bartolomé (2006), demand to be recognised as collective entities. That is, they demand a form of citizenship that will allow them to belong both to the national community and at the same time to their smaller native community.

Guillermo de la Peña (1999) has named as 'ethnic citizenship' the possibility of retaining a diverse cultural identity and social organisation within a state. This is similar to the notion of cultural citizenship posed by Renato Rosaldo (1994) in an attempt to obtain recognition for the right of Latin American communities in the United States to be different. Likewise, Kymlicka (1995) has discussed the rights of diverse social groups within democratic states, based on the notion of multicultural citizenship that should be adopted by multi-ethnic states. This is important to countries such as Mexico, where various living cultures coexist, striving to achieve a form of citizenship that will not exclude their heritage. This is particularly pertinent for the citizenship status of the youth of traditional indigenous towns, for whom factors such as the community, sense of belonging and the ways in which identity is built up integrate both personal and collective influences.

Culture, here, is a key word that refers us once again to the presence of an ongoing living history. In relation to the case we analyse here, we have been able to prove that the cultural logic of the Meso-American traditional peoples continues to guide the social life of the community. Tepoztecan children and young people are proud of their traditions, as a result of the fact that the community has opened up spaces for the new generations to participate in culturally meaningful activities (Corona and Pérez 2007).

Youth participation and testimonies of the younger generation

The youth develop an interest in working for their community because of family tradition, because from an early age they have witnessed community work by others, or because they have been invited by civil organisations to participate in a project or to take a course or workshop.

Another significant factor that leads young people to engage in work for their community is the fact that they get to meet other young people who share their interest in this work, in relation to whom they develop a feeling of identity and belonging. This includes young people who engage in community work as environmentalists (see Plate 13.1), entertainment and cultural promoters, health promoters, and firefighters, or as members of a civil organisation with a particular social role.

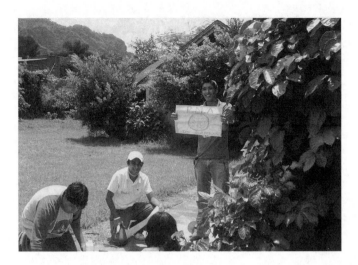

Plate 13.1 Making flyers providing environmental information. Copyright: Julián Hernández

In recent years in Tepoztlán civil associations have been formed for the purpose of contributing certain solutions to the town's environmental, cultural and health problems (see Plate 13.1). These are generally directed by people who have come from elsewhere, but who have involved the locals, including young people.

We can observe that in this type of associations, as well as in community organisations, young people perceive themselves as a sector with an identity of its own, which has enabled them to distance themselves from community forms, to observe the obstacles faced by the community and to analyse the complex role that they are to perform today as actors and articulators of these programmes in relation to their town.

Obstacles, lessons and benefits of youth participation in Tepoztlán

Lack of programmes addressed to them

From the youth's perspective, there are not enough programmes or services addressed specifically to them. Few of the existing ones have shown any interest in having the youth participate in planning; nor do they take into account their main interests, such as environmental care, informal education, technical training, and the promotion of culture, among others.

In the face of this lack of programmes, the youth of Tepoztlán have carried out various projects related to environmental care (Plate 13.2), health care (prevention of drug and alcohol consumption, the promotion of safe sex) and the promotion of culture (cinema forums, courses on crafts or plastic arts, arrangement of spaces for sports), and even the management of spaces for discussion, e.g., for political debates among candidates for municipal presidency.

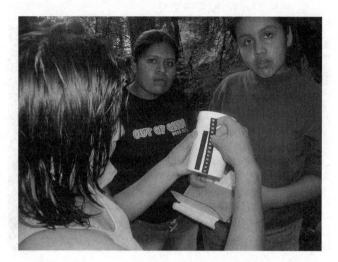

Plate 13.2   Young people monitoring water contamination. Copyright: Julián Hernández

Tensions between youth and adult views

The youth perceive that their way of thinking and of meeting situations differs from that of the previous generation. This disparity of approaches to problems makes them feel that there is no openness towards their proposals, much less any motivation and support from the authorities or from the adults themselves. They also make reference to resistance from the adults, who are used to working within hierarchies where status and authority must be respected, as has been found else-where (see, for example, West 2007). As a 20-year-old youth who participates in environmental and ecological projects explains:

> The young people in my community do want to do things for it, are inter-ested in helping solve the problems; but there are no spaces, there is no one to motivate them. Young people already have a different academic level, we have more open minds, we know about politics, we know who is who, how they work and for whom they work. We are more open and we want to do something for our community, only there is no one to spur us on or to provide us with the necessary resources.

Many local adults and the local authorities see young people stereotypically as apathetic, unreliable and moody, and not sufficiently discerning for decision making. Almost all the young people interviewed pointed to the lack of spaces and programmes geared specifically to them, the lack of financial resources for their projects, and the political conflicts among adults as obstacles to their participation in the community.

> … the assistant gives no support to the youth: he supports only his own people. We are working for the benefit of the environment, and if we ask the

new assistant for help, he will immediately say yes, but he will never say when; so there is an obstacle here, because we will be kept waiting for that day to come, but it just never will.

Difficulties for ensuring the continuity of projects

The main obstacles reported by the youth when engaged in group work within participative projects are: difficulties in negotiating and reaching an agreement when there have been differences among them; inequitable distribution of tasks; failure to keep commitments; distrust among group members; and even romantic problems and separation of couples. They report difficulty in ensuring the continuity of group membership and projects, mostly because they lack time, start high school or college, marry and start a family, get a job, or experience a shift of interests.

> I felt that this issue of having different views hindered us from making progress as a group; besides, there was no equity, because the others did not want to incorporate more young people into the community; plus, there was no balance in the work, because I was doing more [than my share], and sometimes I had to argue with my parents because I had to go water or trim the trees, and that was another reason for my decision to quit: it was beginning to cause me problems with my family ... the group began to disintegrate; one of my workmates quit because of romantic issues with one of the girls in the group and they didn't want to see each other any more.

Civil associations have shown greater interest in training young people in the areas on which they will work in their projects, but not much in helping them to develop the necessary skills for effective organisation and communication, although some succeed in acquiring them with practice.

Learning and identities

In spite of the notorious existence of unequal power relationships between adults and young people, whenever the latter are taken into account, listened to and acknowledged in their ability to contribute to transforming their reality, they develop a feeling of self-confidence, they feel more secure and raise their self-esteem. The 'mutual trust' factor becomes essential to participation. This entails adult facilitators putting trust in young people's abilities and ideas: and the youth trusting that the adults will indeed give them support and take them into account. For the youth, participating in community projects, being listened to, acknowledged and taken into account by the adults is a major experience. Through it they acquire various skills and knowledge, which provide benefits far beyond the aims of the project itself and eventually become a way of life. Gaining awareness of the problems of their community, proposing solutions, managing resources, researching and engaging in team work are actions that develop self-assurance and critical abilities in young people, as well as communication, organisation and negotiation skills.

I am no longer as quiet as I used to be. Before, when there was a meeting, I was unable to speak because I thought I would be silenced immediately. Not any more: now I feel more confident when I speak, I participate more as a citizen within my community. Now, whenever there is a community meeting or whenever there is some community issue, I am there, I participate more, I feel more self-confident, more certain of what I feel, of what I am going to do, and of what I will do for the community.

Alliances with other social actors

Once the youth have organised themselves around an idea or a project, they begin to look for ways to carry it out. For this purpose, in addition to turning to the initial bonds that they have established with adults belonging to civil associations, they seek support from other organisations within their community, from their teachers or from the town hall.

In many cases, resource management, planning and organisation may take a long time before the project can actually be carried out. However, when the youth of Tepoztlán are given the opportunity to create legitimate scenarios for participating in their community according to their own interests, they display a consistent commitment and the intent to work continually on the project. This can be observed in the testimony of a 20-year-old woman who participates in sustainable development projects:

> We were struggling to obtain support for a project that would benefit the people of Tepoztlán. It was the first time that I was engaged in seeking

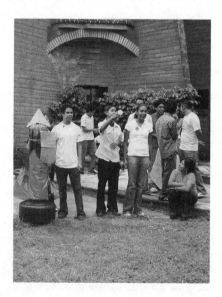

Plate 13.3 Young people meeting about local environmental problems. Copyright: Julián Hernández

resources and support. Four of us, together with an engineer, went to the assistant's office to bring the necessary papers. I thought they were going to say no, because they were totally unfamiliar with dry toilets, but eventually they gave us support, and it was a good feeling because we got help for something that would benefit the community.

As can be observed, the ability to wait for and manage resources contradicts the idea that the youth are impatient, and provides evidence for their ability to persevere with medium- and long-term projects.

Exchange of experiences among the youth

Spreading their projects and exchanging experiences with other young people and adults who are equally interested in participating in their communities turned out to be not only stimulating but also essential to the assessment of their own experience. By realising that there are youth groups that have similar aims and discourses, young people acquire a more global view of their work that provides it with meaning and a social significance.

It was very important for me to meet other young people because I met many different personalities, people who were really interested in solid waste management and environmental issues, and then I realised that I was not alone, that there were many people who shared my interests. I realised that this was really helpful, that it was my thing, that fighting for the environment was great and brought me fulfilment.

The young are no longer limited by the characteristics of the community; because they relate to others they gain a wider, more global perspective of the problems and of problem-solving strategies. They build their identity from their various referents: their own community, their age group, the environmentalist or political groups, and others.

Some particular aspects of youth participation in groups arising from within the community

The testimonies above provide an account of the common issues reported by the young when describing their participation experiences in general. However, after discussing the interviews, we realised that certain distinctive elements mentioned by those young people who participate in collective projects arise from within the community itself and respond to dynamics characteristic of the Meso-American peoples with a Nahua tradition. One of these elements is the transcendent value ascribed to collective work. Beyond the fact of joining forces to attain a goal, collective work in traditional indigenous communities promotes the renewal of bonds among its members, the establishment of alliances and a true intergenerational coexistence.

In this regard, Catherine Good (2000) states that in Nahua indigenous communities the notion of work is complex and is closely related to 'a social system based on

reciprocity and exchange and … a clear sense of their own collective historical continuity … . *Tequitl* or work is a fundamental organisational notion in life; the Nahuas
apply it to all uses of human energy – spiritual, intellectual, emotional, and physical
– for the attainment of a specific purpose.' This can be observed in the testimony of a
young man who belongs to an environmentalist group devoted to fighting forest fires:

> What keeps us all – children, young people, adults and elderly people – working
> for the community is the wish to help selflessly, to engage in team work; actu-
> ally, the group's slogan is: 'my spirit will endure in *cuatequitl*', meaning that my
> spirit will endure through unity, through working together with others, and I
> feel that this is what keeps us together.

On the other hand, in deep connection to this view of work, these organisations are characterised by promoting a form of collective learning that includes an
exchange of knowledge and experiences between generations. This learning takes
place in action itself, through fighting a fire, climbing a mountain, cleaning out
a ravine, or planting trees – young people and adults exchange knowledge that
nurtures their action. In this sense, it is the group that holds the knowledge, and as
they fulfil the task they realise what each has to contribute; for example, children
contribute their agility; the youth, their strength; and the old, their experience.

Equally, this intergenerational coexistence brings about a constant renewal of
the group and ensures its continuity. It is not unusual to find that the young people
who participate in these organisations have done so from a very early age, simply
for the sake of 'being present' in the various activities of the group or because
participation in this type of organisation is a family tradition.

> The group includes very young children who attend grammar school, but
> who engage in reforestation tasks or pick up garbage; and as they grow up
> and learn from those of us who are more experienced, they are allowed to
> help fight fires. Many mothers carry their small children in their arms to our
> meetings, and later on, when these children are older, request that we admit
> them into our group.

As can be observed, young people engage in these kinds of collective actions
originating within the community not as a socially diverse group, but as part of the
community – unlike what happens in activities proposed by civil associations that
include young people among their members.

Final considerations

The testimonies shared by the youth show that there are still various obstacles
they must face in order to be able to follow through on the participative projects in
which they engage and obtain clearer support from adults. At the same time, they
acknowledge the major lessons provided by these experiences and value highly
those instances in which the previous generation opens up spaces for them to have
a bearing on their community.

There is a clear distinction between the more communal manner in which the community incorporates the young and that of the civil associations that see young people as a socially distinct group as they assert their identity in contrast to that of the adults.

These two ways of participating provide evidence for the emergence of new cultural forms that incorporate different realities and thus enrich the community. They articulate traditional elements with innovative resources and technologies provided through their contact with modernity.

Their role attests to Guillermo Bonfil Batalla's (1994) assumption that, among the indigenous peoples, there is a will to endure 'expressed as a tenacious resistance aimed at preserving their decision-making ability and their cultural heritage; in an ongoing, selective appropriation of those foreign cultural elements that they find adequate in order to survive domination, and exercising a ceaseless creativity that enables them to create new cultural elements or to modify the already existing ones as a way to adjust their culture'.

In this sense, the youth, as new social actors, articulate global propositions from elsewhere and adapt them to their own realities by incorporating traditional knowledge. It is the youth who can embody the concerns of their own communities and project them into wider settings. Thus, these actors with multiple identities emerge as interlocutors and promoters of new options for projects for the incorporation of the indigenous traditional communities into the globalised world – as citizens of the world who remain distinctly loyal to their own cultural heritage.

References

Bartolomé, M. A. (2006) *Procesos interculturales. Antropología política del pluralismo cultural en América Latina*, Mexico City: Siglo XXI Editores.

Bonfil Batalla, G. (1994) *México profundo, una civilización negada*, Mexico City: Ed. Grijalbo.

Corona, Y. and Pérez, C. (2007) 'The sense of belonging: The importance of child participation in the ritual life for the recreation of the culture of the indigenous peoples', in T. Wyller and U. Nayar (eds) *The Given Child: Religion's contributions to children's citizenship*, Germany: Vandenhoeck & Ruprecht.

De la Peña, G. (1999) 'Territorio y ciudadanía étnica en la nación globalizada', *Desacatos* 1, CIESAS, Mexico City.

Good, C. (2000) 'Indigenous peoples in Central and Western Mexico', in John Monaghan (ed.), *Handbook of Middle American Indians, Ethnology Supplement*, Austin: University of Texas Press.

Kymlicka, W. (1995) *Multicultural Citizenship. A liberal theory of minority rights*, Oxford: Oxford University Press.

Rosaldo, R. (1994) 'Cultural citizenship and educational democracy', *Cultural Anthropology* 9 (3), 402–11.

West, A. (2007) 'Power relationships and adult resistance to children's participation', *Children, Youth and Environments* 17 (1): 123–35, available at www.colorado.edu/journals/cye.

Commentary 3

Participation in the traps of cultural diversity

Manfred Liebel and Iven Saadi

The chapter by Mason and Bolzan on cross-cultural studies in participation high-lights that it is problematic to take the English term 'participation' as a starting point and then look for semantic equivalents in other languages, as specific conno-tations of the concept are presupposed. Instead, we would favour looking at the practices of young people of different ages without prejudice, and then trying to understand them in their respective social and cultural settings with their respective meanings. All investigations have to reflect self-critically the cultural specificities of every conception of participation, including that formulated in the UNCRC.

In our view, when speaking about participation it is also essential to consider in whose interest and with what intention it is conceptualised and put into practice. Differences between the interests and perspectives of children and adults are to be assumed, notwithstanding the culturally specific patterns of generational relations. As a result, it is necessary to question whether the interests and perspectives of children have actually been put into practice. We assume that a renewal of adults' perspectives on children is necessary in all societies and cultures. We agree with Twum-Danso that this should not imply disrupting cultural order through the participation of children at any cost, but still, children's and adults' interests must be assessed as equally valuable and important. Children are in fact as much a part of society as adults are, and they should have the possibility of contributing to the definition and design of social constructions according to their interests.

With regard to the question focused on in all of the chapters, whether participa-tion is viewed rather as a 'right' or as an 'obligation', we argue that this depends on the existence and explicit differentiation of corresponding ordering principles (rules) in the respective societies or cultures. Applied to children and youth, this also depends on how the pertinent age phases and age groups are constituted within which positions, duties, responsibilities, freedoms etc. are considered appropriate, and how the relation between generations is regulated. For instance, children may have a large number of responsibilities and take part in social activities in a wide sense without explicitly being referred to as right-holders. On the other hand, chil-dren can be entitled to a vast array of rights without their factual contribution to social processes reaching greater dimensions. Rights-based regulations can entail more protection, acceptance and freedom for, or contributions by, children, but in other cases they can result in specific limitations of children's freedom of action and participation, and even in their total exclusion. This effect can be shown when considering legal minimum age provisions regulating the active exercise of specific rights, duties and responsibilities (e.g. ILO Convention 138 on child labour).

What strikes us most in the three chapters under review is the lack of a common understanding of exactly what participation means, making a comparative appraisal of the quality and amount of participation practised by children and youth in their respective social contexts almost impossible. With UNCRC articles 12 to 15 as an entry point, Twum-Danso's use of participation is in line with the Western tradition of conceptualising it as consisting of an individual right to take a role in decision making. Corona et al. base their understanding of participation on the local and indigenous setting being studied, and consider it as 'work for the community'. The chapter by Mason and Bolzan identifies different constructions of participation, conceived according to country-specific uses: thus, in Australia it means 'to take part in activities designed and structured by adults with the educational aim to become a good adult and citizen', whereas in Asian countries the emphasis is on a 'taking part' in social practices embedded in children's obligations and responsibilities towards the family and community.

In many (non-Western) cultures the child is represented as an integral member of the community, maybe with particular characteristics, but not strictly separated from the 'adult' members of his or her community. Depending on real and perceived capabilities (which are not necessarily measured against a chronological age), children are expected to take over specific tasks that are important to the community. These tasks can be of a social, economic or political nature, for example contributing to agricultural work, doing household chores or exercising political responsibility in communal life. At the same time rules giving children control over specific goods (such as arable land, livestock) may exist (for example in West Africa, and in the Andes in South America), for instance in the form of an inheritance when the parents are still alive, or as a contribution by the community. Such expectations and rules can be considered forms of participation (without explicitly being referred to in that way and without being individually obtainable rights). Concerning the children's standing in and their influence on society, such patterns regulating the relations of the child and the community can open spaces for participation by children which takes place outside the narrowed conceptual horizon of a Western notion of participation. Accordingly, children need not wait until they become adults to be considered as responsible and acting members of society. Corona et al. give a good example of such an instance of children's and youth's participation.

However, another notion of childhood prevalent in some non-Western societies, which places children in a relation of total obedience and servitude towards elders (especially their providers) and subjects them to the full extent of adults' decisions, is apparent across these chapters. In these cases, children don't have the right to contradict elders or to demand accountability or reasons for adults' conduct or decisions. Such a pattern of generational order can be called paternalistic or authoritarian. Not only is it deeply incompatible with any type of participation by children based on their will and interest, but it also infringes on children's dignity and potentially poses a threat to their health and life. When reading Twum-Danso's contribution one might be tempted to view the Ghanaian situation as fitting into this bracket, but application of a wider understanding of participation might well have exposed other social practices, giving a more complex view of the position of children in Ghana.

A long-term compromise with paternalism or authoritarianism as described above is not conceivable, and at most could be tactical and/or transient. However, approaching such strict generational hierarchies with an attitude of Western superiority or largesse should be avoided. We have to bear in mind that paternalism and authoritarianism are not restricted to non-Western societies, but are widespread in Western or 'modern' societies as well. On the other hand, the respect for elders expected from children in many non-Western cultures and their obligation to take over responsibility towards 'family and society, the State and other legally recognised communities' (African Charter on the Rights and Welfare of the Child, art. 31) are not necessarily tantamount to paternalism and authoritarianism, but can be interpreted as stressing solidarity and interdependency between generations and can well be reciprocated with respect towards children.

In seeking to understand the quality and scope of children's participation and the extent to which adequate strategies have been devised, it is not enough to state – as is the case with Mason and Bolzan – that all cultures are dynamic and therefore susceptible to social change. The researcher and the practitioner also have to consider the ways in which the social position of children and their treatment by others are determined or conditioned by general economic patterns and forms of life. Widening and enhancing the participation of children presumably cannot be achieved without structural changes relating to and affecting society as a whole. What is at stake is more than 'modernising' 'traditional' societies. More importantly, the question is about how best to define social equality and social justice, and how to bring them into being at societal and global levels.

If participation could be conceived of as consisting not only of speaking and being heard, but also of active and routine inclusion into vital social processes, new prospects could be opened up for the situating of children in society. For example, within the notion of 'protagonism' articulated in the working children's movements and their demand for a 'right to work', the claim to act autonomously is inseparable from willingness to assume responsibility for the community and wider society. Children's participation here is not presented as a specific type of communication with children that is to be punctually arranged for specific purposes, but as a seminal daily articulation of meaningful agency. And because this agency is always embedded into social relations, one challenge is not to consider children as fulfilling orders and expectations imposed on them by adults, but to understand and respect them as independently acting participants with their own rights. And irrespective of how participation is understood, it has to be voluntary, characterised by mutual respect and with the aspiration of engaging meaningfully.

The authors

Professor Dr Manfred Liebel is a sociologist, Director of the Institute for Global Education and International Studies (IGLIS) at the International Academy (INA), director of the European Master's in Childhood Studies and Children's Rights

(EMCR) course at the Free University Berlin, and Vice-president of ProNATs association in support of working children's movements in Africa, Asia and Latin America; he worked for several years as a street worker and consultant for projects with marginalised children and youth in Latin America.

Iven Saadi is a political scientist and a PhD candidate at the University of Münster, and is currently a lecturer of the EMCR, collaborator at IGLIS and member of ProNATs.

This commentary is the fruit of discussions with EMCR students (Alice Knorr, Cornelia Lahmann, Hella Schleef, Ilka Stein) and ProNATs collaborators (Annette Jensen, Franziska Zelina). The authors also took into account comments from students of the Bachelor's in Applied Childhood Studies at the University of Applied Sciences Magdeburg-Stendal (Katharina Barleben, Franziska Blisse, Daniela Pfanne, Lena Siegel, Stefanie Schmidt, Anne Tobiasch).

14 Rights through evaluation and understanding children's realities

Vicky Johnson

Introduction

This chapter looks at how the process of evaluation can be used to promote children's rights by using a participatory approach. The aim is to offer practical learning about preconditions for success, factors that influence the application of rights-based approaches in action research, and issues of accountability and action in evaluation. The examples show the necessity of working pragmatically, using a realistic approach that recognises the complexities faced by evaluators in dealing with different contexts and that allows for flexibility and mixed methods. Ensuring the participation of different stakeholders throughout the evaluation process, including service providers and decision makers, can lead to positive outcomes for children. In particular, it is important to use and value evidence from children and young people: rights-based evaluation can be rigorous and also build on the imagination of children.

Frameworks for evaluation in the 'real world'

The work presented here is located in a framework of rights-based research (Boyden and Ennew 1997; Beazley and Ennew 2006) founded on Article 12 of the UNCRC. The approach incorporates the following elements: developing and adhering to an ethical framework, developing a protocol for research, involving different stakeholders, and using mixed methods including both qualitative and quantitative approaches (Beazley and Ennew 2007). This rights-based approach has informed my work with international NGOs such as ActionAid, Plan International and Save the Children, and has also proved relevant when transferring participatory appraisal methods to a UK context.

An emphasis on participatory monitoring and evaluation in international development since the late 1990s has followed the criticism of conventional monitoring and evaluation for its top-down approach, emphasis on 'objectivity' and quantifiable data, and use of external consultants. In participatory monitoring and evaluation, the emphasis is shifted from controlled data collection to the recognition of stakeholder-based processes of gathering, analysing and using information. The approach seeks to include stakeholders in the different stages of the evaluation process, including determination of what data need to be collected and design of the review process, rather than merely acting as enumerators for external consultants. It also holds that processes should adapt to local circumstances and that learning should promote self-reliance in decision making so that local people's capacity to take action, negotiate and promote change is strengthened (Estrella et al. 2000).

However, the assumption that external evaluation is more objective still influences the perspectives of many service providers and policy makers. Hart and colleagues (2003) discuss the pressure to find indicators that can be applied systematically and consistently across programmes and countries while allowing flexibility to incorporate locally derived indicators, and question whether equal weight is given to these different forms of evidence. They do, however, note the fresh perspective that an external evaluator can provide.

Both external and internal elements were incorporated into the evaluation of the 'Saying Power' scheme for Save the Children UK (Johnson and Nurick 2001). Table 14.1, adapted from Jobes (1997), shows how this participatory monitoring and evaluation differed from more conventional approaches.

In order to gain a child-centred perspective on impact, a wider lens has to be used, rather than just reviewing a set of interventions. Although development targets and individual project objectives may be time-bound and narrow in focus, the ultimate aim of a rights-based approach to programming is to bring about improvement in people's lives, and therefore measuring changes in people's lives

Table 14.1 Approach to participatory monitoring and evaluation in evaluation of the Saying Power scheme, as compared to more conventional approaches

	Conventional monitoring and evaluation	*Participatory monitoring and evaluation*
Who does it?	External experts.	Young people and others involved in the scheme, some facilitation by project workers/ evaluation facilitators.
Why is it done?	To satisfy requirements of funders as one way of ensuring accountability.	To promote young people's control over their own projects and enable them to critically appraise their progress and refine objectives/direction as a result.
What is monitored?	Predetermined and externally driven indicators of success.	Young people identify their own indicators and ways of monitoring them
When is it done?	Usually at the end of a programme or scheme.	Frequently, throughout the lifetime of the project.
How is it done?	Focus on scientific objectives, distancing evaluators from young people, uniform and complex procedures, delayed and limited access to results.	Self-evaluation by young people, participatory and visual methods, open and immediate sharing of results.

is a key aspect of rights-based monitoring and evaluation (Theis 2003). Children's participation in evaluation needs to start at the beginning of the project process and be reviewed at successive stages so as to refresh the strategic direction. There is increasing recognition of Article 12 of the UN Convention on the Rights of the Child (UNCRC), which emphasises participation and a child's right to be heard in all aspects of decisions relating to their lives (Van Beers et al. 2006). There are a growing number of examples in which children participate in an initial needs assessment to identify areas of intervention and to plan services; if this is not done, crucial priorities for children and young people may be missed. However, the changing priorities in children's lives and their changing circumstances over time need to be evaluated. Both children and adults can be treated as respected part-ners, provided that there is transparency in the objectives and process. This can be the case throughout the project cycle, as shown in Figure 14.1, produced by a community artist, Moelyono, during training for Plan International Indonesia.

Rights through Evaluation

'Rights through Evaluation' was the title of a project carried out by Development Focus with partners in Nepal and South Africa[1] (Johnson et al. 2001a; Johnson et al. 2001b; Ewing et al. 2001; Nurick et al. 2001). The project brought to light issues in participatory evaluation that have informed the methodology applied in more recent work, both internationally and in the UK.

The Himalayan Community Development Forum (HICODEF)[2], as local part-ners, embarked on the 'Rights through Evaluation' research to develop more child-sensitive monitoring and evaluation of its community development programmes in order to inform its ongoing work with communities in rural Nawalparasi in a way that would directly improve the lives of girls and boys, taking into account

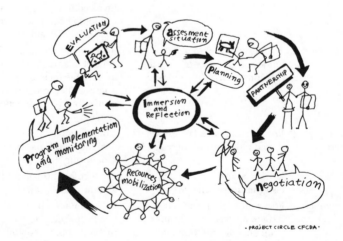

Figure 14.1 'Children can participate throughout the project cycle', drawing by Moelyono when working with Plan International Indonesia

their existing roles in families and communities. At the time it was recognised that much work in the field on child rights was not integrally linked into the broader community development rights-based programming, and there was a lot to share between partner organisations in terms of developing skills in participatory monitoring and evaluation (see Plate 14.1).

For example, children's clubs had been started in local communities in Nawalparasi with HICODEF, but in order for children to realise the potential of the children's clubs a fuller evaluation of the programme was needed. Local children, especially girls, who often spent many hours doing household chores, actually said that they best liked the water and forestry programmes, as these interventions, by reducing their workload in collecting water and wood for the household, gave them more time to go to school and clubs, and to play. Indeed, the children were very animated in showing the kinds of games they could now play. Further evaluation increased their confidence to help other children who could not attend the club or school and to act as a pressure group in the community for issues that were important to them, including keeping pigs in sties, addressing violence when adults get drunk and solving disputes between children and within the community. Before this evaluative work, HICODEF staff had not thought of getting the children to participate in how these broader programmes were implemented, and children had only really been involved in the water programmes as labourers, rather than in planning where taps could be located to save them most time.

The project also showed that methods need to be understandable, fun and engaging. They should therefore be developed and piloted with children, and used flexibly to suit different groups. With HICODEF in Nepal, researchers spent long

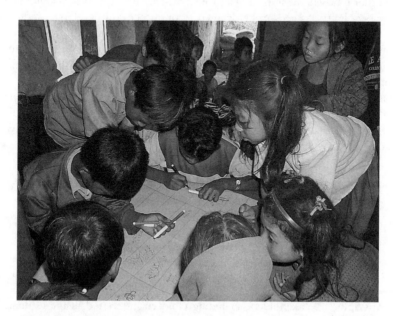

Plate 14.1 Children evaluating HICODEF's community development programme in Nawalparasi in Nepal. Copyright: Development Focus

periods of time working with children to develop visual ways of understanding the impact of projects on the lives of children (Johnson et al. 2001b). Local materials were used and literate children took notes so as to help those who were illiterate to explain their diagrams and drawings. Tools were developed in partnership between children and adult researchers, and modified to suit different situations and settings. Researchers also worked with a smaller group of children to develop tools and indicators for understanding how children's situations were changing in school, family and community; these were then ranked and used with a broader group of children.

In both South Africa and Nepal, staff in government and non-governmental sectors expressed a need for capacity building in participatory processes, including monitoring and evaluation, so that they could implement a more rights-based approach on the ground. Many felt that there was much rhetoric regarding child rights, but that they lacked evidence to show the effect that they might have and the impact on people's lives. Interviews with children and adults in marginalised communities in KwaZulu Natal showed how changes in tourism and resettlement had profound effects on children's lives, and that their indicators for change were very different from those of adults. For example, children, especially girls, expressed the view that safety was a serious concern, with their old networks and community bonds weakened. Previously children had only really been considered with regard to their schooling. For some children this was the first time they had been invited to participate in meetings: a 16-year-old girl said 'We are always overlooked with the excuse that we are too young to understand meetings' (Ewing et al. 2001).

In order to assess the impact of a project or service on the lives of children and young people, time needs to be devoted to the process of developing indicators with them, so that unexpected as well as expected outcomes can be captured. Some indicators may be identified through discussions with funders and commissioners that need to be measured across services and projects; but these should be distinct from those that are developed by service users, including children. Not all indicators will be measured in traditional quantitative ways; one can also use visual ranking methods, qualitative description of change and capturing the direction of change, i.e. whether the service user perceives the change to be positive or negative in the context of their life and why.

Preconditions for successful rights-based evaluation

In trying to establish whether an evaluation can fit into a rights-based framework and whether it can lead to positive outcomes for the boys and girls involved, it may be useful to consider the following questions:

- How has the evaluation agenda been developed, and how were children and young people involved?
- Are different stakeholders, including children, interested in the evaluation, and are they interested in participating or helping to shape the research?
- Is the timeframe adequate?

- Are there resources and mechanisms for follow-up?
- Is there time and scope to develop and agree an ethical framework that will work in the local context, and how will it be adhered to?
- How will a research protocol be developed and agreed, and what will be the input from children?
- Is there space and flexibility in the process to allow for participation of different stakeholders, including children – is there the right to opt out, and how will this work in practice?
- Will the participatory process that is envisaged work in the local context, and do the project staff have sufficient understanding of the context and people?

People may mean different things when they talk of participation, and models have been helpful in unpicking some of this diversity of understanding, such as the ladder of participation (Hart 1992) and circles of participation (Treseder 1997). West (1998) discusses a continuum of approaches, from children being in focus groups, to children carrying out research, to peer research developed by children and adults, to child-led research. The starting point within different organisations, communities and groups of children needs to be taken into account and will affect the levels or degrees of participation that can be achieved in any process (Johnson et al. 1998). Negotiation with the commissioners and other key stakeholders about how evidence gathered in participatory monitoring and evaluation will be placed alongside other forms of evidence, and how decisions will be taken and fed back to communities, should also inform the process. In any project, whether initiated by adults or by children or by both, the commitment of time and interest from children can be critical to how the process can be carried out. Sometimes, children and young people may opt out of the task of developing methods and carrying out research, in favour of being involved in the research as participants, and this also needs to be taken into account in 'judging' how participatory a process is. Sometimes research controlled by children, just as research controlled by adults, may not be inclusive of some of the more excluded or younger children – they may still remain the researched as opposed to the researchers.

Factors that influence the application of rights-based evaluations

Even if the basic preconditions are there for a participatory and rights-based process, there are other contextual factors that will influence the way in which a planned methodology may be applied. This may include the following:

- local power differentials and gender dynamics, including those within households;
- the context of the political economy and how policies are applied nationally and locally;
- children's changing cultures and the changing attitudes of adults towards girls and boys;
- positionality of facilitators;

- skills of facilitators (adult or child) with range of children of different ages;
- interest of key stakeholders, including children, in getting involved or in carrying out the research.

In the local context it is important to understand who can be involved, where, when and how. Children are not a homogeneous group, and there is a need for clarity about which children can be involved and in what roles. Age of children and young people makes a difference, as do gender, ethnicity, religion and such factors as whether children are in or out of school. In each situation there needs to be an analysis of what issues of difference may be important to take into account. An inclusive process will also mean, rather than calling meetings and expecting people to turn up, that facilitators will go out to where people are at times that suit them. This may mean, for example in the case of rural Nawalparasi, going with children while they carry out daily chores, or in an urban UK context waiting outside bowling alleys or fast-food outlets to engage with teenagers.

The local power differentials and dynamics have to be understood – for example, between adults and children, within groups of children, between community members and organisations funding innovations. The organisational or insti-tutional setting of the service providers also makes a difference, as well as how national policies are interpreted and implemented locally. Predominant cultural attitudes towards different groups of children or towards children in general also set the scene, as well as what spaces there are for communication and more inclu-sive decision-making forums in the local setting.

The skills and positionality of the facilitators are important to consider in different local processes, including considering the age, gender, whether the facilitator is an insider or outsider, the language barriers that may exist and the general baggage that we all carry! In 'infusing assessment processes with political consciousness', Guijt (2007a: 54) highlights the requirement for new skills and capacities. This finding resonates with the experience of 'Rights through Evaluation' (Johnson et al. 2001a), where many staff in Nepal and South Africa said that capacity not only in evaluation, assessment and learning, but also in children's participation and rights is key if positive outcomes for children are to be achieved.

Visual methods, theatre techniques and play can be part of a range of strategies that are useful in helping to explore differences in perspective and in exploring power differentials and dynamics, while keeping the process interactive in a fun way. Listening skills are central to assessment and learning, and counselling skills can sometimes be needed in a team situation or by means of referral. Conflict-resolution and negotiation skills are also important in processes that often raise political and sensitive issues. Again, recognising who is setting the agenda is impor-tant, and being transparent about this from the outset, as it may well explain the interest of different parties in the process.

Issues of social change, action and accountability

Key to translating rhetoric into action is communication and dialogue with different stakeholders, including service providers and policy makers, so that strategic decisions affecting service delivery and resource allocation can be informed by the innovative and integral perspectives of children. Some key issues here are:

- involvement of different stakeholders, leading to ownership and a local constituency of support;
- local 'champions' to carry action forward;
- attention to the allocation of resources and strategic prioritisation in response to evidence from evaluations, while still recognising that there may be benefits of the process to individuals;
- continued strengthening of capacity after the evaluation, in order to ensure ongoing rights-based approaches in implementation of action, positive social change and outcomes for children;
- children's indicators can be used in ongoing monitoring of the impact of interventions on children's lives;
- a strong evidence base incorporating children's perspectives allows for pressure for greater accountability downwards.

As with the 'Rights through Evaluation' research, in much of the community-based research and evaluation in the UK it has been useful to set up reference groups where different stakeholders, including service providers and policy makers, are involved from the outset and so have some ownership and understanding of the project, rather than just receiving reports at the end. This can also help to address power dynamics and translate participants' visions into action. 'Dialogue days'[3] with children and service providers can be a useful and constructive way of exploring issues raised in evaluation, although there are risks to children in presenting sensitive issues that affect them to adults in positions of power, and representation or discussion with the children beforehand is vital in order to address this in an ethical and sensitive way.

The roles of different donors, intermediaries and facilitators are important to recognise in terms of their influence on assessment and learning, especially if social change is to be strengthened. Guijt (2007a and 2007b) qualifies social change as 'transformational processes related to distribution of power' and discusses the change in accountability moving from being purely upwards, towards accountabilities that are 'more interactive' and 'downwards accountability'. There has been a growing demand for new approaches and tools, but among social-change groups working on rights-based initiatives there is a move to looking at experiences of social change over time and to recognising that approaches have to be flexible to the context and that there should be transparency in the process of assessment. As Guijt goes on to state: 'In practice, creating an appropriate assessment and learning process requires mixing and matching and adapting from a combination of frameworks, concepts and methods – to ensure that they address information and reflection needs, and match existing capacities' (Guijt 2007a: 5).

Conclusions

Evidence gained through evaluations can inform understanding of how to improve the lives of girls and boys, young men and women, and help to avoid inadvertent negative impact. Evaluation can be seen as an ongoing process of assessment and action rather than a one-off event. Although many people reading this book will already be converted, there are still people 'out there' who need convincing of the value of children's participation in policy and programming; a strong evidence base that includes children's perspectives can contribute to this.

Flexibility is essential: organisations commissioning evaluation must leave space for methods to change, and facilitators must have the capacity to modify their approaches in different settings. Children and adults can be partners in a process if there is transparency in agenda and objectives, and honesty about dilemmas in implementing children's participation in a real world of barriers and constraints.

There are still questions around the value placed on evidence gathered through participatory techniques with children; there is continuing need for debate with policy makers and service providers about the rigour of participatory evaluation showing how new and different insights can contribute to decision-making processes. The challenge is to make it rigorous while still building on the imaginative capacity of children and making processes interactive, responsive and fun.

In order to gain commitment, details of participatory evaluation need to be explained, and involvement and ownership of a range of stakeholders, including service providers and policy makers, need to be built throughout the process: thus also addressing capacity to respond to evidence. More conventional techniques may also need to be employed alongside more qualitative participatory approaches so as to triangulate information and build trust with a range of stakeholders. At the core of the evaluative research described in this chapter lies the belief that children's participation is invaluable in understanding how projects and services can more effectively be delivered and that without their perspectives pieces of the jigsaw are missing. The process of evaluation is a way of providing valuable evidence that can back up this belief and allow more accountability to children. This applies not only to interventions specifically directed at children and young people, but also to broader regeneration and development interventions.

Notes

1. The research was funded by the Department for International Development's (DfID) Innovations Fund. Partners in Nepal were the Himalayan Community Development Forum (HICODEF), supported by ActionAid. Partners in South Africa were the Early Learning Resource Unit (ELRU), Working for Water of the South African government and iMEDIATE Development Communications.
2. HICODEF were recent partners of ActionAid, staff having been working in one of the Development Areas and interest in the research sprung from previous work with ActionAid leading to 'Listening to Smaller Voices' (Johnson et al. 1995a, 1995b).
3. 'Dialogue days' is a term that was used by Vicky Johnson and Barry Percy-Smith in work that they carried out for the YWCA in the UK.

References

Beazley, H. and Ennew, J. (2006) 'Participatory methods and approaches: Tackling the two tyrannies', in V. Desai and R. B. Potter *Doing Development Research*, London: Sage Publications Ltd.

Boyden, J. and Ennew, J. (eds) (1997) *Children in Focus: A manual for participatory research with children*, Stockholm: Save the Children.

Estrella, M., Blauert, J., Campilan, D., Gaventa, J., Gonsalves, J., Guijt, I., Johnson, D. and Ricafort, R. (eds) (2000) *Learning from Change: Issues and experiences in participatory monitoring and evaluation*, London: Intermediate Technology Publications.

Ewing, D., Apelgren, E. and Mathe, M. (2001) *A Land Reform Case Study in Cremin, Kwazulu Natal, South Africa*, Brighton, Durban: Development Focus, iMEDIATE Development Communications.

Guijt, I. (2007a) *Assessing and Learning from Social Change: A discussion paper*, Sussex and the Netherlands: Institute of Development Studies and Learning by Design.

Guijt, I. (2007b) *Critical Readings in Assessing and Learning for Social Change: A review*, Institute of Development Studies, Brighton, UK.

Hart, J., Newman, J. and Ackermann, L. with Feeny, T. (2003) *Children's Participation in Development: Understanding the process, evaluating the impact*, Woking, UK: Plan UK, Plan International.

Hart, R. (1992) *Children's participation: From tokenism to citizenship*, Innocenti Essay No. 4, Florence and New York: UNICEF.

Jobes, K. (1997) *Participatory M&E Guidelines: Experiences in the field*, London: Department for International Development (DfID).

Johnson, V. and Nurick, R. (2001) *Young Voices Heard: Reflection and review of the Saying Power Awards*, Birmingham, UK: Save the Children.

Johnson, V., Hill, J., and Ivan-Smith, E. (1995a) *Listening to Smaller Voices: Children in an environment of change*, London: ActionAid.

Johnson, V., Hill, J., Rana, S., Bharadwaj, M., Sapkota, P., Lamichanne, R., Basnet, B., Ghimimire, S., Sapkota, D., Lamichanne, R. and Ghimire, S. (1995b), *Listening to Smaller Voices: Children in an environment of change (Nepal case study)*, Kathmandu: ActionAid Nepal.

Johnson, V., Ivan-Smith, E., Gordon, G., Pridmore, P., Scott, P. (1998) *Stepping Forward: Children and young people's participation in the development process*, London: IT Publications.

Johnson, V., Ivan-Smith, E. and Nurick, R. (2001a) *Rights through Evaluation: Putting child rights into practice in South Africa and Nepal*, Brighton: Development Focus Trust.

Johnson, V., Sapkota, P., Sthapit, S., Ghimire, K. P., Mahato, M. (2001b) *Rights Through Evaluation: Nepal case study*, Brighton and London: Development Focus Trust and Department for International Development (DfID).

Nurick, R. with August, G., Biersteker, L. and Noemdoe, S. (2001) *Rights through Evaluation: South Africa case study workshop proceedings*, Brighton: Development Focus Trust.

Theis, J. (2003) *Rights-based monitoring and evaluation: A discussion paper*, London: Save the Children UK.

Treseder, P. (1997) *Empowering Children and Young People: Training manual*, London: Children's Rights Office and Save the Children UK.

Van Beers, H., Invernizzi, A., Milne, B. (2006) *Beyond Article 12: Essential readings in children's participation*, Bangkok: Black on White Publications, Knowing Children.

West, A. (1998) 'Different questions, different ideas: Child-led research and other participation' in V. Johnson et al. (eds) *Stepping Forward: Children and young people's participation in the development process*, London: IT Publications, pp. 271–7.

15 Children's participation in school and community

European perspectives

Renate Kränzl-Nagl and Ulrike Zartler

Planning something for children without asking them is absolutely stupid.

(Boy, 11 years, Norway)

Children have ideas which adults don't have! They need our contributions.

(Boy, 9 years, France)

Introduction

The participation and active citizenship of children and young people is a major priority across Europe. The recognition of the children's right to participation has had a long-standing tradition in the Council of Europe[1] legal texts, including the Revised European Social Charter, the Convention on the Exercise of Children's Rights and the recommendations on the participation of children and family integrated policy. Particularly noteworthy are Recommendation (1998) 8 on children's participation in family and social life, which covers a broad scope of areas in which children can participate, including children's associations, work, training and public life; and Recommendation (2002) 12 on education for democratic citizenship. In accordance with the human rights approach of the Council of Europe and the UN Convention on the Rights of the Child, participation means that children have the right to express their views and relate their experiences, and that these be given due weight in the decision-making process.

The increasing priority of children and young people across European national policy agendas has tended to focus attention on contributions *to* children rather than contributions *by* children. However, prevailing models of active democratic citizenship have given rise to an increasing recognition that children and young people can play a more active role in projects in collaboration with adults. In 2003, a cross-European project 'Children, Democracy and Participation in Society'[2] was commissioned by the Council of Europe's Forum for Children and Families in order to promote participation projects *with* children. The aim of the project was to evaluate the implementation and impact of participation projects with children and young people in schools and communities across European countries. This chapter draws on the findings of this project to capture some of the key lessons for successful, child-friendly participatory project design and critically assesses the impacts and benefits that arise from participation projects with children and young people.

The 'Children, Democracy and Participation in Society' project

The first stage of the project identified a diverse range of child participation projects in schools and local communities across Europe through an open call. Sixty-eight project descriptions were received, analysed and selected according to the following criteria: approaches and methods used in each project, gender issues, different stages of the child's development, geographical balance (covering Central/Eastern, Western/Northern and Southern Europe) and a balance between different types of participation projects. Children and adults were then involved in selecting six case-study projects for further analysis, involving study visits to gain a deeper insight into their practical implementation and impact. Special emphasis was given to the participation experiences of younger children (aged 5 to 11), as less information existed about participation experiences of this age group. The following six projects were selected:

1   Stop Child Labour in Albania, Albania

The objectives of this nationwide programme were to provide non-formal educational and psychosocial assistance, as well as tools to exercise the right of participation for child workers and trafficked children (target group: 6 to 16 years old). A major activity was to establish children's clubs that aimed to increase children's participation at the national and local level and reduce the number of child workers and street children. The children were actively involved in the preparation of daily activities, exhibitions, public campaigns and publications, and participated in meetings with local and national authorities.

2   Quality in Schools, Austria

This project aimed at supporting schools to review, monitor and develop their own quality standards and put children's ideas into practice in a creative way. A school development plan was worked out by all school partners (head-teacher, teachers, pupils, parents, non-educational staff and citizens) and served as a guideline and planning tool for educational action. One of the projects, in a primary school, involved pupils aged 6 to 10 years carrying out a survey on the topic 'The school I am dreaming of', which resulted in the implementation of new, child-friendly playgrounds and school settings.

3   Conseil Communal des Jeunes de Brie, France

The Youth Council of the community of Brie consisted of about 20 children (aged 10 to 14) who were elected annually by their classmates. The main objectives were to prepare young people for democracy and citizenship at the community level, to socialise them into the political system, to promote their participation in the community and to encourage them to take on responsibility. The members of the Youth Council managed their own budget (€4,000 per year) and realised projects that they created and initiated themselves.

4   *Children and Youth: Empowerment, participation and influence, Norway*

The core project within this collaboration programme between three regional partners was 'Children's Tracks', which looked for information on children's use of space in their spare time. Working in small groups, supported by a teacher and a professional in the planning unit, the participants (9 to 12 years old) registered local areas of specific value for children. The results were used to inform the municipality planning process. Another initiative involved children's councils, where children aged 11 to 14 years participated as elected representatives and worked in advisory groups for authorities at the local and regional political levels.

5   *The School and the Assembly, Portugal*

This project with pupils aged 10 to 18 was aimed at strengthening children's participation at the national level by offering them the possibility of participating in a special session in the Portuguese Republic Assembly. During these bi-annual sessions at the parliament, children worked together with deputies, ministers and the assembly president, and they discussed subjects related to childhood and youth policies. A main objective was to show young people the values and practices of democracy, and to promote citizenship education.

6   *Playing for Real, United Kingdom*

This consultation programme was designed to meet the needs of children with regard to their play areas in a specific community or school. Through environmental games, model making and discussions, children could express their opinions about their play space, and the equipment and landscaping they would like to incorporate. The participation of children (5 to 14 years) in designing their own environment was considered to be a step towards citizenship education.

Study visits to all six projects were undertaken and contained the following core elements:

*   on-site visits (children's clubs, playgrounds, schools, meetings);
*   focus group interviews with 81 children: age- and gender-mixed groups, with emphasis on the views of young children (6 to 10 years);
*   semi-structured face-to-face interviews and/or group discussions with 47 adults involved in the projects.

Criteria for successful child-friendly participatory projects with children and young people

This section reflects on the key lessons from these projects for successful, child-friendly participatory projects which seek to enhance the active citizenship of young people.

Political context and support

There is considerable variation between European countries, which have different welfare state regimes and distinct forms of relationships between the family, civil society, the state and the market; and different histories with regard to their political systems. Nevertheless, an increasing awareness of children's rights and promotion of children's participation existed in all six countries, regardless of their different historical development. Efforts to promote children's rights on national, regional and local levels, for example, through legal regulations, financial support, awareness-raising campaigns and existing networks, are key to implementing children's participation projects.

Interestingly, we observed different motivations at the political level to push forward children's participation. In 'young' democracies the emphasis is on 'promoting the political socialisation of young people by offering them opportunities to learn the rules and procedures of democracy as early as possible', as pointed out by the president of the Portuguese parliament. In contrast, Norway has a long-standing tradition of promoting children's participation based on human rights principles, but even in this country such projects are always dependent on the good-will of politicians or other authorities. Gaining project support from politicians is essential for successful project implementation. For example, in the Portuguese project an official declaration was signed by members of parliament and children acting as deputies.

Preparatory work / building on existing networks and initiatives

Preparatory work is essential for successful participation projects. This needs to involve securing cooperation and commitment with local partner organisations such as schools and other child-relevant institutions. For example, in the Austrian case the use of existing networks was an excellent precondition for the implementation of the planned project, because numerous activities had been implemented in collaboration with schools, local authorities and children in the past. Projects are more effective and sustainable when they build on existing programmes and networks at national and regional levels.

Involvement of children in all stages of the project

Our findings underline the importance of involving children in all phases of the project. In particular, children need to be involved early on in the planning process. Children were quite sensitive about being ignored in the beginning, in particular concerning the content and objectives of the project:

> The best way to start a participation project is to ask children directly about their needs and interests first!
>
> (Boy, 10 years, Austria)

Because children's participation projects are never static, there needs to be flexibility with respect to project goals, so as to allow projects to change and adapt in the light of learning as the project progresses. Adults need to be open to changing the course of the project as a result of dialogue and reflection with children. This is especially the case with nationwide initiatives, where projects can be trialled, tested and adapted locally before being rolled out nationally, as was the case with the Portuguese project.

Children should be involved in the documentation and dissemination of projects as far as is possible. The Albanian and Austrian projects remind us of the enormous creative potential that children have and the enjoyment they derive from preparing information to share with others and to celebrate their work. Children regard dissemination as an appreciation of their work – for example, cooperation with (local) television or newspapers, organising information campaigns, exhibitions, conferences or seminars.

> We like very much to write small reports or articles or to produce paintings about our experiences.
>
> (Boy, 10 years, Austria)

> It was very exciting to appear on television. My whole family and my friends were very proud of me! They realised that I am an important person.
>
> (Girl, 12 years, Portugal)

When children are not involved in the later stages of projects, it is imperative to keep them informed about the concrete outcomes and the actions taken as a result of the project. For example, in the Norwegian sub-project 'Children's Tracks', children often were not informed whether or not their inputs had been taken into account in the Municipality Master Plan for land use.

> The planners have all our material, but they did not apologise for not sending it to us. That's incredible!
>
> (Boy, 12 years, Norway)

Roles and tasks of adults

The roles and tasks of adults with regard to children's participation projects are manifold. They play a key role in supporting children in their work and ensuring that approaches are child friendly. Adults play a key role at the beginning of projects, for example, by finding partners, establishing networks, coordinating the project and ensuring that organisational arrangements are in place. Adults play only a supportive and facilitative, rather than an intervening role.

> We do not need the advice of adults, but they need our advice and knowledge, because we are the experts for childhood matters and not the adults!
>
> (Girl, 19 years, Portugal)

> Children have to do all the work, and adults can assist and support them.
>
> (Boy, 15 years, Norway)

Due to the fact that participation projects are sometimes huge and complex initiatives, numerous adults are involved who have specific tasks at different levels and stages of the project. The main groups are:

• the coordinators, often highly motivated persons with a 'burning heart' for the project, who play a key role for its success;
• adults working with children in the field, whose core activities are to assist and support the children by putting a child-friendly design into practice, to facilitate meetings, or to assist children in the dissemination of their work. They serve as a link between children and policy makers or other stakeholders. Close cooperation with coordinators is essential in fulfilling these tasks and making project improvements;
• other actors and stakeholders (e.g. politicians, representatives of different authorities or NGOs) may be involved who do not work directly with children, but play an important role for the project's success.

The fulfilment of these tasks requires specific skills and competencies, in particular when working with socially excluded children (see Albanian project). Adults who work with children have to be self-critical, flexible and willing to listen carefully to children. Project workers need to be trained and experienced in project management and community-building skills.

Principles of a child-friendly project design

Every step of the process, from preparatory work to project implementation and dissemination of results, should be designed in a child-friendly way, according to the age and ability of the children taking part. Child-friendly principles are important in ensuring that children can participate meaningfully and effectively alongside adults, as one boy stated:

> The politicians always talk a lot, but it is not easy to understand what they want to say. They are not speaking our language.
>
> (Boy, 11 years, Portugal)

The following are guidelines for child friendliness, based on the case-study projects across Europe.[3]

- Respect children and be honest. Treat children seriously and respectfully. This will help them to feel that their contribution is important and valued.
- Involve children as early as possible, ideally during the preparation phase. This strengthens their motivation and identification with the project's objectives.
- Invite and encourage all children to participate in the project. Stay open to all children, regardless of their social, cultural or ethnic background or their performance at school.
- Ensure that all children are treated equally and all are given the opportunity to express their opinion.
- Ensure that the focus of projects is attractive to children, concrete and closely related to their daily life.
- Take the different time horizons of children and adults into account. For younger children especially, it is important to get at least some results promptly. In children's eyes, visibility of results is a main factor of success.
- Provide sufficient information on the project, easily accessible and under-standable, in a child-friendly format.
- Keep the organisational structures and procedures transparent. The success of a participation project depends on a clear distribution of work between children and adults.
- Use child-friendly settings, methods, formats, language and background material (e.g. paintings, photos, internet resources, varied materials, symbols, smiling faces, moderating cards, amusing games, contests, small working groups).
- Appreciate the children's work and make this visible. Aside from small gifts (stickers, pencils etc.), official documents are of high importance for children (diplomas, personal letters).
- Be self-critical and flexible. If some methods, tools or approaches turn out to be not sufficiently child friendly, original ideas need to be adapted to children's needs and requirements.
- Finally, having fun while working in a participation project is a key principle of a child-friendly project design.

An excellent example for a child-friendly approach was observed in the UK project where a 'James Bond game' for 6- to10-year-old children was used as a way of exploring playground sites. This game was particularly effective, as children enjoyed acting as spies on a secret mission. They explored the area by performing tasks such as looking for something colourful or spiky, and afterwards they were asked what they liked or disliked. This method is more fun for children than being formally interviewed about their preferences.

The French project underlines the high importance of symbols of appreciation and visible signs of sharing power. The elected children on the council participated in all important ceremonies and festivities of the community (e.g. in weddings), delivered speeches in front of an adult audience and were allowed to wear the tricolor sash alongside the mayor, which has an enormous symbolic value for them.

Impact of children's participation projects – who benefits?

Our findings indicate that participation projects can only be successful if there are benefits for children, adults, institutions, community and wider society. Those benefits can be manifold, as shown below.

Benefits for children

On an individual level, children can benefit in various ways from participation projects:

- To be taken seriously by adults is a very positive experience, in particular for younger children. Ideally, children become acquainted with a democratic decision-making culture in which children and adults are equal.

> At the Children's Club I could do what I want to do for the first time in my life. I was very surprised that an adult asked me about my interests and needs.
>
> (Boy, 13 years, Albania)

- Children benefit from opportunities to participate actively in spheres usually closed to them (e.g. decisions on the local policy level). This gives children a sense of importance and builds their self-confidence.

> I have learned that even children have rights and not only adults. I did not know that before.
>
> (Boy, 14 years, Albania)

- Participation in decision-making processes can increase respect for property and common goods. For example, children are more likely to use and look after new play equipment if they have participated in the decision-making process.

> Since we have a newly created playground based on our own proposals and ideas we use it more often.
>
> (Boy, 10 years, Austria)

- Children learn from each other; in many cases older children serve as role models for younger ones (peer education).

> I have learned a lot from the older children! For instance, how to behave in the group, to say 'Good morning' when entering the club and things like that.
>
> (Boy, 13 years, Albania)

• Children learn to work as part of a team, which strengthens solidarity and team spirit, and may help to establish new friendships.

• Children have the opportunity to learn personal and social skills (for example methods of conflict resolution, decision making etc.).

> We have learned to take on more responsibilities.
>
> (Girl, 13 years, Norway)

• Children learn that, in well-implemented projects, participation can be fun.

> Please tell all the children in the world that we have learned a lot about our rights and that taking part in a participation project can be very enjoyable and effective!
>
> (Girl, 10 years, Albania)

Benefits for adults

Participation projects can increase adults' awareness of children's needs, opinions and wishes. Adults learn how to share power with children, how to get in touch with children's views and realise the great potential of the younger generation. They discover how sophisticated, sensible and thoughtful children's views are, and how much knowledge they have on different topics. The active involvement of adults in participation projects leads to more tolerance and respect towards children.

Impact on school, community life and wider society

In addition to informing decisions, children's participation can have an important impact in enriching social life within schools and communities. Children's devotion of their time to community concerns can help to improve their communities while changing their standing within the community as a result of changes to the way adults view children. Participation projects can generate an increased awareness of children's rights within the community, and can strengthen community relations through intergenerational dialogue and shared experiences. Adults reported that they learned more about the conditions of modern childhood as a result of participation with children.

Participation projects raise awareness of children's views and needs on the policy-making level. The whole of society benefits from children's experiences: girls and boys who are empowered to form and defend their own opinions, who are aware of their skills and needs and have experienced practical democratic decision making are competent, responsible citizens who will contribute to a society's development.

Notes

1. For more information see www.coe.int/DefaultEN.asp.
2. This project was part of a series of activities within the Directorate General III for Social Cohesion, supported by the Integrated Project 'Making Democratic Institutions Work'.
3. Based on the outcomes of this study, a toolkit for adults was prepared by the authors: Council of Europe (2004): *Children, participation, projects – how to make it work!* (Available in English, French and Russian.)

16 Building towards effective participation

A learning-based network approach to youth participation

Tiina Sotkasiira, Lotta Haikkola and Liisa Horelli

In search of effective youth participation

Youth is a phase of life during which people acquire culturally defined roles and statuses. These positions are mobile, as young people navigate between different locations of membership and marginalisation. It is vital that young people are supported and encouraged to take part in decision making within their communities, since participative activities may provide new kinds of political agencies, social relations and even societal change.

Previous research (Horelli et al. 1998; Chawla 1999; 2002; Driskell 2002) has indicated that youth participation seldom emerges on its own. On the contrary, it needs systematic support, continuity and persistent application of dynamic enabling techniques. In order to be effective, youth participation requires emotional and intellectual resources, as well as material and social structures that allow young people to navigate in the adult world. In practice, few young people have sufficient skills and resources to influence the world around them.

During our work in various projects with young people and our research on child and youth participation (Horelli, Haikkola and Sotkasiira 2007) we have noticed that participation does not automatically improve the capacity of young people to lead their lives. Instead of empowerment, participation also seems to embody new forms of controlling the use of time and space of young people. Thus, the enhancement of youth participation by adults and professionals is not unproblematic. In order to offer an alternative to the participation that emanates from the adult world, this chapter introduces the concept of 'effective' participation. The latter refers to participation that emerges at the interface of social interaction and political activity. Ideally, it makes space for the meeting of two processes: the transformation of young people's living conditions and the learning of citizenship skills. This context brings forth our research question: how to enhance effective participation?

We argue that effective participation can be promoted through a so-called learning-based network approach to planning (LENA) which we have developed with children and young people (Horelli and Sotkasiira 2003; Horelli 2006). The LENA, which is based on environmental psychology, planning, sociology and youth studies, seeks to integrate networks (resources and know-how) with learning, as well as with youth-based politics. The latter means activities that seek to improve and transform society through negotiations and struggles dealing with values-based goals and the necessary means to achieve them (Ahponen 2001:14).

The aim of this chapter is to present theoretical concepts concerning youth participation and the LENA, as well as its application in an action research study in the context of one of the Nordic welfare states, Finland. The chapter concludes by discussing the constraints and opportunities of effective youth participation.

Youth participation in the Finnish context

The ideas and forms of child and youth participation in Finland have historically followed European and, especially, Nordic developments. In the 1960s, the student movement initiated a radical discussion about power relations in Finnish society. Among other things, it aimed at restructuring intergenerational relations. The democratisation, or even politicisation, of schools opened up spaces for student participation (Satka et al. 2002: 245–7). During the following decades, other forms of participation grew stronger: the environmental movement in the 1980s and the animal rights movement in the 1990s. The notion of citizen participation was also introduced into community planning, which provided opportunities for even children and young people to become visible as capable and creative participants (Horelli 1994; Horelli 1998; Horelli, Kyttä and Kaaja 1998). At the turn of the millennium new forms of activism (Anti-Capitalist and Global Justice Movement) rose, and decreasing electoral turnout led to discussions on the declining political participation of all citizens, young people included. This resulted in the first policy programme of the government to support citizen participation. This gave impetus to several participatory youth projects which drew on the UN Convention on the Rights of the Child and its emphasis on children's right to participate.

A recent comparison of the conditions for youth participation between Finland and Italy revealed that adequate legislation, policy and participatory structures are vital for the successful involvement of young people in significant issues of daily life (Haikkola and Rissotto 2007). Supportive structures concern special measures for involving children and youth in decision making (councils and parliaments), youth organisations (for example, sports associations), participation projects and, above all, municipal youth centres. More than 1,000 youth centres exist in Finland, which are free and open to all children and supported by municipal youth workers. Youth work refers to activities organised out of school. However, it also has a deeper aim, namely the education of children and young people to become responsible citizens. Currently, participation has become, to some extent, an accepted method in youth work (Horelli et al. 2007).

Nevertheless, youth participation almost always embodies a contradiction between control and freedom. In the recent Finnish debate, youth participation is often associated with the education or rearing of children and young people. An assumption exists that if young people are involved in participative projects and activities, their personal and social skills are enhanced, and thus they are better qualified to come to terms with the needs and challenges of society. The notion of participation gets entangled with educational or controlling goals. Thus, the recent emphasis on participation can also be interpreted as a reflection of 'risk politics' (Harrikari and Satka 2006: 211). Risk politics refers to a shift in the welfare policy in which children and young people have come to be seen as societal risks. Perceived risks can be managed by interventions and control, not by supportive measures or policies, such as participatory means that enhance children's agency (ibid.: 212). The tendency to regard participation as an intervention and control method is visible in the second Finnish government participation policy programme on youth, which dealt with the prevention of social exclusion, rather than systematically supporting youth participation.

Youth participation – a fuzzy concept

Participation is a fuzzy and multifaceted concept that needs clarification. First, the distinction between *participation as social activity* and *participation as influencing or creating change* in political or societal processes needs to be recognised. 'Influencing' means that certain transformation has been achieved in the processes or through decision making (Anttiroiko 2003: 19). The interface between the two interpretations can be labelled as effective participation. Second, participation is a normative concept. Whether in education, youth work or planning, participation always involves implicit or explicit aims that concern individual or societal change. In order not to be trapped in the contradiction described above, the aims of a project or a measure in question should always be openly negotiated. Normativeness is closely connected to power, which is a prerequisite of change. Power *per se* is neither good nor bad, rather, its nature emerges from the way in which it is used. Depending on the context, power can be control (power over), empowerment (power to) or power in structures, practices and networks (see Allen 2003). Participation in its ideal form may increase youth empowerment. Supportive structures and networks may also enhance the position of young people.

Third, participation can be applied to different contexts and activities, such as urban planning, budgeting or even to complex systems such as waste management. Participatory endeavours may extend from the micro level (design of playgrounds or youth centre activities) to the meso level (neighbourhoods) and even to the macro level (Bronfenbrenner 1993; Horelli 2002). Thus, the whole community or region can be the target of participatory planning and politics. The participation processes of children and young people have, in fact, grown more complex in recent years (Horelli 2003; Francis and Lorenzo 2002).

We claim that, while acknowledging the educational aims of youth participation, it is equally important to recognise that youth participation can have other meanings. If participation is used only as a tool for citizenship education, a great deal of resources and creativity may be lost. Successful youth participation has also to be effective in terms of being able to create change in the lived realities of children and young people.

Modelling the learning-based network approach to youth participation

Research literature on 'children as urban planners' reveals that young participants are both able critics of their environments and producers of new ideas for
implementation, but their participation has not become part of accepted child
policy, nor a praxis in European planning systems (Horelli 1998; 2001; Chawla
2002). The problem remains of how to bridge the gap between competent young
people (aged 7 to 18) and the adult gatekeepers of urban planning and development. The provision of resources and methodological supports to children, such
as internet-assisted urban planning (Horelli and Kaaja 2002; Kyttä et al. 2004),
might alleviate the gap slightly, but as long as the participation of young people
takes place within the traditional top-down, hierarchic planning paradigm, little
progress seems to occur (Booher and Innes 2002).

On the other hand, the network approach to development and youth participation indicates that even young people can improve their position when they
are members or even partners in the networks of social cohesion (Horelli 2003).
Actor networks may provide a context and arenas where young people are treated
not in terms of their age, but on the basis of their skills and knowledge. This,
in turn, enhances the opportunities for collaboration in local and even regional
development.

Managing and improving everyday life in complex network societies in which
people struggle with 'glocal' problems requires multilevel and multidimensional
approaches, as well as new concepts. These include the notions of place-based
politics (Harcourt and Escobar 2002), a variety of strategies and knowledges, environmental competence, and an approach that is called the learning-based network
approach to planning (LENA), which enables young people and adults to take part
in interdependent actor networks (Latour 1993; Booher and Innes 2002).

The LENA

The LENA can be described through a tripartite schema that consists of:

- a model of planning
- specific tasks of development, and
- a collective monitoring and self-evaluation system.

The model of planning (Figure 16.1) comprises a core idea (for example the
construction of innovative arenas of empowerment), contextual analyses, collective
envisioning of the future with the participants, as well as a few shared principles
of implementation. The latter gradually crystallises into strategies of implementation. In the case of the North Karelian young people's project, described in the
next section, the strategies of implementation comprised the constant creation of
meaningful events (buzz), participatory networking, capacity building, application
of ICT, marketing integrated into all interventions, application of art and creative
methods, and ongoing collective monitoring and self-evaluation (Horelli 2003).

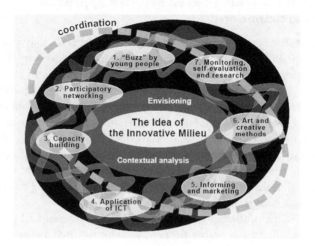

Figure 16.1   The model of the learning-based network approach to planning: nodes and
their links emerge through the implementation of the chosen strategies and
sensitive coordination

The chosen set of strategies encourages the stakeholders to create and reproduce
nodes and links of the network that eventually provide the supportive infrastructure of everyday life (Horelli 2007; Haikkola et al. 2007).

Gender- and age-sensitive coordination of the planning and development process
is, according to the Finnish experiences, not about enforcement but about constant
negotiating and interacting with different partners. This presupposes that special
attention is paid both to the time dimension (present and future) and to the necessi-
ties and contingencies of everyday life. The matrix of these dimensions discloses four
types of tasks that are important in the implementation of participative youth projects
when applying the LENA. The tasks are daily problem solving, shaping of structures, organising of 'buzz' and nurturing of hope (Figure 16.2; Horelli 2006). The
latter is particularly important in the unpredictable 'glocal' contexts of diminishing
resources in which young people often find themselves (see also Snyder 2002).

The third part of the schema is the collective monitoring and self-evaluation
system which comprises tools for ongoing monitoring at the operational level
(weekly assessment sheets, work plans, the budget etc.), tools for collective self-evaluation of the network as a whole (metaphoric and analytic assessment of the nodes
and links), as well as the thematic and summative evaluations of the project results
which are discussed with both young and older stakeholders (Horelli 2003).

Application of the learning-based network approach to youth participation

In order to enhance effective youth participation, the LENA was applied in the
North Karelian Youth Forum project (Nufo), which took place in the easternmost

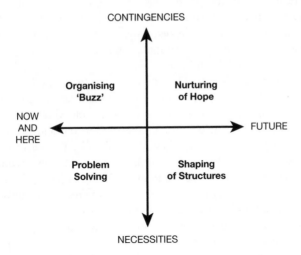

Figure 16.2 The tasks of the learning-based network approach to planning: problem
solving, shaping of structures, organisation of 'buzz' and the nurturing of hope

region in Finland during 2000–3. Its goal was to create a supportive network with
young people that could provide arenas of empowerment and dialogue between
adolescents and adults (Horelli 2006). For two reasons, we will focus on one of its
sub-projects, which aimed at providing rehearsal facilities for local bands. First,
the case study illustrates how social interaction is linked with the concrete aim
of transforming the everyday life of young people. Second, the key objective in
this case was to explain how the success of effective participation depends on
networking, for example, the imperative of connecting young people to the actors
who have the resources to support them.

North Karelia (170,000 residents) is a sparsely populated region with vast areas
of forests and lakes. This former agrarian region has several clusters of forestry and
metal industries as well as numerous high-tech centres. The unemployment rate
is high (18 per cent), and alarmingly high among young people, who are increasingly moving to the more prosperous parts of the country. Although the Regional
Council had been aware of the youth problem for a long time, it took nearly
three years to negotiate a special project that would seek to create supportive local
and regional networks for and with young people. In 2001, Nufo was granted
€500,000 from the European Social Fund and three municipalities (Joensuu,
Kitee and Lieksa). This made it possible to hire four young people to coordinate and manage the project for two years. The vision of the project, which was
created together with the participants, crystallised as 'A joyful North Karelia with
survival opportunities for young people'. The objectives implied the creation of a
supportive network for and with young people, as well as possibilities for work and
local initiatives through their own sub-projects, enjoyable events and having a say
in regional development.

The practical work of the project was launched by organising participatory workshops in the schools of the three municipalities. During the workshops, pupils worked in small groups and addressed issues and problems that they faced in their everyday lives and discussed possible solutions with local decision makers. In Joensuu, the capital of North Karelia, one of the main complaints was the lack of rehearsal facilities for bands. The city is known for its lively rock scene, but newly formed bands lacked appropriate spaces for rehearsing. Nufo started to solve the problem by setting up a team of young people who began to search for suitable locations, with the help of adult mentors. The participants were pupils of the schools, their friends and acquaintances, united by the wish to improve the situation for local bands. After numerous phone conversations, meetings and the inspection of properties, a flat was found in the centre of Joensuu which could be converted into rehearsal rooms. In order to sublet the rooms to bands, an association was set up to administer the necessary formalities.

The process of searching for a suitable property was an educational experience which demanded a lot from the young people and adults involved. The young participants formed the soul of the team. They defined the goals of the project and provided expertise in terms of what kind of facilities the bands needed. The young team members also linked Nufo with musicians and formed the board of the future band association. From the very beginning it was clear that the young team members could not succeed on their own, because they lacked credibility in the eyes of the potential landlords. This was why Nufo joined forces with the local Live Music Association, which has developed a position of 'reliable intermediary' in cultural disputes. Through organising a successful rock festival, the Association has gathered funds, which it uses to support local and regional bands and performers. Once the suitable property was found, the Association paid the guarantee, financed a major part of the renovation work and also assisted the team of youngsters in organising concerts and band nights to raise money for their activities.

The role of Nufo in the process was manifold. First and foremost, the project workers supported and guided young people and encouraged them to continue the search, even when no solutions to the problem seemed to be available. Nufo also helped the youngsters to fill in fund applications and acted as a link between decision makers and the young people. It required sensitivity to figure out when it was time to push ahead with the project and when young participants needed to 'let their hair down' and have fun. Even though the financial gains from band nights were modest, several events were organised to boost the morale of the team and to give the musicians a chance to display their talent. On the other hand, young people were serious about getting the work done. In line with the model of effective participation, the goal was to enjoy the experience of working as a team, while keeping their eyes on the target.

The use of city-owned properties and the distribution of resources among cultural actors is an ongoing battle in Joensuu. Over the years, the young members of the band association have met with the city authorities several times to convince them to subsidise the rent for the bands. So far all negotiations have failed, although the young activists are not too concerned, as they feel that the city can dictate the rules of the association if it starts financing its activities. While relying on the support of certain adults, the young activists do not want to depend too much on formal authorities or outside financing. The main point is that the rules have to be defined by the young people themselves. This is a top priority, even if it means in practice that all board meetings start with complaints about the untidiness of the place and the difficulty of getting the bands to pay their rent on time.

We claim that the platforms for action, such as the band team, are also political spaces (Eyerman and Jamison 1991), since they enable young people to articulate their ideas. Their voices are, however, frail and in need of constant nurturing. The band team was one of the many teams set up by Nufo. Despite the setbacks, the young board members have managed to keep the activities running for the past five years. Fifteen bands are currently using the rehearsal facilities. A reason for its success is the combination of buzz (ongoing stream of events and happenings) and the clear and concrete vision: the need to find suitable premises for bands. The application of the learning-based network approach to development was crucial, especially in the initial stage. It mobilised the right partners to realise the project and assured that the project never got out of the hands of the young team members.

Conclusion

Young people are growing up in increasingly globalised and intricate contexts. It is therefore crucial to pay attention to the complexity of social and political situations in which young people strive for empowerment and the betterment of their living conditions. It is also essential to focus on the dynamics and conditions of participation, as the role of participation is wider than educating well-behaved citizens.

In this chapter we have defined some core concepts of participation and claimed that participation is a fuzzy concept with normative implications. Participation can be applied to many fields and on many levels, from large platforms of empowerment, such as Nufo, to concrete, small-scale youth projects carried out in schools, youth clubs etc. As the enhancement of young people's participation by adults and professionals is not unproblematic, we introduced the concept of effective participation. It means that participation should have an impact on the transformation of young people's living conditions and the learning of citizenship skills. We have argued that the learning-based network approach to planning is one way of enhancing effective youth participation.

The tripartite schema of the LENA, consisting of the model itself, specific tasks of development and a collective monitoring and self-evaluation system, seemed to fare well in the Finnish context, in which young people and adults succeeded in creating space for self-organisation and in generating a culture that supported young people rather than silencing them, at least for a certain period of time. The LENA did have a meaningful role in assisting young people to fulfil their dreams and aspirations and in connecting them with actors who have resources to help. The network approach seems to be a necessary prerequisite of survival even in other complex contexts, such as in the world of social media and in synthetic or virtual communities.

The changing role of adults is important. As young people also seem to yearn for adult contacts, grown-ups, and especially professionals, should provide the platforms and tools with which young people can express themselves and generate their own outcomes. Effective participation requires dialogue with young and old, provision of spaces and room for the self-governance of young people's own plans and activities. This leads to an improved understanding of the needs and demands of young people and enhances the identification of a wider range of solutions for the dilemma at hand. Furthermore, effective participation may have intrinsic value as a form of collective decision making and involvement of young people in community development.

References

Ahponen, P. (2001) *Kulttuurin pesäpaikka. Yhteiskunnallisia lähestymistapoja kulttuuriteoriaan* (The habitat of culture. Social approaches to cultural theory), Helsinki: WSOY.

Allen, J. (2003) *Lost Geographies of Power*, London: Blackwell Publishing.

Anttiroiko, A.-V. (2003) 'Kansalaisten osallistuminen, osallisuus ja vaikuttaminen tietoyhteiskunnassa' (Citizen participation in the information society), in P. Bäcklund (ed.) *Tietoyhteiskunnan osallistuva kansalainen. Tapaus Nettimaunula* (Citizen participation in the information society. Case Nettimaunula), Helsinki: Helsingin kaupungin tietokeskus, 11–32.

Booher, D. and Innes, J. (2002) 'Network power in collaborative planning', *Journal of Planning Education and Research* 21: 221–36.

Bronfenbrenner, U. (1993) 'Ecology of cognitive development: Research models and fugitive findings', in R. H. Wozniak and K. W. Fischer (eds) *Development in Context. Acting and thinking in specific environments*, Hillsdale, NJ: Lawrence Erlbaum, 221–88.

Chawla, L. (1999) 'Life paths into effective environmental action', *The Journal of Environmental Education* 31: 15–26.

Chawla, L. (ed.) (2002) *Growing Up in an Urbanising World*, London: UNESCO and Earthscan.

Driskell, D. (ed.) (2002) *Creating Better Cities with Children and Youth. A manual for participation*, London: UNESCO and Earthscan.

Eyerman, R. and Jamison, A. (1991) *Social Movements. A Cognitive Approach*, Pittsburgh: Pennsylvania State University Press.

Francis, M. and Lorenzo, R. (2002) 'Seven realms of children's participation', *Journal of Environmental Psychology* 22: 157–69.

Haikkola, L. and Rissotto, A. (2007) 'Legislation, policy and participatory structures as opportunities for children's participation? A comparison of Finland and Italy', *Children, Youth and Environments* 17(4): 352–87.

Haikkola, L., Pacilli, M. G., Horelli, L., and Prezza, M. (2007) 'Interpretations of urban child-friendliness: A comparative study in two neighborhoods in Helsinki and Rome', *Children, Youth and Environments* 17(4): 319–51, available at www.colorado.edu/journals/cye, accessed 12 December 2007.

Harcourt, W. and Escobar, A. (2002) 'Women and the politics of place', *Development* 45: 7–14.

Harrikari, T. and Satka, M. (2006) 'A new regime of governing childhood? Finland as an example', *Social Work and Society* 4(2): 209–16.

Horelli, L. (1994) 'Children as urban planners', *Architecture et Comportement* 10(4): 21–5.

Horelli, L. (1998) 'Creating child-friendly environments: Case studies on children's participation in three European countries', *Childhood* 5: 225–39.

Horelli, L. (2001) 'Young people's participation: Lip service or serious business', in H. Helve and C. Wallace (eds) *Youth, Citizenship and Empowerment*, Aldershot: Ashgate Publishing Ltd, 57–71.

Horelli, L. (2002) 'A methodology of participatory planning', in R. Bechtel and A. Churchman (eds) *Handbook of Environmental Psychology*, New York: John Wiley, 607–28.

Horelli, L. (2003) *Valittajista tekijöiksi* (From complainers to agents: Adolescents on the arenas of empowerment), Espoo: Helsinki University of Technology.

Horelli, L. (2006) 'A learning-based network approach to urban planning with young people', in C. Spencer and M. Blades (eds) *Children and Their Environments: Learning, using and designing spaces*, Cambridge: Cambridge University Press, pp. 238–55.

Horelli, L. (2007) 'Constructing a framework for environmental child-friendliness', *Children, Youth and Environments* 17(4): 267–92, available at www.colorado.edu/journals/cye, accessed 30 December 2007.

Horelli, L. and Kaaja, M. (2002) 'Opportunities and constraints of internet-assisted urban planning with young people', *Journal of Environmental Psychology* 22: 191–200.

Horelli, L. and Sotkasiira, T. (eds) (2003) *Töpinäksi! Nufon itsearviointi- ja menetelmäopas* (Self-evaluation manual for Nufo), Joensuu: Pohjois-Karjalan nuorten foorumi-hanke.

Horelli, L., Haikkola, L. and Sotkasiira, T. (2007) 'Osallistuminen nuorisotyön lähesty-mistapana' (Participation as an approach in youth work), in T. Hoikkala and A. Sell (eds) *Nuorisotyötä on tehtävä. Menetelmien perustat, rajat ja mahdollisuudet* (We must do youth work. Methods, basis, limitations and possibilities), Helsinki: Nuorisotutkimusverkosto, julkaisuja 76, pp. 217–42.

Horelli, L., Kyttä, M. and Kaaja, M. (1998) *Lapset ympäristön ekoagentteina* (Children as ecoagents of the environment), Helsinki: TKK, Arkkitehtiosasto, 98/49.

Kyttä, M., Kaaja, M. and Horelli, L. (2004) 'An internet-based design game as a mediator of children's environmental visions', *Environment and Behavior* 35(10): 1–24.

Latour, B. (1993) *We Have Never Been Modern*, Cambridge, MA: Harvard University Press.

Satka, M., Moilanen, J. and Kiili, J. (2002) 'Suomalaisen lapsipolitiikan mutkainen tie (The winding road of Finnish child policy) *Yhteiskuntapolitiikka* 67(3): 245–59.

Snyder, C.R. (2002) 'Hope theory: Rainbows in the mind', *Psychological Inquiry* 13(4): 249–75.

17 Getting the measure of children and young people's participation

An exploration of practice in Wales

Anne Crowley and Anna Skeels

Introduction

The Children and Young People's Participation Consortium was set up in 2003 to coordinate the strategic development of children and young people's participation in Wales. One of its first challenges was to establish 'easy to use' mechanisms to improve the quality of participatory practice across Wales and to collate evidence of the benefits and impacts of children and young people's participation. This chapter reviews the ongoing process of establishing a set of national standards for children and young people's participation in Wales and developing a framework (and accompanying tools) for assessing and measuring the impact of participation on children or young people themselves, on institutions, on related policies and services and on communities.

It has been argued that standardisation risks abandoning participatory practice to the ravages of consumerism, and that instead a more empowering perspective should be adopted which locates the young citizen as a public actor who may desire to act in many varied ways that do not necessarily conform to any standards (Harry Shier, personal communication). We argue, however, that in the UK at least, the time has passed when just 'doing' participation 'any old how' is good enough. We acknowledge that in other global contexts there will be a different story to tell, but, without losing sight of the need to encourage and support a diverse range of approaches and methods, in Wales, among young people's organisations, practitioners and policy makers alike there is broad agreement that more must be done to drive up the quality of participatory practice. At the same time, in an age focused on evidence-based practice as a key determinant of funding and government support (Cabinet Office 1999), the need for evidence about the *impact* of children and young people's participation is becoming ever more urgent.

Credibility with donors is vital, but so too is credibility with children and young people. Concerns have been raised by children, young people and practitioners that children's participation in decision making in the UK can be tokenistic, a 'box-ticking' exercise that fails to deliver any substantive change (Sinclair 2004). Understandably, this perception can turn off many would-be beneficiaries who arguably have better things to do with their time. The debates about children's participation now stretch beyond the mere recognition that children should participate, to demand that participation results (and, perhaps as importantly, is seen to result) in 'political' change (Tisdall and Bell 2006). As Lansdown argues (this volume) we now need a stronger focus on application to embed participation in all areas of children's lives, identifying indicators against which to evaluate whether the necessary legislative, policy and practice provisions are in place and establishing the means by which to measure the extent, quality and impact of the participatory activity that children are engaged in.

After setting out the specific Welsh context for children and young people's participation, we outline the development and contribution of the national standards in Wales and the ongoing development of an impact assessment framework tool. The aim is not only to highlight some of the many challenges of translating these developments into effective mechanisms for improving quality and increasing institutional support, but also to argue that addressing these challenges is not insurmountable and that the process promises rich rewards.

Children and young people's participation in Wales

There is a clear and strong commitment in law, policy and practice in Wales to children and young people's participation in decision making. Taking stock of developments in children's policy and practice since the establishment of devolved government in Wales in 1999, Thomas and Crowley (2007: 177) conclude that

> The 'participation agenda' really does seem to have caught on, in that it is much better understood by many more professionals – social workers and doctors, civil servants and chief executives – and that participation by children and young people is increasingly becoming an accepted part of practice.

There is not enough space here to list all relevant developments in Wales (for a more detailed review see Butler 2007; Croke and Crowley 2006), but against a backdrop where the National Assembly for Wales has adopted the United Nations Convention on the Rights of the Child (UNCRC) as the basis of all its policy making (National Assembly for Wales 2004), there has been strong Assembly Government support for the strategic development of children and young people's participation across Wales. The Assembly Government funds structures to support and enable participation in policy and service development, including: Funky Dragon; the Children and Young People's Assembly; the Participation Unit hosted by Save the Children, which supports the work of the Participation Consortium; and a 'participation project' within the Assembly Government itself, which supports and encourages children and young people's participation within the government's policy-making processes. Participation in schools has been given a statutory basis, with regulations requiring school councils to be established in all primary, secondary and special schools across Wales (Welsh Assembly Government 2005). Guidance on the production and implementation of local participation strategies has been issued to the 22 local strategic partnerships that oversee children and young people's service development in Wales.

Undoubtedly, there is much still to be done. The funding of participation structures remains short-term and opportunistic. There is only a limited statutory basis and the government still has no overarching strategy for developing and supporting children and young people's participation. Children and young people are not routinely informed about their rights, and often are only asked to give their views and opinions on matters where adults decide to ask them. Support for the development of participation by younger children (10 and under) in public policy is woefully inadequate and the inclusion of 'hard to reach' young people remains a key issue. While there is clear commitment, supporting structures and many examples of good practice, there is still a need for cultural and organisational change to truly embed participatory practice across Wales. Concluding their review of the evidence on implementation of Article 12 of the UNCRC in the most recent NGO 'alternative' report, Skeels and Thomas argue that evidence of the benefits of participation is urgently required to push forward the agenda (2007: 20).

This is the background to the two developments that we set out below. The first, establishing a set of national participation standards and the second, the development of a framework for assessing the impact of children or young people's participation in public policy and service development.

National standards

The National Children and Young People's Participation Standards for Wales relate to the quality of the process of participation. As with other examples of practice standards in this field, for example 'Hear by Right' in England (Badham and Wade 2005) and the International Save the Children Alliance's practice standards (Save the Children 2005), the Welsh standards reflect commonly agreed principles of good practice, such as respect, diversity, choice and benefits for the children and young people involved (Cutler 2003). The seven standards – 'information', 'it's your choice', 'no discrimination', 'respect', 'you get something out of it', 'feedback' and 'improving how we work' – provide benchmarks for assessing the quality of participation processes. Each standard is expressed in terms of an *explanation* and a *commitment*. For example:

> INFORMATION
> This means:
> • Information that is easy to understand for everyone
> • Adults working with you who know what is going on and are up front and clear.
> We will:
> • Ensure everyone has enough information to get properly involved
> • Let you know what difference you being involved will make
> • Inform you about who is going to listen and make changes.
> (Save the Children, 2007)

Development of the National Participation Standards in Wales has been inclusive. They were drafted, designed and piloted through workshops with children, young people and practitioners. The children and young people involved have included primary school council members, looked-after young people, young people from youth forums and 'at risk' youth groups. The standards have been endorsed by Funky Dragon and the Welsh Assembly Government, and were launched at a national seminar in January 2007 to a large range of agencies and young people from across Wales.

The development is a deliberately chosen path, with its own rationale. While standardisation is not always viewed as positive, with the risks of stamping out diversity and imposing one dominant view over others, the standards are seen as essential to driving up the quality of children and young people's participation in Wales. The aim is to 'raise the bar' in terms of the quality of the process, in order to create an environment that enables diverse and varied participation practices and methods to flourish. It is hoped that the standards will provide a meaningful, reliable 'core' to children and young people's participation and capacity building with adults, while positively reaffirming their experience of participation. Without this, there is the danger that children and young people will 'vote with their feet' and become more and more reluctant to be involved in activity that has less and less credibility among their peers (Sinclair 2004).

This path chosen in Wales is different from developments in England. 'Hear by Right' provides a standards framework primarily for practitioners to support the development of children and young people's participation and organisational change (Badham and Wade 2005). It is an optional framework for practitioners, and is relatively complex in structure. The Welsh standards are deliberately simple because the aim is to make them as inclusive as possible and to get all parties on board. However, the two approaches are not mutually exclusive. Once the crucial baseline in the Welsh standards has been established, the 'Hear by Right' methodology can assist organisations to map out in more detail how they might move further forward in their practice.

The National Standards in Wales have been called for and developed 'bottom-up' by children and young people in Wales. The standards are 'owned' by them (young people in Funky Dragon call them '*our* standards'); they have been piloted by children and young people, who will also be involved in using the standards to inspect services.

The Participation Consortium is concerned to ensure that the standards work to improve the quality of participatory practice and make a difference to the experiences of children and young people. Operationalising the standards and integrating them into the relevant frameworks and tools is key, and work has begun to incorporate them into:

- inspection frameworks across social care (Care and Social Services Inspectorate for Wales; education (Estyn) and health (Health Inspection Wales);
- quality assurance schemes, e.g. those covering regulated services for the under-8s;
- policy assessment tools e.g. the Welsh Assembly Government's Policy Gateway and Equalities Impact Assessments;
- self-evaluation and performance management frameworks, e.g. the National Service Framework self-assessment tool;
- kitemarking schemes,[1] e.g. Clywed, a peer-led scheme operating in Gwynedd

in North Wales.

A self-assessment pack takes organisations through the standards and explores what evidence they will need to collate in order to demonstrate compliance. Feedback from users indicates that the pack helps organisations acclimatise to the notion of standards and gets them used to critically self-assessing their practice. Funding has also been secured to develop mechanisms for *externally* assessing against the standards, ranging from the development of a new independent 'kitemark' to a quality assurance process that is firmly tied into existing national inspection regimes, for example those of the Care and Social Services Inspectorate for Wales. Links have now been established for this purpose with local participation inspection and quality assurance schemes across Wales, a number of which are peer led, as well as with national inspectorates. Through joint exploration, a range of issues will be considered, including how best to set performance indicators against the standards, whether there should be different 'levels' (bronze, silver, gold) that can be achieved or simply a baseline, and how to effectively train up young people so that they have the confidence and critical skills to take part meaningfully in an inspection process. A pilot external inspection of the Participation Unit against the National Standards by an independent team of young people in December 2007 has begun to help us address these questions. There are many more challenges ahead, in particular how to drive up quality without stifling diversity, achieve robust inspection without alienation and run a national scheme effectively at a local level.

Impact assessment

We argued at the beginning of the chapter that, as well as integrating quality standards into the practice of engaging children and young people in decision making, we need to be clearer about what impacts can be achieved and identified. If sustained commitments are to be made to invest in the necessary legal, social and economic supports to make it a reality for children to participate in decisions affecting their lives, then we need to do more to demonstrate the positive impacts of children's participation for them, for organisations and institutions and for communities as a whole (Lansdown 2006).

A review for the Carnegie Young People's Initiative (CYPI) of evidence for the benefits of children's participation revealed surprisingly little empirical data on the impact on children or on their communities (Kirby with Bryson 2002). The authors conclude that, while young people are increasingly being involved in various projects, the evidence so far is that this is having little independent impact on outcomes. The review found some evidence that youth participation work could help to increase dialogue and relations between young people and adults and between peers, and that young people benefit from good quality participatory practice which enhances their confidence, self-esteem, knowledge, understanding and skills attainment. The authors call for more participatory research to evaluate work that seeks to involve young people in policy and service development, but suggest that qualitative approaches should be complemented by quantitative, longitudinal and control studies.

A subsequent discussion paper prepared for the International Save the Children

Alliance Child Participation Working Group (Kirby et al. 2004) identifies in a global context areas where there are measurable impacts that are central to most participation work, which the authors suggest could be researched using context-specific indicators. These core impacts focus on three dimensions of change:

- Impact on services, policies and institutions: suggested indicators include children's inputs leading to improved laws, policies and practice, and improved structures, policies, resources and mechanisms for involving children.
- Impact on social and power relations: suggested indicators include enhanced dialogue and support between children and adults (including professionals, family, decision makers and wider community, as appropriate), and children having greater self-efficacy (belief in their ability to affect the world).
- Impact on children's personal development and well-being: suggested indicators include improved well-being of children with respect to one or more of the following: health, education, environment, protection from violence and abuse; and children's enhanced critical thinking (including the ability to analyse their situation, incorporate other evidence, reach a decision).

Plan UK/Plan International, in their review of work on evaluating children's participation, identified four realms of impact and sought to develop understanding on the kind of changes that will be meaningful for children themselves as well as for their families and communities. The four realms (individual, familial, communal and institutional) are broad enough, the authors suggest, to have some validity across cultures within a framework that is flexible enough to allow for local understandings (Ackerman et al. 2003).

Lansdown (2006: 152) suggests three dimensions to be addressed when exploring how children's participation is measured and evaluated:

- Scope: what degree of participation has been achieved?
- Quality: to what extent have participatory processes complied with recognised standards for good practice?
- Impact: what has been the impact on the young people themselves, families and the supporting agency, and on the wider realisation of young people's rights within families, local communities and at local and national government levels?

Arguably, scope can be considered with reference to existing frameworks for understanding 'degrees' of participation, for example, Hart's ladder (1992); Treseder's circle (1997) and Shier's pathways (2001). Quality can be benchmarked using practice standards such as the Welsh National Standards or the 'Hear by Right' framework. But as yet, there is only very early exploration of just how we can assess and measure the impacts or outcomes of children and young people's participation. For example, the 'Spider Tool' developed by Feinstein and O'Kane (2005), piloted in seven countries including Wales, provides a valuable self-assessment and planning tool for children, young people and adult supporters reflecting on the strengths of child-led initiatives and organisations.

Initial work by Lewis and Thomas (2006) on developing an impact assessment framework in Wales took Kirby et al.'s (2004) 'core impacts' as the starting point, consulted with a wide range of children and young people, practitioners and policy makers as to the possible impacts of participation practice within the three domains, and piloted a self-assessment framework containing a set of statements that organisations and service users were asked to score themselves against 'before and after' with supporting evidence. The second phase of the impact assessment project is focused on delivering 'fit for purpose' instruments and tools to capture the relevant evidence (ideally both qualitative and quantitative data from a range of sources). Links have been established with a Welsh Assembly Government initiative that is aiming to set indicators for assessing young people's progress under the new arrangements for the education and training of 14- to 19-year-olds in Wales, as well as to develop tools for measuring 'soft' outcomes for young people, such as increased confidence and motivation (Welsh Assembly Government 2006). Capturing evidence of these soft outcomes of children and young people's participation is crucially important. The interim report on an evaluation of the development of young people's participation plans in two Children's Trusts in England identifies the overriding value young people place on the personal benefits of their participation, for example, the impact on their learning and development and on their confidence. Interestingly, the adults interviewed in the two Trusts identified the ability to gain messages about more effective services as the key benefit of young people's participation (Percy-Smith 2007).

The next phase of the impact assessment project is to conduct extended pilots of the impact assessment framework and a number of supporting data collection instruments with a wide range of organisations. Training and support will focus on 'what works' in terms of application and, in time, contribute to consistency of approach. Subsequently, the Participation Consortium will be seeking support for a national roll-out of the framework, so that evidence of impacts can be gathered across Wales and thereby inform strategic planning processes and resource allocation at a national as well as a local level.

The hope is that, with training and support, the framework will encourage organisations to reflect on their own participatory practice and maintain a focus on positive impacts and beneficial outcomes. It should also provide a means of highlighting work that is tokenistic or work that has no (or even negative) impact. Ultimately, the impact assessment framework will enable us to gather evidence that can be used to challenge the participation agenda and move it forward to garner increased (and more sustainable) institutional and financial support.

There are major challenges ahead. The aim is to produce a framework, with supporting training and guidance, that is applicable in all relevant settings in Wales and that can be used by adults and young people alike. The Participation Consortium has determined that the impact assessment framework must be simple to use and must promote participatory practice rather than put people off. Mirroring success criteria reflected in the National Standards, the framework has to be positive, inclusive and owned by key stakeholders. It needs to avoid duplication and read across to the performance management and outcome measurement systems already in use in particular contexts, for example in schools, local councils, hospitals, GP surgeries and youth offending teams. Inevitably, the impact assessment framework (and the accompanying tools) will have to be revised and updated in the light of experience and remain formative and developmental for some time to come.

Conclusion

We have argued, with reference to our experience in Wales, that a set of national standards for children and young people's participation and a framework and tools for assessing and collecting evidence on the impacts of participation both have critical roles to play in ensuring the necessary endorsement and institutional support for children and young people's participation in public policy and service development. These initiatives will of course only make a difference if and when they are fully operationalised and integrated into existing generic and specialist systems for improving public services. All too often, as those who work in public services will be aware, these things gather dust on some office shelf. Encouraging and supporting ownership by key stakeholders, including children, young people and practitioners, is crucial.

The materials would inevitably need adapting to any other local context, for example with context-specific indicators of impact and evidence in support of each of the standards, but we would argue that they could have resonance in a global context. Perhaps they could be especially useful in countries where the debate has moved on from just 'doing' participation to asking just how good an experience it is for children or young people, and what exactly does it achieve.

Note

1. In Britain, the Kitemark is a symbol which is put on products or services that have met certain standards of safety and quality.

References

Ackerman, L. Thomas, F., Hart, J. and Newman, J. (2003) *Understanding and Evaluating Children's Participation*, London: Plan UK / Plan International.

Badham, B. and Wade, H. (2005) *Hear by Right* (2nd edn), London: National Youth Agency.

Butler, I. (2007) 'Children's Policy in Wales', in Williams, C. (ed.) *Social Policy for Social Welfare Practice in a Devolved Wales*, Birmingham: Venture Press.

Cabinet Office (1999) *Modernising government*, London: HMSO, available at www.archive.official-documents.co.uk/document/cm43/43104310.htm.

Cutler, D. (2003) *Standard!* London: Carnegie UK Trust Young People Initiative.

Croke, R. and Crowley, A. (eds) (2006) *Righting the Wrongs: The reality of children's rights in Wales*, Cardiff: Save the Children.

Feinstein, C. and O'Kane, C. (2005) *The Spider Tool: A self assessment and planning tool for child led initiatives and organisations*, London: International Save the Children Alliance.

Hart, R. (1992) *Children's Participation: From tokenism to citizenship*, Florence: UNICEF International Child Development Centre.

Kirby, P. with Bryson, S. (2002) *Measuring the Magic*, London: Carnegie UK Trust.

Kirby, P., Laws, S. and Pettitt, B. (2004) 'Assessing the impact of children's participation: A discussion paper towards a new study' (unpublished paper), London: Save the Children.

Lansdown, G. (2006) 'International developments in children's participation: Lessons and challenges', in E. K. M. Tisdall, J. Davis, M. Hill, and A. Prout (eds) *Children, Young People and Social Inclusion: Participation for what?* Bristol: The Policy Press.

Lewis, G. and Thomas, N. (2006) *Report on the Development and Piloting of the Impact Assessment Tool*, Cardiff: Children and Young People's Participation Consortium for Wales.

National Assembly for Wales (2004) *Record of Proceedings/Cofnod* for 14 January.

Percy-Smith, B. (2007) *Evaluating the Development of Young People's Participation Plans in two Children's Trusts (Interim Report Year 1)*, Leicester: National Youth Agency.

Save the Children (2005) *Practice Standards for Children's Participation*, London: International Save the Children Alliance.

Save the Children (2007) *National Standards for Children and Young People's Participation (Wales)*, available at www.savethechildren.org.uk/en/docs/wales_nat_standard.pdf.

Shier, H. (2001) 'Pathways to participation: Openings, opportunities and obligations', *Children & Society* 15: 107–17.

Sinclair, R. (2004) 'Participation in practice: making it meaningful, effective and sustainable', *Children & Society* 18(2): 106–18.

Skeels, A. and Thomas, E. (2007) 'Participation', in R. Croke and A. Crowley (eds) *Stop, Look and Listen*, Cardiff: Save the Children.

Thomas, N. and Crowley, A. (2007) 'Children's rights and wellbeing in Wales', *Contemporary Wales* 19: 161–79.

Tisdall, E. and Bell, R. (2006) 'Included in governance? Children's participation in "public" decision making', in E. K. M. Tisdall, J. Davis, M. Hill, and A. Prout (eds) *Children, Young People and Social Inclusion: Participation for what?* Bristol: The Policy Press.

Treseder, P. (1997) *Empowering Children and Young People: A training manual*, London: Save the Children and Children Right's Office.

Welsh Assembly Government (2005) *The School Councils (Wales) Regulations 2005*, available at www.legislation.hmso.gov.uk/legislation/wales/wsi2005/20053200e.htm.

Welsh Assembly Government (2006) *Young People: Youth work: Youth service*, available at http://new.wales.gov.uk/docrepos/40382/4038232/403829/Consultations/2006/YS-strat-consultation-v1-e.pdf?lang=en.

Commentary 4

Methods and frameworks

Janet Batsleer

Crowley and Skeels direct their focus towards the increasingly pertinent issue of assessing the 'impact' of participation. Over and over again, it has been my experience that for adults, young people's participation is about shaping the services, policies and institutions that adults have provided in the first place. We value the insights that young people bring. At Forty Second Street, the young people's mental health project in Manchester where I have been in various roles, including Chair, on the Board of Trustees for nearly 20 years, we have continually struggled with our understanding of young people's involvement and participation in the life of the organisation, and it is on this experience, as well as on my wider knowledge of youth and community work, that this commentary draws.

One of the biggest issues in participation is the risk of it being seen as 'tokenistic' both by young people themselves and by adults; a replacement for real adult power. The arguments of this chapter are important because they suggest ways in which this fear of tokenism might be addressed, so that children, young people and adults all see the results of their involvement.

Young people tend to emphasise the impact of participation on their personal and social development, the confidence and increased hope that participation brings. Of course, this may be recognised by adults, but its importance is often not really appreciated. If young people are involved, for example in appointing staff and having an equal say in the voting on appointments, this may seem to benefit the organisation most. But the experience of being trusted to make a decision may have a very important impact on the life of the young person. The question of how and why particular young people are encouraged to participate and get involved is an important one too. Facilitators may be wary of involving certain young people. I think about the young people who self-harm who use Forty Second Street, either because they are concerned that they will not be able to cope or because they themselves are frightened that they will not be able to cope, as adults, with mental health issues. Who should be the best judge of the impact of participation on young people themselves? If we create standards and try to generalise the impact of participation through standard bureaucratic and quality control methods, can we be completely confident that this will not have a 'dead hand' effect on a potentially joyful and life-enhancing experience?

Evaluation is necessarily a key element of understanding impact, and the contribution by Vicky Johnson sharpens the focus on the tension between the need to find indicators that can be applied systematically and consistently across programmes and countries and the insights generated when children and young people develop their own examples. By working in ways that are based on the recognition of meaning in the whole lives of children and young people and not just in the aspect which requires assessment, evaluators and researchers can create a fuller understanding of the context for interventions, but they need to develop a very different approach to research processes from those traditionally associated with the distance and objectivity of the researcher. They need to develop styles of facilitation that can be imaginative and fun, and above all dialogic. It is in the 'dialogue days' developed by researchers as a way of developing a deeper understanding of the concerns children have in collaboration with service providers and decision makers, that the challenging and empowering potential of participatory evaluation can be seen. Although the researcher/evaluator in this case uses many of the same skills as the youth and community worker, the role is a different one. But the availability to young people's projects of such researchers and evaluators, with a role sustained over time, while rare, is clearly potentially a source of advocacy for achieving the meaningful participation of young people with adults, and another guard against the charge of tokenism in the processes of participation.

In the chapter by Kränzl-Nagl and Zartler, the lessons from an international project concerned with children's participation in school and community are discussed. Here it is the range of sites of intervention that is so impressive. One of the fears, alongside tokenism, that I have about the 'participation agenda' is that agendas are in the end always the pre-existing agendas of the organisations that seek participation. The involvement in schools, in decision making about budgets for young people's participation in particular communities, the involvement in play; all these attest to the ways in which the places and experiences of immediate significance for young people can be influenced by them, through participation. Most movingly, the cry against child labour from young people in Albania demonstrates the power of participation as a vehicle for self-advocacy. It is important that adult facilitators investigate the frameworks for participation that they offer to young people and do not impose false limitations. Young people have things to say about their lives on a local and a global scale. They both can find ways to improve access to their own project, school or village: be participant members of learning organisations; and can act as members of wider communities, seeking peace, justice, wholeness. I remember a member of a local lesbian and gay project launching a passionate defence of the project at a demonstration challenging Section 28 (which was in force in England at the time, apparently prohibiting the discussion of homosexuality and homosexual relationships in schools). She said, to thousands of people, that it was the weekly support that the project offered, just by being there and enabling her to be a member that had kept her alive. The intensely personal and the broadly political are intimately entwined.

The role of adult facilitators is strongly emphasised in this chapter and the adults involved demonstrate the skills of good youth and community workers (in terms of our UK traditions). They are adults with a 'burning heart' and passionate commitment to young people, who understand children and young people's rights and who can assist, advise and support children and young people who are competent actors in their own lives. Appreciation and recognition of children and young people's competence are fundamental in any challenge to children and young people's invisibility and powerlessness. This is the informal education tradition which emphasises 'starting from strengths'.

This issue of the role of adult facilitators is developed further by Sotkasiira, Haikkola and Horelli. How can we avoid the dangers of developing participation projects which already have a built-in model of what it means to be a good citizen, simply channelling children and young people into a prescribed adult future? Meaningful change needs to be recognised as change in the here and now and on young people's agendas and their terms as well as nurturing hope for the future. The young people's call, reported in this chapter, for 'A joyful North Karelia with survival opportunities for young people' raises once again that interface between the social and political and the personal, and the role of the adult facilitator, the youth and community worker as modelling and enabling the connection between the here and now and the future. The concept of hope offers the bridge between the here and now and the future and it is the practice of arts- and creativity-based work that enables the visions and dreams which are the substance of hope. Creating possibilities where there were no possibilities before must be at the heart of participatory practice which can do more than shore up existing structures, which can melt and dissolve old power relationships in order to create the space for 'the new' to emerge. And 'hope' – which is 'in things not seen' – is also the condition for survival. This is familiar from the work in a young people's mental health project in which, responding to young people's attempted suicide, the role of workers can be understood as creating the conditions of hopefulness, where they have been lost, representing a possible future life to young people when they have lost belief in the possibility of such a future. The development in this chapter of a theoretical model which enables an understanding of systemic change processes as built into participation rather than as a possible outcome is immensely valuable. And it is heartening to an informal educator that it is a 'learning theory' – 'learning-based network approach' – which underpins the model.

The author

Janet Batsleer is currently Principal Lecturer in Youth and Community Work at Manchester Metropolitan University. She has been involved in youth work since the early 1970s and has been involved with young people on the Board of Trustees at Forty Second Street, a community-based resource in Manchester for young people with mental health difficulties, since the early 1990s.

18 'No one ever listens to us'

Challenging obstacles to the participation of children and young people in Rwanda[1]

Kirrily Pells

> We have great resilience to keep going despite everything that has happened. This gives us hope for the future. We have resilience inside. We do not want people to do things for us. We can do it ourselves.

Enshrined in Article 12 of the Convention on the Rights of the Child (CRC), participation is both a right in itself and a means by which other rights should be realised. Despite increasing attempts to mainstream the discourses of rights and participation by non-governmental organisations (NGOs), insufficient attention has been paid to how these principles play out in practice, especially in environments where the concept of child participation is highly complex.

This chapter analyses the ways in which participatory approaches to child and youth programming are operationalised within three Rwandan programmes: CARE International's Nkundabana[2] Initiative for Psychosocial Support (NIPS); Save the Children Fund's (SCF) (2005) rights-based training toolkit; and the NGO–government collaborative National Summit for Children and Young People. First, the chapter considers the barriers to youth participation, internal and external to NGOs, in an environment that is constrained by cultural conservatism, social hierarchy and requirements imposed by donor agencies. Second, it explores how participation is conceived from the perspective of children and young people, and questions how these understandings are translated into practice by the three programmes. Third, in evaluating the different strategies employed by NGOs in meeting these challenges, the chapter argues that success in challenging external obstacles is dependent on the extent of, and importance attached to, child and youth participation within programming cycles and its 'rootedness' in the everyday lives and communities of participants.

'We have life without living': children and young people in post-genocide Rwanda

The impact and enduring legacies of the 1994 genocide and the HIV/AIDS epidemic upon Rwandan children and youth are well documented (Human Rights Watch 2003). Estimates state that 10 per cent of children have lost one or both parents, 110,000 orphans are living in child-headed households (CHHs), 7,000 children live on the streets and 65,000 of 12- to 14-year-olds are affected by HIV/

AIDS (UNICEF et al. 2006). The shattering of social relations has destroyed traditional protective structures, meaning that children are left inadequately supported
in their daily struggles of survival, compounded by the emotional distress caused
by the loss or imprisonment of loved ones.

To address this situation, the government of Rwanda, with the support of international and national NGOs, has incorporated the CRC into national legislation
(in 2001) and created a National Policy for Orphans and Vulnerable Children
(OVC), implemented through the National Plan of Action. Reflecting the international drive towards rights-based programming, which views rights as both the
means and the end of the development process, the National Policy for OVC
endorses a community-based approach to address the situation of the most vulnerable children through involving 'the community and children in the research of
solutions and decision-making' (MINALOC, 2004: 7).

The mainstreaming of participatory language by both the government and
NGOs stands in stark contrast to the country's sociocultural context. Rwandan
society is strongly hierarchical and lacks space for public debate. Rights discourse
is accompanied by an emphasis on obedience to authorities, reflective more of the
African Charter on the Rights and Welfare of the Child, in which children's rights
are counterbalanced by responsibilities to family, community and nation, than of
the CRC.

Within communities there is recognition that children have rights, but these are
not seen as absolute. There is a greater acceptance of survival and development
rights than of rights to participation and decision making (UNICEF et al. 2006:
42–4), which are viewed largely as the prerogative of being an adult. Economic
constraints and emotional problems are also cited:

> The CRC is irrelevant on the ground because of poverty and people do not
> have resources. Parents know what children need but they are not able to
> provide it. Also they are wounded and not able to take care of their children,
> they do not see that their children need attention, as they are withdrawn in
> their own hurts.
>
> (Pastor)

Yet children identify the right to participation as the most important to
implement (Save the Children Rwanda 2005). Participation is seen both as a
right in itself and, more importantly for the young people, as a means to access
other rights.

'They come, talk with us, leave, then we never hear from them again': children's understandings and experiences of participation

Individual interviews and focus group discussions with children and young people
revealed that the majority felt they did not have the opportunity to participate:
'They can bring you a jumper when you don't even have an exercise book! They

decide for us without having asked.' This was more pronounced among rural youth – 'Development is taking place so rapidly that many are being left behind. Western donors could play a role in helping rural areas to participate in the process' – and children living on their own – 'Our rights are not fulfilled because of poverty and being orphans. No one listens to us.'

Interestingly, children did not use the language of participation directly, in terms of wanting 'to participate'. Instead, emerging from the discussions were two distinct forms of participatory practice. The first I have called 'performed participation'. This is drawn from children's portrayal of participation as an activity extraordinary to their daily lives, often taking the form of consultation and involving the language of listening and being heard. 'There were workers who came and asked us if we had mosquito nets, if we had a radio, if we ate meat … .' The majority of young people were in agreement that this was a one-off event, rarely followed up:

> They come, talk with us, leave, then we never hear from them again.

This lack of follow-up, or being really heard, has promoted a level of scepticism among the young of the motives of those using the language of rights and participation. 'Are the UN people here to help or for business?' asked one focus group participant. It also ignores many children's desire to have a greater say in the running of programmes and to build collaborative relationships with NGOs:

> People should come to ask for our opinions. NGOs which assist children can come to consult us, we are ready to give our contribution of ideas …

stated one girl, in a sentiment echoed across the focus groups.

However, 'performed participation' is not without value. Children worldwide argue that adults do not listen to them, but in post-genocide Rwanda the adults are often not actually there at all. This creates an ambiguous position. Children have 'adult' positions – caring for siblings by being heads of households, but without involvement in the community decision-making processes to address the problems that they are facing. This is exacerbated by stigma towards orphans and CHHs. The lack of participation in the community is reflected within households, where younger siblings report not being consulted by older siblings: 'Alice is my mother and my father. I am like a baby as Alice is the parents.' For the head of the household, however, this position as decision maker is frequently burdensome: 'It is hard as I must always be the strong one. My sister is always crying, but crying does not bring solutions.'

Therefore, being visited and consulted by outsiders is important. Yet, as will be argued in the following section, this form of participation is open to manipulation and is not entirely suited to addressing the everyday realities faced by children and young people. Instead, children advocate a second type of participation, which I have termed 'lived participation'. Rooted in the structures and activities of daily life, 'lived participation' is part of an ongoing series of supportive relationships and is used as a means of accessing other rights, so enabling those who have been marginalised to achieve an oft-repeated desire of becoming 'like the other children'.

'The participation of children should be the central strategy'[3]

Three programmes have been selected here, to illustrate how, despite each one advocating the use of participatory approaches to securing children's rights, the framing of the programmes (in terms of language and design) and their operationalisation (in terms of programme direction and types of activities) differ greatly. In addition, the three programmes represent the two types of participation identified from the focus group discussion reported above: the National Summit embodying 'performed participation'; NIPS demonstrating 'lived participation'; and the rights-based toolkit forming a hybrid of the two.

The National Policy for OVC established that there should be an annual National Summit for children and young people.[4] It is organised by the Ministry in Charge of Family and Gender Promotion (MIGEPROF) in conjunction with a steering committee headed by UNICEF and comprising international and national NGOs. One child from every sector is peer-elected to attend a series of preparatory meetings followed by a two-day event where delegates are given the opportunity to present their opinions, ideas and concerns to various government and NGO representatives. Each year has a theme for discussion and the 2007 summit focused on the participation of children and young people in the economic development of Rwanda. The language of rights and participation was at the forefront of the summit. The minister opening the summit stated that 'children are not beneficiaries but partners' in the development of the country and delegates were encouraged to 'speak up for yourselves, advocate for your rights. Don't expect others to come and do it for you as they might not do.'

NIPS, implemented by CARE Rwanda, is framed by a mixture of rights-based and psychosocial language. Children are asked to identify CHHs in the community where the oldest sibling is under 21.[5] Those children then nominate persons in the community whom they trust to become *Nkundabana*. Trained as volunteers, *Nkundabana* provide guidance and care for children living without adult support through regular home visits. The participants receive sensitisation on health matters and the dangers of HIV/AIDS, empowerment on rights issues, and economic and social support through youth associations and guilds. The associations of CHH, supported by the *Nkundabana*, meet regularly with local authorities to present their problems. CARE uses a participatory monitoring tool where participants are asked questions every four months to give feedback on the project, contribute ideas and suggest future directions (Jones 2005).

SCF's rights toolkit provides training for children and youth, as well as for adults (parents, community members and those in positions of authority at local and national levels). Using participatory methods, the toolkit aims to adapt rights concepts to the Rwandan reality and the situation of participants. Children and adults are trained in using the toolkit by SCF staff and voluntary child rights facilitators. The children (peer-elected) then form child rights forums and the adults establish child protection committees. The latter support the former in devising their own strategies to secure their rights and make their voices heard. Although the creation of forums is more akin to 'performed participation', because these take place in the local community and involve children, adults and those in authority from the community, I have described this as a hybrid of 'lived' and 'performed' participation.

'Authorities didn't care about our problems but today they do listen to us': evaluating participation

If programmes are truly rights-based and participatory, then the perspectives of the child and youth participants must be prioritised in evaluating the outcomes. In comparing the three programmes discussed here it is questioned whether one form of participation is more successful than the others. The focus is on three intertwined, central issues: agency and meaningful engagement; relationships and the community; accountability and transparency.

Meaningful engagement

All three programmes created spaces in which children could be listened to, but whether they were engaged meaningfully and really heard was another matter. Despite the heavy use of participatory language at the National Summit, the children sit in rows, listening to very long presentations by government officials and then have the opportunity to ask questions at the end. However, this is until the children express something contrary to government rhetoric. One child stated: 'We children who have our parents in prison we do not like the Government of National Unity. We want the government to help us like the others.' This child was severely rebuked for a long time by the representative of the National Commission of Human Rights for propagating genocidal ideology. By speaking against the government and advocating on behalf of those with parents held in prison either charged with or sentenced for committing acts of genocide, the child was being accused of invoking the divisionism which led to the 1994 genocide. Likewise, when children reported that parents were selling their children as slaves to other households, they were rebuked firmly by ministers and told that slavery did not exist in Rwanda. Thus there was a feeling among some children that this type of event is just a performance; as one said, it is a substitute for 'real action' as 'talking does not bring change'.

This highlights not only the great discrepancy that can exist between participation in theory and in practice, but that participation should not be considered as an aspect of programming or an isolated strategy, but as an integral aspect of daily life, whereby through participating in a programme children can gain more control over their everyday lives. In turn, this means giving ownership of and control over programme direction to the young participants. This requires that NGOs are flexible in terms of management, which can clash with donor requirements for predetermined outcomes. For example, CARE had to determine resources, participant numbers and strategies before knowing the amount of work and resources needed within the programme. Yet, where possible, CARE has attempted to build in flexibility in the allocation of key resources, through community consultations. Thus, meaningful participation facilitates the agency of children.

Relationships and community

Regarding relationships and the community, SCF's approach achieves the greatest flexibility among the programmes in engaging with community problems on the ground, as they arise. Children have direction over the programme, as they decide what to work on and how to go about it. However, the forum places additional burdens on children's already limited free time, and children need to be supported in what they are doing. At the moment the child protection committees are not showing as much initiative as the child rights forums. So far, the children have managed to get some out-of-school youth back into education, provide rights training to their peers and report abuse to local authorities. One forum was even approached by parents who were having difficulties in getting their children to help around the house. Forum members explained to these children their rights and responsibilities, and it was reported that they are no longer idle around the home!

Members of the rights forums encountered resistance from some parents in allowing their children to attend the peer-led child rights training sessions. As noted earlier, suspicion is rife in Rwandan society. This illustrates the importance of involving the wider community in a programme, not just the target group. Moreover, children cannot secure the protection and fulfilment of rights on their own. At the National Summit a number of delegates reported abuse in their communities but were told to go to their head teachers. Yet, as one child commented:

> We fear head teachers more than the army, police and parents. We want a free phone line to report what we see.

In contrast, NIPS demonstrates that engaging the wider community through the programme can bring about a shift in attitude towards child rights and participation, reduce resentment towards participants, and create local ownership and programme sustainability. A participant reported 'most of the times when one had a problem and she told it to neighbours they didn't help, but today they help us'. Involving the community in the selection of participants helped to prevent jealousy, as it ensured that the criteria were clear and that there was agreement over who were the most vulnerable. A *Nkundabana* commented that 'initially people wanted integration of their children in the programme. But when they got explanations, they understood that the project concerned only vulnerable children.' However, there is room for improvement, as participants were described by some community members as 'CARE's children' and a participant explained that 'since we are in this *Nkundabana* programme, people don't give us anything. They say we have become rich. They used to give us food.'

Accountability and transparency

The importance of relationships to young people has already been discussed, but in evaluating the programmes the critical factor was not just the existence of relationships, but their quality in terms of accountability and transparency. Greater attention needs to be paid to the nature of relationships between NGOs and children, particularly in terms of better communication and transparency in decision-making processes and resource allocation. This was demonstrated clearly by NIPS. Several participants stated that CARE 'promised to build us houses but they did it to only some of us others we are still waiting'. According to CARE staff, this was never an integral part of the NIPS programme, but for participants it was not clear why some children received houses and others did not. In contrast, when children were involved in the decision making and understood the actions undertaken, there was less resentment:

> Even though they gave radios to girls alone, they explained to us that they are more at risk to have problems than boys, especially when they come from neighbours where they go to listen to radio at night, because they can be attacked and raped.

Youth participants also suggested reforming the selection criteria for NIPS, arguing that some households might have one parent but be just as vulnerable, due to poverty, alcoholism, HIV/AIDS etc., as those without adult support. Incorporating the concerns and ideas of youth in programme design and operation makes it more relevant to the priorities and needs of these young people. In addition, the meetings with local authorities give children and young people opportunities to call to account those responsible for respecting and fulfilling their rights:

> We used to have problems of where to go to claim our rights, but now the authorities listen to us and help us.

'We want to be the creators of solutions'

Children are agents of social change and desire greater scope for participation within their daily lives. Participation is viewed as a skill that can be used in daily life to access other rights and create space for voices to be heard. The most successful context for this to occur is in building protective and participatory relationships in the community through 'lived participation'. Participatory practice cannot be imposed from the top downwards, or it will be met with resistance from the community. Nor is successful programming focused on children in isolation, but rather in their everyday environments and relationships. While there is scope for consultations to provide a platform for children's ideas and opinions, to avoid becoming 'performed participation' they must be rooted in everyday life and relationships, such as regular meetings between local authorities and youth, rather than one-off events that are not followed up. Finally, there is a need for a greater linkage between participation as means and end. This not only achieves more successful outcomes, as children are experts in their own lives, but it also overcomes resistance if communities are involved in devising solutions. NGOs must be clear in communicating what are the aims and objectives of programmes, so as to avoid raised expectations and disaffection, and should be aware of the dangers of participatory rhetoric.

Acknowledgements

The author wishes to thank the School of Advanced Study for funding the doctoral research, and the Central Research Fund, University of London, for partially funding fieldwork in Rwanda. In addition, the author offers sincere appreciation for the cooperation and support of Save the Children UK; CARE International and colleagues Tonya Thurman and Joseph Ntaganira with whom NIPS was evaluated; Professor Paul Gready for his valuable comments and support; and, above all, the children and young people of Rwanda for their warmth and generosity. Opinions expressed here are those of the author and do not necessarily reflect those of the organisations listed.

Notes

1. All quotations are taken from interviews and focus groups conducted in Rwanda, March–May 2006 and July–August 2007, unless otherwise stated.
2. A Kinyarwanda word meaning 'I love children'.
3. NGO staff member.
4. So far, due to logistical constraints, summits have been held in 2004, 2006 and 2007.
5. The age of majority in Rwanda is 21.

References

Human Rights Watch (2003) *Lasting Wounds: Consequences of genocide and war*, New York: Human Rights Watch, available at www.hrw.org/reports/2003/rwanda0403, accessed 1 September 2004.

Jones, A. (2005) 'The case of CARE International in Rwanda', in P. Gready and J. Ensor (eds) *Reinventing Development? Translating rights-based approaches from theory into practice*, London: Zed Books: pp. 79–98.

MINALOC (2004) *National Policy for Orphans and Vulnerable Children*, available at www.unicef.org/southafrica/SAF_resources_ovcrwanda.doc, accessed 30 August 2008.

Save the Children Rwanda (2005) *The Right to Protection. Training and mobilisation kit for child rights and protection. Toolkit for children, toolkit for adults and trainers guide*, London: Save the Children.

UNICEF and The African Child Policy Forum (2006) *What Children and Youth Think: Rwanda. A statistical presentation of opinions and perceptions of children and youth in Rwanda*, Nairobi: The African Child Policy Forum, www.africanchildforum.org/Documents/Rwanda.pdf, accessed 30 January 2008.

19 Child reporters as agents of change

Lalatendu Acharya

Introduction

Nila Chalan has an infectious smile and an indomitable will – which helped her to become the second girl from her village to study in 7th grade, an achievement in itself. Nila is well known too, in the higher echelons of the district's official circles, as the girl who made her village a success in sanitation and hygiene programmes. Nila, leading the team of child reporters, talked with the villagers and campaigned for total sanitation and hygiene in her village (Plate 19.1).

The villagers were defecating in the open fields. The child reporters discussed, reflected on and understood the importance of cleanliness and they approached the villagers to construct toilets in the village. After repeated persuasion, the villagers constructed toilets in their houses. These child reporters paid regular visits to the construction sites and encouraged their completion. The child reporters also wrote reports about the village's sanitation in their newsletter and spoke about it in conferences. Soon, Nila's village had a toilet in every house. No wonder Nila and the child

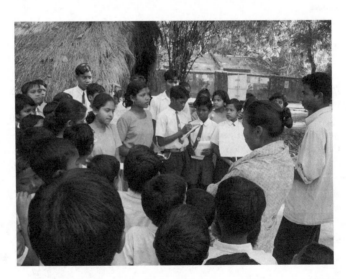

Plate 19.1 Nila and other child reporters in the field. Copyright: Lalatendu Acharya

reporters are consulted in matters of their village's development. There are many stories of change, with girls like Nila and her friends in the village of Koraput. What binds them together is that all of them are *child reporters* from Orissa in India.

Child participation has become the focus of a multitude of initiatives for and with children, as a result of the Convention on the Rights of the Child. Involving children as democratic citizens has been a long journey, and still continues. The importance of children as decision makers has achieved acceptance in the corporate world of consumer marketing and advertising, where agencies design their ads primarily to influence children. But involving children in social sector development programmes is still at a rudimentary stage. Development professionals acknowledge the rationale for children's participation, but building it into work plans has been harder to realise. Understanding of child participation differs widely across the spectrum. And so does the actual process of involvement, as work plan priorities, funds, goals, outcomes, objectively verifiable indicators and impact analysis take centre stage. It is also increasingly common in many organisations, both governmental and non-governmental, to involve children as poster material to attract media attention, only for children to be relegated to backstage once the purpose has been accomplished.

As a result, in 2006 the chief minister of the state of Orissa in India banned the involvement of children in welcoming ceremonies for visiting dignitaries. The involvement of the state chief did bring changes in Orissa, but bringing about social and organisational change needs much more by way of concerted effort from the people themselves. One of the challenges involves organisations and programme managers reflecting upon and clarifying the purposes of involving children and the roles that adults and children play.

For the development worker with a mandate for children's development, certain questions crop up regularly:

- As communicators, programme managers, knowledge workers, do we listen to children?
- Is it important that we listen to them?
- Do children know their needs, or do they need us as experts for a safe and healthy life?
- Can our communication campaign and programme deliverables be exclusive of children?

To address these questions and to help children participate in a meaningful way, the child reporters came into being. The child reporters are an intrepid band of children, 5,000 strong and growing, who report on development issues in their villages, and monitor and communicate about the process of development – or lack of it – in their milieux.

The child reporters write about their homes, their villages, people in their villages, their understanding of the world around them and their dreams. These cadres of child reporters have developed into a growing force to be reckoned with in the development landscape of Orissa. The initiative, which started with 100 children in the remote tribal district Koraput, has spread across the state of Orissa.

The concept of child reporters

The Child Reporters project was conceived with children in Orissa. The leading concern in framing the idea of the child reporter was to ensure the meaningful participation of children. There have been numerous projects involving children across the spectrum of development activities in different regions of the world, with varying degrees of participation and engagement. Children and women form the most vulnerable sections of society and are invariably at the weaker end of the power equation. Experience in regular and emergency programming situations reveals that it's the children who suffer most.

The challenge was not only to support the participation of children, but also to ensure genuine participation of children from marginalised groups and families who are poor, who live in difficult circumstances and who have little access to mainstream resources. The context in Orissa posed unique challenges. If we examine the development paradigms, it is usually the wealthy or the better-educated who have access to better resources. They are the first to pick up new services or subsidies, and the first to take up opportunities to influence plans. The poorest children are most likely to be denied the right and opportunity to make their views heard. In conceiving the Child Reporters initiative, the challenge lay in this important question of inclusion: how do we involve the poorest and most under-privileged children in the process of child participation?

The child reporter concept evolved from an initiative with children that the author undertook while working as the communications officer for UNICEF Orissa in 2004. The process involved training groups of children from different schools in basic news reporting skills, involving them in discussions regarding development, and inspiring their thinking on development issues (Plate 19.2).

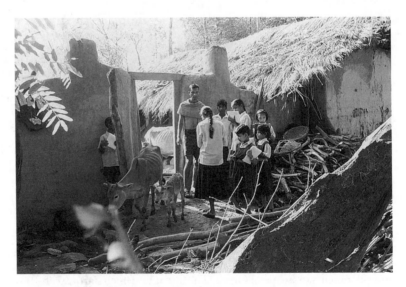

Plate 19.2 Exploring development issues in the village. Copyright: Lalatendu Acharya

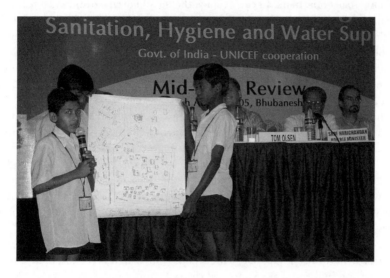

Plate 19.3   Child reporters presenting their findings. Copyright: Lalatendu Acharya

Five schools – both private and government administered – were selected in the state capital where the medium of instruction varied between English, Hindi and the local language Oriya. The mix was purposely designed to involve children from different backgrounds and environments and with a variety of skill sets. The children's groups from the five schools were given orientation and training by media and development professionals. They then developed topics and went out on reporting assignments. Finally, the children presented their reports in front of a high-level group comprising the Chief Minister; the Senior State Secretaries for Education, Women and Child Development; the Chief Secretary; the media and other stakeholders (Plate 19.3). The children had a platform to air their views on issues and topics they had thought of themselves rather than as part of an adult-led organisational agenda.

The children developed their thinking about the issues and, through their analysis, were able to bring different perspectives. It was fascinating to experience the level of empowerment in the children when they were given the freedom to choose their subjects and report on them. This was the early development of the Child Reporters initiative. In 2005 the Child Reporters project became located in Koraput, following an agreement between UNICEF and the district administration to carry out development projects there.

The development of child reporters as agents of change

The Child Reporters project started by selecting 100 children, ten from each of the ten schools and villages in Koraput, in consultation with the district authorities and civil society partners. In each village the ten children constituted a team with a team leader, supported by a capable local teacher from the village school. The children were from primary (Grade 1 to Grade 5) and upper primary (Grade 1 to Grade 7) schools, in the age group of 8 to 14 years. All the children were selected from their respective schools by the teachers, the parent teacher association of the school and the children themselves. The selection process was facilitated by the local NGO partners.

The children had two orientation workshops on the broad issues of development in Orissa: their district, their village, their life; and on journalism and reporting. After the initial orientation, each month, there were re-energising/reinforcing visits and discussions with the teams in their villages. The children noted down their daily observations and thoughts in detail in diaries. All the child reporters had writing skills, albeit of different levels. They proactively collected and noted down the views and thoughts of other children in the school who were not part of the team and who could not express themselves in writing.

The diaries were collected and the best writings were put together in the form of a monthly newsletter, 1,000 copies of which were circulated to the top decision makers of the state and district, to the media and to key NGOs. The selection of writings for the newsletter was done by the local facilitating group, which was careful to ensure that most reports were given a place in the newsletters. These reports, their content, quality and selection were constantly discussed with the child reporters during the facilitators' re-energising/rein-forcing visits. The children made special presentations of their reports in different forums. A group of interested children from the teams was selected, given basic information about audio-visual equipment, and provided with a cameraman to document a developmental process called Village Based Planning.

In 2005, the 100 children wrote their daily diaries, published five issues of their bi-monthly newsletter, interviewed a variety of people and made one film documentary on the village-based planning process. They participated in numerous conferences, represented the state at national conferences and represented the country at an international conference in China.

The most important point to note is that all of this was accomplished mostly by tribal children from a remote part of India where they had never seen a train or a television, or stayed at a hotel, and who had never been to any big places outside their villages. For children who were shy and unable to speak fluently at the initial sessions, developing and making independent presentations was a huge achievement. The process gained support, appreciation and the gradual involvement of many stakeholders, notably the media and government function-aries. Government support in these processes was vital in providing sustainability. Government resources were the largest in India, and the involvement of the Education Department meant that there were opportunities for incorporating the child participation process into regular school activities, contributing to the development of participatory learning processes in the schools. In 2006, the process expanded to all fourteen blocks of Koraput, with participation by around 1,500 children from over 200 schools.

In addition to writing their diaries, the children also began to communicate by postcard so that their reports would reach the district administration in time. In July 2006 the child reporters group established a blog to air its views on a wider platform (www.childreporters.blogspot.com). In 2007, the initiative expanded to include out-of-school children (25 per cent of total), and it grew further to include more than 5,000 children across 519 villages and two local urban areas, involving 539 schools in Koraput.

One imperative was to get the buy-in of an increasing number of stakeholders to the process of listening to children and children's participation, and to move up the ladder of participation from tokenism towards real participation. The other imperative was to create a framework in Koraput whereby the ownership of the process rested with multiple stakeholders and the children themselves, so that it was sustainable.

Reports from the intrepid child reporters of Orissa

The child reporters' reports provide us with insights that we would not have had in the normal course of work. They span perspectives from their schools, their homes, their villages, on government schemes, on incidents near their villages, on their trips to nearby towns, on issues that impress them, on issues that irk them and so on. Some examples are provided here.

> The roof of our school leaks in the rainy season. There is no toilet or play-ground in our school. We face problems.
>
> (Sunita Gemel, 11-year-old girl, Maliput village)

> There are many children in our village. But half of them do not go to school. Parents send them to guard the cattle. Children are punished if they do not obey them.
>
> (Kumar Muduli, 10-year-old boy, Murkar village)

> People in our village do not use mosquito nets. They also suffer as there is no hospital in the village.
>
> (Sibaram Pangi, 11-year-old boy, Deopottangi)

> The Government planted saplings in our village, but they did not survive as they were planted towards the end of the monsoon.
>
> (Chinmayi Subudhi, 9-year-old girl)

> I was taking the cattle herd up the hill for grazing when I came across this old man. He was from Sanatalguda village. He said since he is single and stays with his nephews, they are exploiting him. They take away all his old age pension. Earlier, he used to weave fishing-nets to earn some money but can't do it now as his eyesight is getting weaker by the day.

So reports Bibhuti Majhi, a 10-year-old boy from Gangrajpur village, adding:

Is sacrifice necessary to appease the gods? I feel for the animals that are sacrificed. Today the villagers have gone to Pottangi hills to give offerings and pray to goddess Gangma with hens, goats and pigeons. Does the goddess really seek sacrifice?

I learnt from the villagers that a few days ago a woman and her new-born baby died after not getting the proper diet. Girls do not go to schools in this village. Our village is in a forested area but roads are bad. Infant mortality is high here. The health workers can help curb it.

(Shankar Muduli, 10-year-old boy, Murkar)

And the reports continue to flow. By reading them, programme managers, NGOs, media, government functionaries, parents and teachers listen to the voices and learn. As it was aptly put by the then District Collector of Koraput, 'The child reporters' reports give us feedback as to how the government programmes are faring at grassroots level.' The reports are discussed in many of the government coordination meetings. As narrated by Santakar, a media person and one of the key civil society collaborators of the Child Reporters initiative, 'A child was seriously injured in an accident in Maliput village of Pottangi Block. The parents had left the child in the hands of local traditional healers. But the child reporters were not convinced and they called us. Based on the request of the child reporters, the administration treated the child free of cost. The Chief District Medical Officer of the district also took note and acted on other reports from the children of diarrhoea, malnutrition and disabled people in their villages.'

The child reporters demonstrated that there was much that we did not see or address in our programme design and delivery, and that did not find space in our

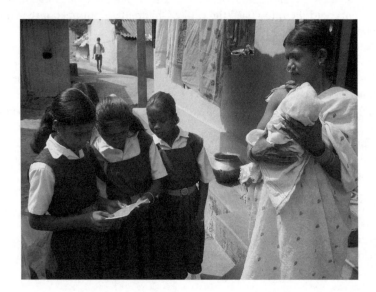

Plate 19.4 Collecting news with a mother and baby. Copyright: Lalatendu Acharya

---

Box 19.1 Pollama's story and the blind boy from Dangarpaunsi

The child reporters of Sunki Primary school in Koraput district persuaded a girl to resume her schooling after she had discontinued her studies for two years. The girl, Pollama, had left school after her father died in order to help her mother with the work of the household. Slowly, she forgot her studies and did not want to come to school any more, as she felt ashamed. The child reporters of Sunki got to know about her, talked with her, and by convincing Pollama and her mother ensured that she began to attend school again.

The children from a school in Dangarpaunsi village visited Koraput to attend a child reporters' workshop. They saw a school for the blind near the workshop venue and they talked to the children and the authorities, including the teachers, about the process of admission. When they returned to their village they visited the home of a child who had been blind since birth and had never been to school. They talked about the facilities that were available for blind children in the special school at Koraput and urged the parents to enrol the child. The parents enrolled their child in the school.

---

work plans, forecasts and outcome statements. The child reports highlighted the basic necessity of our listening to the voices of children if we wanted to make a difference in their lives.

This case study reveals that there are many points in both Pollama's returning to school and the blind child being enrolled that the teachers and programme managers could not have addressed in the yearly back-to-school campaigns. As Upendra Banka, a fearless 11-year-old boy child reporter from remote Gangrajpur village, related of his best report:

> The best was that when we had written on the bad condition of our village road and the road connecting our village with block headquarters Pottangi. It had come to our mind when one of our friends fell and injured himself on the muddy road. We all wrote the same report and wished if it could be repaired. Our BDO [Block Development Officer, equivalent to the chief government officer of the block administrative unit] read the news and we also spoke to him when he visited our village. He was nice and repaired the road. We felt happy as everyone in the village had said Child Reporters *Jindabad* [Hail the child reporters!].

Reflections on the child reporters: success and limitations

The Child Reporters initiative experienced significant successes, but also had its share of challenges. The process had significant impact for the children, the community, the government and wider society. The schoolteachers and parents found that the children benefited individually by being child reporters. Their school attendance and interest in their studies improved, and so did their handwriting, speaking skills, inquisitiveness, outlook, knowledge about the outside world and, most importantly, confidence. The children learned the art of asking questions, and more children in the schools were interested in becoming child reporters.

One particular teacher reflected on the experience of the child reporters by relating the story of Nilambar. Nilambar (a boy aged 12) was a passive and below-average student, and many had worried whether he would be successful in the public examination. But somehow he was chosen to become a child reporter. The child who used to sit in the back row came to the front, asked questions and came forward to lead the work in the school. He had heard in some meeting of the child reporters that in order to write ten words one has to read at least fifty words. That created a great impression on him. To write his report in the most correct manner, he started reading the textbooks aloud, asking fellow children to identify his mistakes. One visit to Delhi to meet with other children was enough to kindle even greater hope for his progress. He graduated from school with fairly good marks in the Grade 7 public examination.

At the governance level, the district authorities treated the child reporters' news-letter with respect, as a feedback tool. Some remarked that it served as a monitoring tool and gave them a first-hand account of their schemes and of their work at the village level. The children's reports found a place in the district and block review meetings. District programme managers such as the Chief District Medical Officer, the Executive Engineer (Water and Sanitation), the District Education Officer and the District Social Welfare Officer (responsible for mother and child nutrition and development) read the reports and factored them into their ongoing activities. The Executive Engineer sent supplies and repaired many village hand-pumps on the basis of the children's reports. At a societal level, the process impacted on all pillars of society. The media persons in the district felt the project had been highly successful in highlighting the situation of children and women, and of village development in general, and developed their own stories based on the child reporters' reports.

Recognising the potential and effectiveness of the child reporters, the UNICEF India country office replicated the initiative in 2006 in all UNICEF-supported states in India. Three other government district managers have also initiated the child reporters process in their own areas in Orissa.

However, there continue to be some tough challenges. Many of the reports get lost on the way to the desks of the district managers or in the course of the work. Frequent changes of government programme managers also affect the child reporters, as new incumbents have to learn about the initiative. Schoolteachers are important partners, but are also overburdened with administrative duties. The process is weakened when child reporters graduate to higher classes and enter other institutes of learning apart from the schools. The reports are also noticeably thin during examination time and summer/winter breaks.

A key challenge involves factoring the children's participation as reporters into development agency programme planning and implementation. Child participation is often viewed as a secondary objective in comparison to immunisation, sanitation and hygiene, education and emergency response. This has been a critical

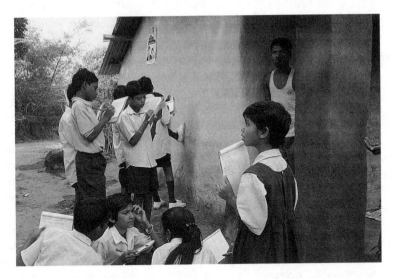

Plate 19.5   Investigating and discussing issues in the village. Copyright: Lalatendu
   Acharya

challenge, and efforts have been made to integrate child participation into the
achievement of all other programme goals.

Two critical issues from the very beginning have been those of the child
reporters' security and the sustainability of the process. Many of the children's
reports put them at risk both at school and also within their communities. There
have been instances where the schoolteachers have felt threatened by the children's reports on the quality of education and the overall condition of the schools.
Similarly, community members have felt threatened by reports of alcoholism
and the improper use of community and school funds. While it has been good
to get the real picture, from a transparent source at grassroots level, the child
reporters' security raises a challenge. Finally, there is the critical issue of sustaining
momentum when funds from UNICEF cease.

To address these issues, there was a concerted effort from the beginning to
house the child reporters process within a supportive network based locally in
the district. The network that was formed, the PGCD Koraput (People's Group
of Children's Development), consisted of local professionals (teachers, doctors,
government programme managers and local politicians), other NGOs, youth and
children. The network spans the district and the individual villages. The PGCD
strengthens itself by constantly learning about and discussing meaningful child
participation and advocating for it across district forums. The network has also
recruited other child advocates to ensure that the child reporters are supported
and protected. Additionally, for security reasons, the child reporters' reports are
published anonymously. Over time, the PGCD has grown and organisations
other than UNICEF have expressed an interest in funding or supporting the
Child Reporters initiative. One of the greatest achievements has been gaining

the buy-in of the district Education Department to strengthen child participation activities.

Conclusion: the way ahead

The Child Reporters project provides a way for children to be active participants in the development of their communities. While not without difficulties, the Child Reporters initiative has provided important learning about ways forward in meeting the challenges of child participation. The most important aspect of these experiences has been to build on small successes within village communities. In Orissa, the process has been replicated in three other districts by the government Education Department, in partnership with local organisations, and these offer further advocacy and opportunities for child participation. So far, the child reporters process has been unable to tap into the tremendous potential of children who are out of school, of street children, or of children in other vulnerable circumstances. Ultimately, the child-reporter approach can provide all children with a forum for participation that can accommodate their different faculties and skills of expression. Increasing access to the internet in remote areas provides an opportunity to connect worldwide, and enables a unique forum for child reporters to present their reports and interact with the wider world.

20 'Pathways to participation' revisited

Learning from Nicaragua's child coffee workers

Harry Shier

Introduction

Work on children and young people's participation in the UK (and other northern countries) has tended to focus on one specific aspect, namely consulting children and young people around their use of public services. Much analysis has focused on labelling different modes and models through which such participation may be facilitated. The author's own 'pathways to participation' model is an example (Shier 2001; see also Kirby et al. 2003; Sinclair 2004).

By contrast, organisations working with children and young people in the global south, where there are few if any public services to access, have often taken different approaches, coming up with different models of practice, supporting and promoting more varied and developed forms of participation. In this context, children and young people are widely recognised as 'public actors', capable of influencing development (see for example Liebel 2007; O'Kane and Karkara 2007).

My experience of working with child coffee-plantation workers in Nicaragua for the past seven years (2001–8) has revealed how narrow was the concept of child participation that I had brought from my previous work in the UK.

This chapter will describe how children and young people organise and participate in Nicaragua's coffee plantations and surrounding rural communities, and how the team of community education workers at the local NGO CESESMA (Centre for Education in Health and Environment) supports and facilitates them. Analysing this experience can help us to identify some of the elements needed to construct a more comprehensive model of children and young people's participation and, as a result, be able to implement and facilitate a wider range of participation processes.

Children's life and work in Nicaragua's coffee sector

Some of the world's finest coffee is grown in the remote mountains of northern Nicaragua, where extreme poverty and dependence on coffee production lead to a high incidence of child labour and associated social problems. The Nicaraguan coffee industry employs many thousands of child workers who work long hours in difficult and dangerous conditions, receiving little or no payment for their efforts. Almost all drop out of school early, while some have no opportunity to go to school at all. The globalised coffee market has little respect for the rights, much

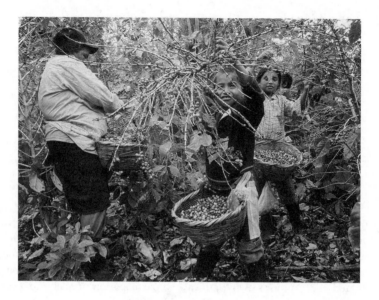

Plate 20.1 Children picking coffee at Hacienda La Isla. Copyright: CESESMA

less the dreams, of these children. The consequence is a cycle of dependency, hunger and destitution in these remote mountain communities.

Nicaragua has, on the face of it, a legislative framework well constructed to support children and young people's participation, starting with the constitution, which gives full legal force to the United Nations Convention on the Rights of the Child. This is further institutionalised in the Children's Legal Code (1998), and the Citizen Participation Law (2003). These laws provide for children and young people to have voice and representation in various local governance spaces, including school councils and municipal children's and youth committees. In Nicaragua, however, what the law permits and what the people in reality have access to are very different. Children's right to participate may be guaranteed in law, but, for this to be meaningful, it must be actively demanded and defended at every turn.

CESESMA

CESESMA is an independent non-governmental organisation working with children and young people in this region. It was founded in 1992 as an environmental education action group and incorporated as a not-for-profit voluntary organisation in 1998. All CESESMA's management and staff are Nicaraguans, with the sole exception of this author, and most are local people.

CESESMA's mission statement is 'To promote and defend the rights of children and young people, through processes of awareness-raising, reflection and action in partnership with rural children and young people, and other members of the community.' CESESMA has also adopted a statement of shared vision which is of: 'Children and young people with greater self-esteem; with opportunities for an integrated education; taking control of their own development; capable of organising themselves to defend their rights and able to contribute to finding solutions for the social, environmental and cultural problems affecting their communities.' Important elements here are that children and young people are 'taking control of their own development' and are considered 'capable of organising themselves'. If they aren't already doing so, this vision implies a firm belief that they have the potential to do so, given a facilitative and supportive environment.

CESESMA's strategy of training and development of Young Community Education Activists (*promotores* and *promotoras*)

At the centre of CESESMA's strategy is the training and support of young community education activists (*promotores* and *promotoras* in Spanish). *Promotores/as*, typically aged 12–18, are young people trained to run out-of-school learning groups with younger children in their communities. This gives them a leadership role and a platform for active organisation and engagement in community development activities and direct action in defence of children's rights, through which they influence political processes at different levels.

The process of training and development of a *promotor/a* typically has five stages which are described below. To bring them to life, we will follow the personal stories of two young people, Deybi and Heyling, both of whom picked coffee on the plantations from an early age, and were aged 16 when interviewed in November 2007.

Stage 1: Children from age 6 upwards join out-of-school activity groups in their village community, which are run by already-trained and experienced promotores/as

Groups currently active are:

- organic farming and environmental action groups
- folk-dance groups
- mural-painting group
- young radio reporters' team
- youth theatre groups
- crafts groups: sewing and dress making, crochet, macramé
- girls' groups (all the other groups are mixed; the girls' groups exist specifically to give girls and young women their own space to work on issues of identity, gender, sexual and reproductive health and women's rights).

School is generally during the mornings only. Although most children work on coffee plantations, on family small-holdings, in domestic work or all three, they can generally organise their time so they can participate in activities that interest them. All activities are free and all participation is voluntary. There is no advertising, as village communities are small and information spreads by word of mouth. Children who join these groups and attend regularly gain new skills, build friendships and grow in confidence and self-esteem. There are often noticeable improvements in their school work. It is important to stress that all the above-mentioned groups are organised and led by the young people themselves, not by adults, the only exception being two newly formed theatre groups.

CESESMA encourages the *promotores/as* who run these groups to talk with children about their rights: how, where and by whom their rights are not respected, and what they, as children and young people, can do about it.

Following the personal stories of Heyling and Deybi: in 1999 Heyling, then aged 8, joined a folk-dance group run by a friend of hers in her home village of Samulalí. In 2002 Deybi, aged 11, joined CESESMA's children's radio project and became a local radio reporter, sending in regular stories from his village of Granadillo.

Stage 2: Children join a promotores/as' training course run by CESESMA, and thus themselves become promotores and promotoras

Children who are active members of these local activity groups learn quickly and, as their confidence and self-esteem increase, soon many of them decide that they too want to be *promotores/as* and share their skills with the other children of their community. At this stage they can sign up for one of CESESMA's three training programmes:

FOCAPEC: Training and Development Programme for Community Education promotores/as

This is a one-year course of monthly two-day workshops, with practical tasks and projects in between. The curriculum combines key issues and key skills. The key issues are: children's rights, participation, identity and self-esteem, leadership, gender equality, non-violence, environmental conservation and health. The key skills are: group work, group organisation and leadership, communication skills, conflict resolution, community appraisal, community organisation, and influencing decision making.

FOPAE: Training and Development Programme for Ecological Agriculture promotores/as

This is similar to FOCAPEC, but with an emphasis on the environment, nutrition and sustainable agriculture.

Girls' and Young Women's Network training programme

This programme has an emphasis on women's rights, gender equality, and sexual and reproductive health. This is the option for those girls and young women who want to work with other girls and young women in their community on these issues.

The target age-group for all three programmes is 12 to 16.

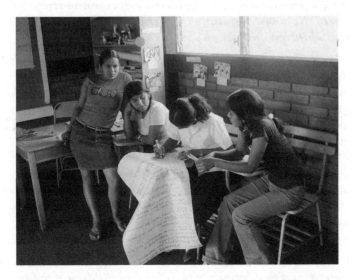

Plate 20.2   Girls' and Young Women's Network training programme, Samulalí.
Copyright: CESESMA

The educational approach of the *promotores/as*' training programmes is based on a four-stage learning cycle model, derived from Kolb (1984) and adapted by CESESMA to emphasise collective action for social change (Figure 20.1).

Both Deybi and Heyling soon decided that they were ready to share their knowledge with others, and so opted to join FOCAPEC courses in their home districts: Deybi in 2003, aged 12, and Heyling in 2004, aged 13.

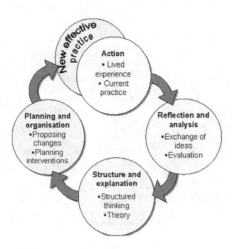

Figure 20.1   Four-stage learning cycle (after Kolb 1984)

Stage 3: New promotores/as, organised in a community Promotores' Network, multiply their skills and knowledge with other children and young people in their communities

At this stage, typically aged 13+, some work alongside more experienced *promotores/as*, while others quickly form new groups. All become members of the district Promotores/as' Network, where CESESMA provides support and back-up, and ongoing training and development opportunities. However, our aim is to reduce their dependence on us as much as possible, in its place encouraging autonomy and mutual support among the network of *promotores/as* in the area.

By 2006, Heyling was active in the local Girls' Network, helping organise a girls' group in her village. About the same time she also started a dress-making course. Deybi organised a local children's group in his village to share the skills and knowledge he had picked up on the FOCAPEC course. He also learned macramé from local *promotores* and started teaching this craft to children in his group.

Stage 4: Promotores/as become active in community action for development, and in advocacy and defence of children's rights

Organised in the Promotores' Network, aware of the key issues, with developed skills and confidence, the young *promotores* get involved in a wide range of development and campaigning activities including:

- participation in school councils, community children's and youth committees, and as student representatives on school management committees;

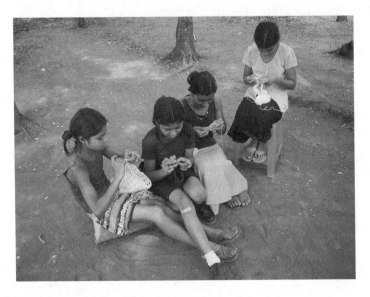

Plate 20.3   Children's crochet group organised and taught by a young *promotora*.
Copyright: CESESMA

- participation as youth representatives in adult-dominated groups such as Municipal Children and Youth committees and Municipal Development committees;
- environmental campaigns: for example reporting illegal logging to the authorities, anti-burning and reforestation campaigns;
- awareness raising on child-labour issues on the coffee plantations: the aim is not to abolish child labour, which is considered unrealistic, but to defend the rights of working children; for example reducing children's involvement in harmful work such as spraying pesticides;
- the theatre groups devise, produce and present original plays which expose issues of violence, abuse and exploitation to get communities talking about them;
- through its young reporters' network, the children's radio team raises awareness of children's rights abuses, encouraging and publicising action in defence of children's rights.

Deybi, at age 15, was elected co-coordinator of the Promotores' Network in his community. 'It's a big responsibility,' he explained, 'being in charge of all the work that has to be done: organising, promoting, mobilising, supporting, instructing.' He also became active in national initiatives, including the National Children and Young Workers' Movement (NATRAS). Heyling continued to play a lead role in the Girls' and Young Women's Network in her district, helping to organise women's rights workshops with local girls' groups.

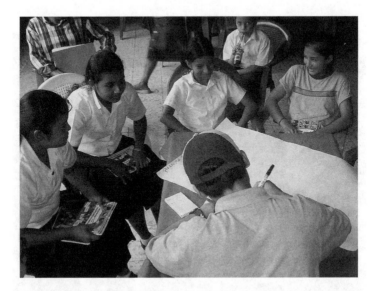

Plate 20.4   Children and young people participating in a district Education Planning Forum in La Dalia. The forum was a key step in drawing up the Municipal Education Development Plan. Copyright: CESESMA

Stage 5: The most capable and committed promotores/as join CESESMA's area teams.

The three area teams, one in each of the districts where CESESMA works, are the main coordinating bodies, responsible for planning, organising, monitoring, follow-up and evaluation of CESESMA's work in the district. The teams are made up of young *promotores/as*, their ages currently ranging from 11 to 20. The three team coordinators are themselves local young people, currently aged 20 to 23, employed by CESESMA as full-time Community Education Workers. The teams themselves seek new members from among the active *promotores/as* in their district. They try to maintain representation of all the village communities that make up the district, and also a balance between the different ages, interests and activity groups.

All the work of the young *promotores/as* is voluntary, including the responsibility taken on by the area teams, whose commitment is often virtually full-time. This presents complex issues for CESESMA.

We do not pay them a salary. This is partly because we don't have the resources, but more importantly because we have always insisted that they do not work for us. What they do, they do for the good of their community and for the defence of their rights as children and young people.

On the other hand, as they grow up, they need to survive and this means earning a living. For most this means agricultural work on a coffee plantation or a family small-holding, while for others it means moving to the city in search of work. Thus, by relying solely on voluntary commitment to fuel development, the communities are losing some of their most valuable human capacity.

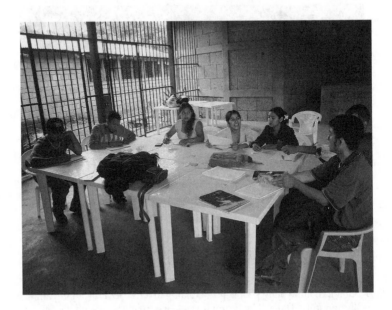

Plate 20.5   Area team meeting, La Dalia. Copyright: CESESMA

CESESMA responds to this in two ways. Where young *promotores/as* want to pursue secondary or technical education, we can sometimes provide them with a small bursary to make this possible. Another option is our programme of support for small production initiatives, or micro-businesses. Here we support young *promotores* in setting up their own small enterprises in the community. These currently include poultry farming, bee-keeping, and dressmaking. This enables many young *promotores*, who would otherwise emigrate or drop out, to remain in the community, dividing their time between their own small business and their community work.

Heyling joined the Samulalí Area Team in 2007, aged 16. At about the same time, with CESESMA's help, she and two other young women started a small dress-making business. Deybi joined the La Dalia Area Team the same year, and became one of five partners in a poultry farm.

These five stages explain CESESMA's central strategy. It is a renewable and sustainable cycle, with children constantly joining, many going on to become *promotores/as*, and involving new groups of children in community activities. While this work with children and young people is the heart of our work, its success depends on the adoption of an integrated or 'whole community' approach. Therefore CESESMA works in parallel to build alliances with parents, teachers, community leaders and local officials.

Reflection: ten key learnings

How can this experience contribute to our understanding and conceptualisation of children and young people's participation, and what can it offer to practitioners in the UK and other contexts?

1   It is a long-term process promoting personal development

The CESESMA approach is a process of personal development over years. We can see this process unfolding in the stories of Deybi and Heyling. It is not a hit-and-run 'Let's get a group of young people together for a participation project' approach. Therefore we should not be surprised that, over time, participants develop impressive levels of competence, awareness, confidence, organising ability and communication skills; in short, empowerment.

2   Recognising children's capability and competence is a good starting point

We start from an unshakeable belief that children and young people are capable and competent. They have expert knowledge about their lives, their families, their communities, their hopes and fears. The tools they have available for analysis of this information may be limited to start with, but this is due to lack of educational opportunities, not lack of capability, and their local knowledge is no less valid and valuable.

3   *Children and young people's roles as educators in the community*

A *promotor* or *promotora* is an educator, organiser and activist, and for many the emphasis is on the role of community educator. Young people form and run activity groups, sharing their knowledge and skills with others, leading to what we call the 'multiplier effect'. In this, CESESMA's approach has much in common with 'child-to-child' or peer-learning models. These peer-learning groups are the platforms that lead to community action for change, and the collective defence of children's rights.

4   *Children and young people as community leaders*

CESESMA's work is leading to a growing recognition that children and young people can have a leadership role, an element rarely seen in Northern contexts. At the same time, it is challenging traditional leadership styles with new ideas about who is a leader and their role in the community.

5   *Children and young people as advocates and defenders of their rights*

Central to this approach is a strong children's rights focus, which implies moving from a needs-based to a rights-based approach (see Save the Children 2002). It also implies organised action by children and young people in the promotion and defence of their rights. Among the rights local children and young people identify as priorities are the right to quality education, the right to live without violence, the right to participate and have a say in their community, and the right not to be mistreated or exploited at work (the need to work, at least part of the time, being taken for granted).

6   *Self-organisation, proactivism and autonomy*

CESESMA promotes models of self-organisation, joint organisation, and children and young people's engagement in adult-dominated spaces; all of which have a role to play in the promotion and defence of children and young people's rights.

7   *Capacity to influence decisions in adult-dominated spaces*

Young people increasingly take on roles as elected representatives, delegated to represent their peer group in adult-dominated decision-making spaces, which inevitably involves challenging adult attitudes. When participation becomes fashionable, the tendency is for adults to permit young people's participation without believing in its value. This is the road to tokenism. For this type of participation to be effective and non-tokenistic, the young people need to be empowered to set and pursue their own agenda for change.

8   Direct action: campaigning, protest actions and using the media

When children and young people are supported in taking a lead in direct action, there is always a risk of manipulation by adults. Marches and protests are fun, so it is easy to persuade children and young people to lend their numbers to a cause that is not theirs, to hand out T-shirts and baseball caps, or to provide flags to wave. On the other hand, if children and young people have their own organisation and leadership, including spokespeople who can handle the media and make it clear that it is a cause they believe in, direct action can be hugely effective in working for change.

Young people's community theatre is a powerful communication medium in campaigns and protests. Youth theatre groups supported by CESESMA have performed original plays in support of local and national campaigns against child abuse, corporal punishment and exploitation of child labour on the coffee plantations.

Children and young people can also take control of the media in an organised and effective way; for example, the young people's radio project that CESESMA supports. Their weekly programme *Children and Young People's Voices Heard*, has been running continually for five years on local radio.

9   Adult roles in facilitating and accompanying these processes

The adult support role needs to be handled sensitively and skilfully so as to offer appropriate support with the aim of encouraging autonomy and reducing dependence on adult facilitators. In order to do this the facilitator needs to know:

- When do I tell the young people what to do?
- When do I help them to decide what to do?
- When do I back off, so they can facilitate the process themselves?

Adults working in these processes need training, specifically looking at their own attitudes and learning practical techniques of process facilitation.

10   Adult recognition and valuing of children and young people's action

CESESMA's impact evaluation (CESESMA 2003) shows that adults recognise the contribution children and young people are making to the community, and this is the biggest factor in winning adult support for the promotion of children and young people's rights. What is even more striking is that adults are also recognising that learning is a two-way process; that sometimes they might even learn things from their children.

This contributes to changing adult attitudes so that respect for children and young people's rights is no longer seen as a threat to the established order, but rather as bringing real benefit to the community as a whole.

> My children have developed. Now they can relate better to other people, adults as well as other children. They take responsibility for the workshops

they run and they all participate. One runs a dance group and the others are involved in the organic farming workshops. They relate better to the community.

(Parent, Samulalí, quoted in CESESMA 2003)

Conclusion

The CESESMA experience shows that 'participation' is bigger, broader, more varied and more complex than previous analyses have suggested. One of the big challenges for adults aiming to facilitate non-tokenistic participation beyond a limited local level is to ensure that children and young people are not manipulated into serving adult agendas. CESESMA's experience suggests that one way to achieve this is to support children's gradual 'bottom-up' processes of learning, sharing, organising and mobilising, so that when children demand a voice in the big decisions that affect their lives, they arrive at the table as a force to be reckoned with.

To illustrate this final learning, I present the following visualisation of children and young people's participation, drawn up by a group of Nicaraguan participation workers in 2007 (Figure 20.2). This is followed by a visual account of their work produced by the Young Consultants Team of Santa Martha coffee plantation (Figure 20.3).

References

CESESMA (2003) *Evaluación de Impacto 2000–2003*, San Ramón Matagalpa: CESESMA.
Kirby, P. et al. (2003) *Building a Culture of Participation: Involving children and young people in policy, service planning, development and evaluation*, London: Department of Education and Skills.
Kolb, D. (1984) *Experiential Learning: Experience as the source of learning and development*, New Jersey: Prentice-Hall.
Liebel, M. (2007) 'Paternalism, participation and children's protagonism', *Children, Youth and Environments* 17(2): 56–73.
O'Kane, C. and Karkara, R. (2007) 'Pushing the boundaries: Critical perspectives on the participation of children in South and Central Asia', *Children, Youth and Environments* 17(1): 136–47.
Save the Children (2002) *Child Rights Programming: How to apply rights-based approaches in programming*, Stockholm: Save the Children.
Shier, H. (2001) 'Pathways to participation: Openings, opportunities and obligations', *Children & Society* 15: 107–17.
Sinclair, R. (2004) 'Participation in practice: Making it meaningful, effective and sustainable', *Children & Society* 18: 106–18.

The Participation Tree

By the "Building a Children's Rights Culture" working group, CODENI, Nicaragua, August 2007
Translated from the original Spanish

To understand the tree, start at the roots.

The fruits: Respect, equality, respect for human rights, development, peace

The leaves of the tree: Children and young people empowered

- Children and young people as community educators
- Children and young people in community development
- Children and young people supporting others in difficulty
- Children and young people as defenders of children's rights
- Children and young people reporting abuse and exploitation
- Children and young people in educational policy and planning
- Children and young people as renewers and defenders of traditional culture
- Children and young people as spokespeople and representatives in local democracy
- Children and young people as protectors and defenders of the environment
- Children and young people in their own groups and organisations
- Children and young people in direct action for social change
- Children and young people in media and communications
- Children and young people as mediators of conflict
- Children and young people as a new generation of community leaders.

The branches of the tree are the various activity groups and spaces in which children and young people gradually develop their active and pro-active participation in tune with the growth of their knowledge and experience

The seed from which the tree grows is the family home: the first setting where the child learns to participate and be a part of the community

The trunk: The strong central trunk that holds up the whole tree is made up of all the learning processes through which children and young people gain awareness of their rights, raised self-esteem, awareness of themselves as members of society and rights-holders, as competent and capable of achieving anything in life; ability to express themselves and to organise.

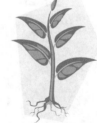

The growing seedling is strengthened by attendance at organised activities outside the home: That's to say, the child becomes a "Participant".

Roots and earth: Participation is rooted in the children's rights focus and the legal framework that guarantees these rights: Children's Rights Code, UNCRC

Figure 20.2 The participation tree

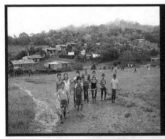

The Young Consultants of Santa Martha coffee plantation investigate the problem of violence

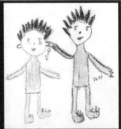

We are 11 children and young people from the community of Santa Martha. Now we are from 12 to 18 years old but when we became consultants a year and a half ago we were aged from 10 to 17. We were all attending the primary school in our community and were in third to sixth grade. Now two of us are in secondary school.

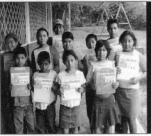

Our community, Santa Martha, is a coffee plantation. It is in the area called Yasica Sur, which is part of the municipality of San Ramón in the Department of Matagalpa, Nicaragua.

NICARAGUA

During the coffee harvest we all work on the plantation.

Some of us work all year round looking after the coffee plants.

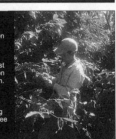

This is the story of how we became Consultants and presented the findings of our research at the National Conference "Violence against Children: A global problem, a Nicaraguan response" in the capital city Managua in August 2007.

To start off we had a meeting with our mums there so everyone was in agreement about the work we were going to do as consultants. The mums gave their permission and chose three of them to accompany us to Managua. At this stage we didn't really know what it meant to be a Consultant.

Mum, please can I go?

Meeting about the journey to Managua

At the start of the first workshop we did drawings of violence we've experienced in the community. Then we showed each other our drawings and each of us talked about the different kinds of violence we had drawn.

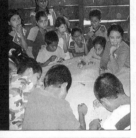

Then we read and discussed a booklet about the 'United Nations Special Report on Violence Against Children',

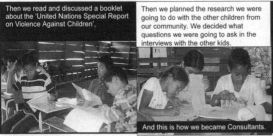

Then we planned the research we were going to do with the other children from our community. We decided what questions we were going to ask in the interviews with the other kids.

And this is how we became Consultants.

The agreement was that each of us would interview at least five other kids about their experience of violence. We asked them about the violence they had experienced and the types of violence they knew about. We interviewed a total of 59 children and young people

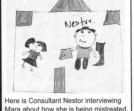

Here is Consultant Nestor interviewing Mara about how she is being mistreated.

Then we met for a second workshop to discuss the findings of our research and agree on conclusions about the children's experience of violence in the community, in school, in the coffee fields, in the home etc.

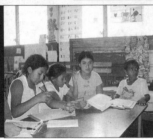

We drew up our recommendations to reduce violence: What each group in the community should do: parents, community leaders, teachers, plantation overseers and foremen, the government, and ourselves the children and young people.

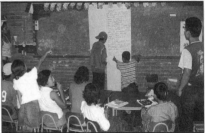

Figure 20.3 Young Consultants Team of Santa Martha coffee plantation investigate the problem of violence

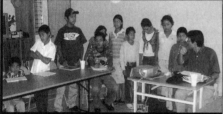

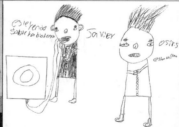

We practised the presentation we were going to do in Managua with the computer and projector. Each of us took a turn to practise our part using the microphone. Then we made plans for the journey to Managua.

In the last workshop we went to the CESESMA office in San Ramón to put together our final report.

The day of the journey we met in Santa Martha. Richard, the driver, took us as far as La Praga in the pick-up truck. There we changed to the minibus.

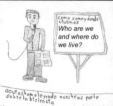

We had lunch in Matagalpa town. We arrived in Managua in the afternoon and went to look at the Crowne Plaza Convention Centre where we were going to make our presentation the next day. We had dinner and slept in a hotel

The next morning we got up and had breakfast.

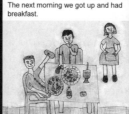

Then we went to the national confernece.

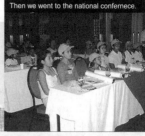

We did our presentation; each one took the microphone to read their part.

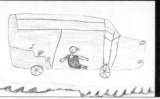

Here we are, reading our parts about violence

Who are we and where do we live?

Then Arlen presented three questions on cards to the Minister for the Family. The questions asked her what she was going to do to reduce violence against children.

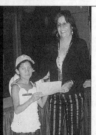

Later we gave the same three cards, of different colours, to every-one. Then we collected the cards to make a display of the commitments that the adults had made with the children and young people of Nicaragua.

We closed off the side doors so when the adults left the conference hall they saw the commitments they had made in writing.

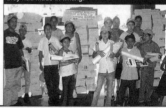

We slept another night in the hotel in Managua and the next day we went home to Santa Martha.
A couple of weeks later we had an evaluation meeting to think about the experience. Here are our reflections about the experience of being Consultants.

What did we learn from the experience?

We learnt to do things that adults do, like being Consultants. We learnt to speak in public without being embarrassed. We learnt how we can all help to reduce violence, and who we can turn to for help. We learnt that we are all equal: nobody is bigger than me. And we learnt about how people live in the capital, for example eating with knives and forks.

Did the adults take us seriously?

We think they did, because they gave us the opportunity to do our presentation, and the adults were paying attention when we made the presentation. Even the Minister for the Family took us into account, because she accepted the three cards and answered our questions. Also our parents let us participate in the workshops and go to Managua. Although the people at the conference in Managua took us seriously, we realise that the problem of violence continues in Santa Martha. There's a lot of work still to do to eliminate violence in Santa Martha.

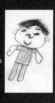

What would we say to those adults who say that children can't be Consultants because they don't know anything and will be manipulated by the adults?

We would tell them they are very much mistaken, because we can too. They should stop abusing their power and give us the space. Put us to the test and they'll see if we can or not.

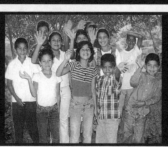

How did we feel when it was all over?

Happy because of all the new things we saw and all the things we learnt, and because we had contributed to the reduction of violence. Sad because it was over and we weren't going to meet again.

Our message to other children and young people who want to be consultants:

They should join the groups that CESESMA runs. They should speak out about those who violate their rights. Tell the truth and don't be scared.

Axel
Roberto
Nestor
Osiris
Junior
Jorling
Arlen
Brenda
Scarleth
Brenda Yadira
Ervin
Jossabeth

21 Students as professionals

The London Secondary School Councils Action Research Project

Hiromi Yamashita and Lynn Davies

Introduction

School councils[1] are often mentioned as a vehicle for promoting and practising student participation in decision making at school. Although it is not compulsory to have a school council in England, unlike in other countries such as Germany, the Netherlands (Davies and Kirkpatrick 2000), Japan (Yamashita and Williams 2002) and, most recently, Wales (Crowley and Skeels, this volume), setting one up is often highly recommended, both by the government and by various charitable organisations, as well as by movements promoting citizenship education or the implementation of the Convention on the Rights of the Child (Davies et al. 2006). School inspections have also started to make more detailed notes on student participation activities at school and often use as their starting point the activity of the school council.

However, some practitioners fear that ineffective school council activities not only are less constructive but also can have a negative impact on pupils by sending messages that participation is 'a waste of time'. Is the school council an effective way to promote student participation, or just a convenient body to 'tick the box' for the school inspection? What kinds of elements do practitioners really need in order to ensure real and meaningful school council activities?

In this chapter, we wish to discuss three key elements that appear to make school councils more meaningful: including all students; dealing with serious issues that matter to students and staff; and shifting the culture towards 'students as professionals'. This model emerged from a three-year action research project with eight secondary schools in London.

Background to the project

The London Secondary School Councils Action Research Project (LSSCARP) began in 2004, initiated by the NGO School Councils UK (SCUK) and funded by Deutsche Bank and the Esmée Fairbairn Foundation. The aim of the project was to work with a small group of selected secondary schools to develop their school councils, investigating the process of such intervention and the impact of the school councils. Some schools had school councils already, but felt that they needed development; others did not yet have a system of student participation. A project manager from SCUK, Lois Canessa, worked intensively with the schools, providing training and support to students and staff. The councils were also encouraged to network with each other.

The research identified a range of factors which made a difference to effective school council work. These included the role of the head, the inclusion of school council work in staff job descriptions, representation from different groups of students, links with other areas of school life, communication and feedback, the time dedicated and the timing of the activity, budget, dealing with student frustration, breaking cycles of complaint, continuity and monitoring. However, the three elements mentioned below seemed to be of key significance, and will be the focus of this chapter.

Inclusion of all students

School Councils have been accused of being beneficial only for those on the council itself, often seen as an elite group. This view was apparent in our research schools, especially at the beginning of the project. This is linked to the ways in which the school interprets 'participation' and puts that interpretation into practice. If student participation is understood simply as involving a few student representatives at meetings or enabling councillors to discuss student issues and feed them into school management, this may be enough. However, if participation is seen as ensuring that the voice of every child is heard and valued, or as a practical part of everyday life in the school, then a more inclusive approach is crucial.

The LSSCARP project worked towards involving every student in the school. To achieve this, at the beginning of the project each school worked to agree and set up a structure of class or form councils leading into year-group or house councils, in turn leading into an executive (Figure 21.1). Meetings were to be organised in more systematic ways than previously, and each tutor group had two councillors, who chaired meetings with their classmates every week, so that every student

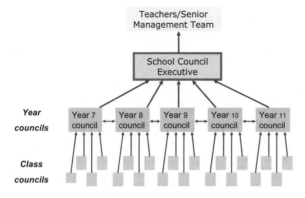

Figure 21.1 School council structure proposed by LSSCARP

would have a chance to know about the work of the school council – and, more-over, have a chance to voice their opinions.

This sounds simple, but for some schools even to make the commitment to provide systematic meeting opportunities proved to be difficult (often with the common refrain of 'no time'). Gradually most schools saw the benefits of this structural approach, yet, even after the structure was put into place, we found that the real inclusion of all students depended on two things.

The first was feedback or communication, going not just in one direction (students making demands or requests up the system, or teachers consulting students downwards about school policy), but in continuous cycles – students hearing the *results* of their requests or suggestions, and everyone building on these, horizontally as well as vertically (Figure 21.2).

The majority of complaints from students (both councillors and non-councillors) were about not knowing what happened to what they said and contributed. Even at the most successful schools in terms of participation, it was often forgotten to ensure and protect the time slot in class for the class councillors to feed back what had been agreed and rejected in the year or executive council. The project manager said in a field note:

> I think all staff underestimate the contempt with which students hold token-istic school councils that are only there to serve the purposes of the adults. They also resent the amount of time they invest in these attempts only to be disappointed time after time when they are not taken seriously, or nobody had the decency to explain to them why a particular decision has been made.

The second point is that this structural approach to ensure all students' partici-pation needs, in turn, the very active and informed engagement of form tutors to run class councils on a regular basis. Previously, in past research, which rightly had stressed the important role of the head, this had not come up much. We

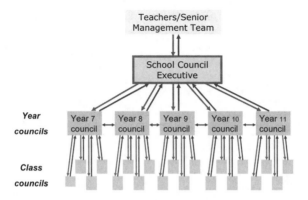

Figure 21.2 Communication flow within the school council structure

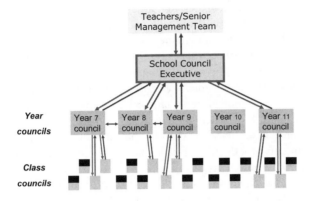

Figure 21.3 When the class council meetings do not happen ...

discovered that form tutors needed training and support to run class councils and to use and protect tutor time or form time effectively, not getting side-tracked into other issues of the day. They needed to be clear about what 'representation' meant. In some classes, student councillors were saying: 'It feels like we're supposed to be the voice of the students, but we don't actually have a voice of our own at the moment.' If some class councils were not meeting, or were meeting sporadically, the discussion at the school council executive would not represent or reflect all the students' voices (Figure 21.3).

This structural approach was originally introduced to make sure that every student had an opportunity to participate. However, the model appears hierarchical, and power could remain in the hands of tutors. The aim of the project was that once a systematic mechanism for student involvement was in place, the other offshoots of students' participation meetings could operate with or without the help of the existing structure and commitment of particular 'gate keepers' towards student participation. Indeed, as we discuss later, in some schools a variety of 'offshoot' committees developed (e.g. teaching and learning committee, environment committee, behaviour committee) which were not directly related to school councils or councillors. These provided students with additional feedback and participation spaces which were run by different groups of students and supported by different members of staff.

Agenda of serious issues

Even when the system is up and running, there are often limits on what kinds of decisions students can be involved in at school. At an early stage of the project, we conducted an activity with school councillors and teachers from participating schools to establish the boundaries of student participation in various aspects of school life. The students and the teachers individually worked on card-sorting activities and later compared their notes, focusing on four areas: where pupils make the decisions; where pupils discuss and make suggestions to staff; where pupils and staff make decisions together; and areas which are currently off-limits to pupils. The decisions that were identified by students across different schools as being 'off-limits' included: lessons; homework; appointment or induction of staff; discipline/punishment; school rules; code of behaviour; discussing individuals (staff or pupils); uniform; and school dinners. For some schools and their students there appeared to be not much left to decide on. Even from the same school, many areas were identified in which teachers thought students contributed to decision making, but students thought they did not, especially around teaching and learning, school rules, codes of behaviour, discipline and punishment, and appointments or induction of staff. This was a genuine surprise for the teachers participating in the activity, and they were eager to know the reasons for the students' perceptions, which were often based on negative past experiences of 'participation' attempts, or indeed a complete lack of these.

After identifying the danger of school council meetings only talking about 'soft' and uncontroversial issues (most commonly toilets, school dinners and student parties), the project manager encouraged class, year and school councils to use a four-part agenda covering four main areas that impact on students' life at school: teaching and learning; environment; peer issues; and extra-curricular issues. This meant that important, serious areas of school life were not neglected, and one did not have a whole meeting just talking about the toilets (important though they are). For each area, the agenda sheet had two columns – issues raised, and suggestions/ action points – to encourage thinking about what actually could be done either by the students or by others, rather than just 'whingeing'. In this way, a complaint about 'boring teaching', for example, became an issue of wanting teachers to have a wider variety of teaching styles, which under 'action points' became a request to teachers to make more use of the interactive whiteboards as visual aids. Student council work then becomes not just about 'voice', or giving a view, but about activity, 'inquiry' and proposing solutions to problems, and students having their own tasks and contributions in core areas. These suggestions were often taken to staff meetings and various departmental meetings (Figure 21.4).

Linking back to inclusion, this also meant the establishment of working committees or sub-councils (learning and teaching, behaviour, environment etc.) to bring in even more students who were not on the executive, sometimes being given a budget for school improvement in this area. Schools were engaged in different activities, but the most innovative schools were two that set up a Behaviour Panel and a Teaching and Learning sub-council.

The Behaviour Panel at the one school identified sites of classroom disruption through observation and surveys, and then worked directly to mediate with specific problem students and to set targets for improved behaviour. These types of involvement gave students new insights into the task of teaching and directly benefited classroom processes. Teachers were very positive about such initiatives.

At the other school the Teaching and Learning sub-council ran a six-week pilot programme of lesson observations with ten teachers across three departments. Initially, the project worker identified some common misconceptions: some teachers did not believe that their students felt much responsibility for, or interest in, their

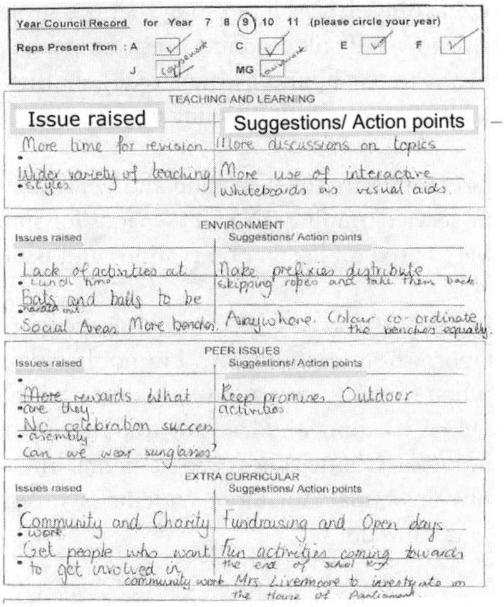

Year Council Record for Year 7 8 9 10 11 (please circle your year)

Reps Present from : A ✓ C ✓ E ✓ F ✓
J MG

TEACHING AND LEARNING

Issue raised	Suggestions/ Action points
More time for revision	More discussions on topics
Wider variety of teaching styles	More use of interactive whiteboards as visual aids.

ENVIRONMENT

Issues raised	Suggestions/ Action points
Lack of activities at lunch time	Make prefixies distribute skipping ropes and take them back.
Bats and balls to be handed out	
Social Areas More benches.	Anywhere. Colour co-ordinate the benches equally.

PEER ISSUES

Issues raised	Suggestions/ Action points
More rewards What are they	Keep promises Outdoor activities
No celebration success assembly	
Can we wear sunglasses?	

EXTRA CURRICULAR

Issues raised	Suggestions/ Action points
Community and Charity work	Fundraising and Open days
Get people who want to get involved in community work	Fun activities coming towards the end of school Mrs Livermoore to investigate on the House of Parliament.

Figure 21.4 Council meeting record. This example is a summary of a Year 8 council meeting, although each class council and the school council executive use the same document format

education; while students felt that teachers were not interested in listening to their experiences of teaching and learning. Students on the Teaching and Learning sub-council received training from the project manager in conducting systematic lesson observations and providing feedback to the teachers, in a non-threatening and constructive way, about various aspects of teaching, such as the balance of interaction with different types of students or styles of questioning. The English department chose to focus on the use of questions; this related to open and closed questions, how often students ask questions, and different methods of getting answers rather than just 'hands up' (one class banned hands up). In the Art department, one teacher focused on the use of questioning with regard to the gender of the student.

Both parties clearly found the endeavour fruitful. One Teaching and Learning committee member said: 'I think the staff think that we're doing quite a good job to help them with their learning,' and a teacher commented: 'Students really understood what it was like really to be a teacher.' 'Helping teachers with their own learning' is a very sophisticated concept, and one that really captures the spirit of the 'learning organisation'. The project manager noted that:

> Findings from the observations were quite enlightening. One teacher found that a pupil in their class had been 'off-task' for 38 minutes of a 55 minute period. Another found out that her class thought she liked the pupils sitting on the other side of the room more – when in fact she was favouring a position next to a warm radiator. All those involved agreed the exercise had been

useful, initially in improving relationships in class and latterly in improving specific aspects of teaching. It was interesting that the student observers said they never realised how difficult teaching was. So we have teachers really sharing what it means to teach, and learners really sharing what it means to learn; and both sides of course both teaching and learning.

Using PowerPoint presentations, the Teaching and Learning sub-committee in one school did three in-service training (INSET) sessions for staff, delivering their 'top ten tips' for teachers based on lesson observations and issues taken to school councils.

Unsurprisingly, other schools were less keen. A classic response was from a teacher in another school, who said in horror, 'I'm not having the kids watching me teach!' However, when students were allowed to deal with the serious and core issues of the school, such as teaching and learning and behaviour, their participation truly became meaningful. Change and improvement in the ways that teachers taught was the most obvious impact for those students involved in the process of advising on this. One student said:

> In our classroom we've improved the way it goes, so the way the teachers teach, that's probably the biggest. The observation of teachers and giving them feedback, trying to help them out. Not giving them criticism, just helping.

It was encouraging that even in schools that had not yet gone down the observation route there were perceptions that teaching had improved because of feedback through the school council. In another school, where the school council had been consulted about teaching and learning policies and what makes a good teacher, the non-school-council students had a revealing discussion around teaching methods:

Male 1:   The school council have made a difference to what you're learning in lessons and stuff. Obviously they must have changed the lessons, before the lessons were boring and that.

Female 1:   It's OK, but I'm not here to have fun, I'm here to learn so I don't really mind if the lessons are boring. As long as I learn something.

Male 2:   But obviously if the lessons are boring they need to find more interactive ways to get to the children, else they're just going to be bored.

Female 2:   But yeah, they have found more interactive ways. I don't know about your classes, but my school council have come to our class and talked about it. I think that if you were more proactive like, you're saying 'oh they don't do this, they don't do that', but if you actually went to them and said, instead of sitting and moaning, then maybe something would be done. I don't know what goes on in your class, but I know what goes on in mine. And my school council people speak to me.

What is happening is a shift in discourse – students have always complained about lessons being boring, but now they are relating this to their own learning, and using words like 'interactive' and 'proactive'. The discussions within the school council do seem to have permeated thinking more widely.

Students as 'professionals'

A key term to emerge from the research was 'students as professionals', providing a new image of students and a change of culture. Significant achievements occurred when students were accepted as authorities who made a professional contribution to the school, with their experience and expertise used on teaching and learning, on behaviour and on school climate. What is important is recognition of the expertise of students – they are not just recipients of knowledge or policy from other professionals, or there to be controlled, but 'professionals' in their own right. We know that students do have long-term experience of teaching and learning, and they have in-depth, first-hand recognition of what makes a good teacher; they are also experts in behaviour, and in what makes students behave in certain ways. They simply have different experiences, viewpoints and knowledge from those of teachers.

The phrase 'the students were so professional' started to come up in discussions with teachers. For example, in their involvement in the appointment of staff, a teacher said:

> Recently, the school council were involved in selecting Directors of Study for our school … [Students] were absolutely professional, they asked questions that were straight to the point, if they needed further detail they asked for that as well. If you weren't actually watching the students, and you were just listening to them, they could actually be mistaken for adults.

To make this shift of culture easier, teachers and students at some schools in the project made sure to advertise what students and their participation activities had achieved whenever possible, including at assemblies and at staff meetings. The teachers interviewed said that one of the barriers to this cultural change was the fact that some members of staff did not know the abilities and the levels of contribution students could make to their learning and environment. One teacher described how staff who were initially reluctant to get involved were beginning to change their minds. His feedback sheet for the project read: 'changed several people's [teachers'] opinions: they were very pleasantly surprised by the maturity and level of understanding that the students on the student council showed'.

Students can professionally organise, communicate and even provide INSET sessions for staff, which, as noted above, did happen. They can train others, and some of the councils in the project were training feeder primary schools in participation work, or were organising exchange meetings for councils from other schools to share their experiences. The classic example of this skill and professionalism was a school council running a conference for all local borough schools to help them to develop their council work. Schools can seriously underestimate the capabilities of students; to treat them as professionals means treating them as adults, and that is very hard for some schools and teachers, and means a shift in culture.

It is a question not just of instantly involving and consulting students, but of thinking through what using – and extending – the professionalism of students means. This might involve training, whether in lesson observation, in giving constructive feedback, in chairing meetings, or in leading discussion with diverse and conflicting groups (training which teachers say they would themselves find beneficial). This training would need to be designed in a way that included students with different areas of interest, and to address different levels and styles of student participation. Some schools used online voting, for example, the establishment of which requires technical skills. Training is not just about making confident students even more confident. If it included various ways into participation activities (e.g. computer voting, discussion, budgets and finance, working with younger children, organising network events), it could reach different groups of students. The LSSCARP project provided this, but in the end such training needs to be routinely part of the school development plan; and investing in student professionalism should not stop at periodic training for selected groups. As in our earlier discussion of involving *all* students, it is a question of trying to build and capitalise on adult, participatory relationships across the school, with students recognised, individually and collectively, as authorities in their own learning. It would be nice if all students could be 'mistaken for adults'.

Conclusion

We argue, therefore, that there are three basics, like the three legs of a stool, each of which is crucial for school council impact and indeed for other student participation activities: that *all students* are involved, in *serious issues*, as *professionals* (Figure 21.5).

One thing to stress is that a token, partial, fragmented or indeed one-legged school council is worse than useless, leading to frustrated and alienated students who quickly see through hypocrisy around the issue of 'voice'. Similar to any aspect of school development, if one were to introduce a new curriculum area, like citizenship, one would put planning, time and money, and cross-school sharing of ideas into it. It is the same with a school council; it needs investment. School councils could usefully be made compulsory in English schools, but only if a number of conditions were set

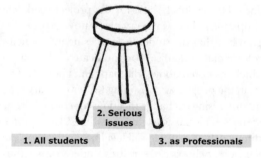

Figure 21.5 Student participation stool

which ensured that they were not token democracies and that they fully engaged in the core business of the school, which is teaching and learning.

Done properly, our view is that a school council may be the best investment a school can make for real school improvement and student development. If one were designing a participation policy for a school, then one would need to find something that:

- could involve everyone in knowledge and decision making about school management;
- could convince teachers that students were able to take responsibility;
- could give teachers first-hand systematic feedback about their teaching and give students greater appreciation of the teaching task;
- could generate sensible and adult codes of conduct which were accepted by the students;
- could give direct experience in skills related to democratic participation and citizenship for later life, and where students can see the results of their actions.

The conclusion from the LSSCARP project is that a solid school council structure can be an effective and efficient way of simultaneously achieving all these objectives.

Further information:

The project report: Davies, L. and Yamashita, H. (2007) 'School councils – school improvement: The London Secondary School Councils Action Research Project', and other resources for teachers and students are downloadable at the School Council UK website at www.schoolcouncils.org. We wish to acknowledge the invaluable assistance from School Councils UK and teachers and students at the participating schools. Our special appreciation to Lois Canessa, LSSCARP project manager, for her continual enthusiasm for student participation and for our research. Any inaccuracies remaining in the study are of course solely our responsibility.

Note

1. A body of representative students whose role is to discuss issues that matter to students and to work with members of staff to improve the learning environment and school/ local communities. Sometimes called 'student council'.

References

Davies, L. and Kirkpatrick, G. (2000) *The EURIDEM Project: Pupil democracy in Europe*, London: Children's Rights Alliance.

Davies, L., Williams, C. and Yamashita, H. with Man-Hing, K. (2006) *Impact and Outcomes: Taking up the challenge of pupil participation*, London: Carnegie Foundation, available at www.participationforschools.org.uk.

Yamashita, H. and Williams, C. (2002) 'A vote for consensus: Democracy and differences in Japan', *Journal of Comparative Education* 38(4): 277–89.

Commentary 5

On strategies and practices

Maha Damaj, Rachel Henderson, Alan Sarraf,
Hana Sleiman, Lelia Abu Jawdeh, Nehme Hamadeh,
Thurayya Zreik, Neal Skinner, Kirsty Jordan
and Owen Hammet

This section was reviewed by one team in Devon, UK, and by one in Beirut, Lebanon. The members were quite diverse in terms of their ages (ranging from 15 to 20), backgrounds and prior experiences or exposures to elements and practices in participation. This review combines the main discussion points raised in each group.

The diversity of their documented experiences in participation, in terms not just of location, but of the actual models drawn, was very valuable in discussing and pinpointing which elements were attractive, which worked, and which need to be taken into account and avoided.

A couple of common issues emerged from the perspectives of both groups, namely in terms of the roles and capacities needed for adults and children to take part in 'meaningful' rather than tokenistic participation, and in terms of the setting up of structures that allowed for follow-up and continuous information sharing. Not surprisingly, these are raised in the chapters.

> The only way to convince children and youth that participation is effective is by linking their suggestions to actual consequences. Only then will they appreciate the value of participation and really understand why it is their right. Once they see the potential of what their participation can achieve, they will start recognising it as an important right. This doesn't mean that they have to be granted whatever they suggest; but at least they should hear back from 'decision making adults' that their input was taken seriously, discussed, and decided upon.
>
> (Young commentator from Beirut)

The experience of the child reporters in India stood out as the most exciting and empowering for the children and young people involved. The group of young reviewers in Beirut called it the 'Secret Agent' chapter and could not stop talking about it, unleashing numerous ideas. Like their counterparts in Devon, they felt that the young people could make a big difference across an area, given the broad target audience of the media. Giving the child reporters a space to express their views was seen as quite powerful, more so as the project took into account political realities.

[The child reporters project] is really empowering and gets the government to notice – young people have proper freedom of expression and the press and young people are working together to get straight to the heart of the problem.

(Young commentator from Devon)

The frustration that the child reporters faced in not knowing what steps would be taken after their reports were disseminated to the decision makers, however, spoke to the need for also installing systems that would allow for feedback and accountability.

Another favourite was the experience of the child coffee-workers in Nicaragua. When previously thinking of child workers, thoughts of abuse would come to mind. However, this chapter gave a brilliant system for participation. The fact that this was taking place in a developing country made us realise how much we could learn from others. It was also interesting that the project was built into learning from the age of 6 and therefore becomes a part of who the children are, and taught skills feeding into life skills and careers, giving the young people options to get out of the coffee fields should they wish to.

The idea of children managing a group and doing everything is very good, I never knew that could happen. It also helps them become more adult-like and responsible, make wise choices. Also, as young trainers, they get to interact with all the other kids, so they hear all points of view.

(Young commentator from Beirut)

This project seemed to interpret all core values of meaningful participation in its structure, including an intrinsic respect for the individuality of children, who could choose whether they took part or not, whether they became *promotores* or not, recognising that not everyone is, or needs to be, a leader. It was also respectful of an existing way of life, working within it rather than superimposing change.

What is special about the Nicaraguan experience is that the project did not try to change the way of life of the people or superimpose new concepts alien to the society. It worked with the children and youth of the community on issues of importance and incorporated the participation process as a means to work on other issues vital to their lives. The project is fascinating, for it managed to help the society develop in areas its people are already working with rather than areas it thought should be developed. ... Applying a real participatory approach, identifying what those children and youth want, and including them in the process of change is the only way to real development or success among these communities.

(Young commentator from Beirut)

The experience in Rwanda, it was felt, was heavily laden with history and political complexities. The Devon review group wondered 'how much history had got in the way of empowerment, and whether revenge and inherited fear played a role'. The Rwandan children's reality was quite difficult and the projects introduced did not seem to ease that by much. Additionally, the project gave the children adult roles, but not the skills to play them fully. It felt as if the children were being forced to take on roles, as if this was an emergency situation rather than development, and there seemed to be a tremendous fear on the part of adults of young people expressing their views. Thus, the chapter provided much insight into the assessment and evaluation of how much 'participation' actually takes place in such projects, which are not uncommonly 'quick-impact' projects in post-crisis situations.

The experience of the London Secondary School Councils was familiar ground for both groups. The intricate structure to ensure representation and participation was impressive, an adult-type model treating the young people as professionals, business-like and preparing them for business skills. Participation is, after all, not just about making a difference but also about learning. But the structure alone clearly did not guarantee success, either in terms of equipping the students to succeed or in terms of promoting the adults' faith in them.

> Children can act on their own when given a chance, but also: they don't know how to do anything! ... They have been marginalised from the participation process for so long that they do not recognise ways they can affect, or the power they hold. This is very dangerous, for little by little this marginalisation has come to be a norm.
>
> (Young commentators from Beirut)

One interesting indicator was how the students highlighted more issues as 'off-limits' than did their teachers, raising the question whether the young people had become accustomed to being marginalised and censored in their participation. This was, however, the only experience that introduced training opportunities for adults to support children's participation. The chapter brought home the point that participation cannot succeed without adults, that young people rely on them and that adults can learn from young people. This interplay could bring about the flexibility in the system that would allow for better involvement of young people, and lead to change.

This specific point was very clear in the discussion of both review groups; participation cannot be solely run by young people, and much needs to be done to encourage adults to listen to and work alongside young people. Any project aiming for meaningful children's participation must take this into account.

> In our situation we don't think participation could be solely run by young people (or at least the projects that we have been involved with). We don't think we would have achieved so much without working alongside adults.
>
> (Young commentator from Devon)

One lone thought that came out of one of the discussions also wondered what influence donor agencies would have on defining participation in these projects.

As mentioned earlier, the two favourite projects were the experience of the child reporters in India, and the child coffee-workers in Nicaragua. It was harder, however, to agree on what would or would not work in our respective contexts, the UK and Lebanon. The Devon young review group could see the child reporters' experience taking off in the UK, with young people having proper freedom of expression and the press and the young people working together to get straight to the heart of the problem. They also felt:

> It would be good if the student council experience involved more students; it would be good to implement proper systems so that EVERYONE can take part.
>
> (Young commentator from Devon)

The Beirut young review group was not so optimistic:

> While reading the chapters, many aspects of participation were brought to my attention, issues that I had not thought of before. This drove me to conclude that our view and understanding of participation in Lebanon is incomplete. We lack the comprehensive understanding of the long participation process, its importance and its impact.
>
> (Young commentator from Beirut)

They could basically see all of the experiences happening in Lebanon in one way or another, but were wary of the lack of interest of young people and adults alike in taking part, and of the constant risk that, if any of these projects were to be implemented, they would quickly have political or religious views imposed on them.

> The country is totally diverse, children in many areas 'live in a box' and think nothing else exists. When approached with some ideas, the reaction would frequently be 'so what?'... If any of these were to be implemented, they would quickly have political or religious views imposed on them. ... Besides, in Lebanon, families are more involved in everything (which would hinder participation). In other countries, developing countries, children already have more duties, and perhaps are better prepared to participate.
>
> (Young commentators in Beirut)

Overall, both review groups found this exposure to experiences in other countries and contexts quite enriching, perhaps more so in realising the global commonalities. The problems with promoting meaningful participation are similar everywhere; adults don't listen to young people, and creating spaces/channels for children's voices to be heard is essential. Similarly, given the opportunity and support, the participation of young people can bring about exciting change and creative solutions.

The authors

From Beirut, Lebanon

Alan Sarraf and Nehme Hamadeh are high school students who have been involved in sports and media activities, but have never taken part in regular participation projects.

Hana Sleiman is an International Affairs university student concentrating on development. She has been involved in programmes of the Arab Resource Center for Popular Arts/Al Jana for ten years and is currently working there.

Lelia Abu Jawdeh is a high school student who spent the early years of her childhood in Ghana. She has been in the Lebanese Scouts for a number of years, and is an active volunteer in community initiatives undertaken in her mountain village.

Thurayya Zreik is a 10th-grade student. She is part of the Model United Nations and has actively worked on fundraising activities for the St Jude's Children's Cancer Centre, as well as participating in relief work during the 2006 war on Lebanon.

Maha Damaj is a child rights activist who has been promoting and training on children's participation in the Arab region since 1997. To date, her work on meaningful participation has included contributions to publications by the Arab Resource Collective, Save the Children Sweden, UNICEF and issues of *Medical Sociology News* and *Children, Youth and Environments*.

From Devon, England

Neal Skinner was elected to the Young People's Shadow Executive of Devon County Council, England, in 2005. In 2006 he set up a Youth Council in his home town and was elected its first chairman. In 2007 he represented Devon as a European Youth Ambassador. He is currently at university and continues to be involved in participation projects.

Kirsty Jordan was the member of Youth Parliament for Devon between 2005 and 2006. She worked with young people from around the county and still has a very keen interest in supporting people to have their voices heard.

Owen Hammet was a member of Youth Parliament for Devon in 2004 and also worked in other councils and organisations. He is currently studying for a degree and has been an active member of a number of committees, councils and societies.

Rachel Henderson is the lead participation worker for Devon Youth Service. Her professional interests are in the voice and influence of young people and how children and young people can be involved in research and development processes in empowering ways.

22 Children's participation in citizenship and governance

Sara L. Austin

Introduction

In many countries around the world children represent the majority of the population; globally, they represent approximately 30 per cent of the population. Yet children's voices are largely absent from political processes, and they have little influence over the development of legislation and policies and the allocation of resources to programmes that directly impact on their lives. Children's interests are often ignored by those in power; they are not regarded as full citizens, and are thus excluded from many of the political processes that would enable them to participate fully in society.

This chapter will address the concept of children as citizens, and the opportunities and challenges they face in exercising their rights as active participants in society. The analysis will draw on case studies of children's citizenship projects that utilise a rights-based approach, emphasising children's civil and political rights as enshrined in international and regional human rights law. Particular attention will be given to the rights of all children to participate, with emphasis placed on the participation of those who tend to be the most marginalised.

Children as active citizens

Fostering children's capacity to be active citizens includes supporting their participation in political processes at local, national and international levels. In so doing, children are able to identify their own concerns, find potential solutions, and engage in the development of legislation and policies that will affect their lives. World Vision is committed to promoting the rights of children to participate in political processes so as to enable children to influence the laws, policies and programmes that directly impact on their lives. Moreover, World Vision also recognises the need to foster children's capacity to be active citizens and to strengthen their enjoyment of their rights during their childhood and as they reach adulthood.

Children's citizenship can be exercised at different levels and for different purposes. At the community level, children have the opportunity to become engaged in matters concerning their family, schools and workplaces, in community affairs and in local-level governance. At the national level, children can participate in influencing the development and implementation of legislation and other policies that impact on them, for instance on issues related to access to education and health care, protection from violence and exploitation, poverty alleviation, and in holding their governments to account for their obligations to children. Internationally, children have a critical role to play in influencing regional or global processes, such as the development of treaties and declarations, and in influencing the implementation of such agreements.

Efforts to foster children's civic engagement must not be an exclusive activity that is reserved for the most highly educated and articulate children. Participation is a right that must be accessible to every child, and particular attention must be given to including those who are most easily excluded, for instance on the basis of gender, disability, economic status, ethnicity or religion.

The following case studies provide tangible examples of methods that World Vision has used to support the inclusive participation of children in civic engagement at local, national and international levels.

Children's community parliaments in northern India

In India, World Vision has been supporting children's empowerment in local-level political processes through the establishment of community parliaments in the State of Uttranchal. The initiative seeks to empower children to assert their constitutional rights, and its motto 'with the children, for the children and by the children' espouses a philosophy in which the children work together to advocate for their own rights.

The Children's Parliament is intended to act as a catalyst for them to develop leadership skills, and then provide the forum in which they can put those skills to use. One of the major goals of the initiative is to enable children to identify challenges in their personal, family or community life, and then advocate for their rights.

The Uttranchal Children's Parliament was developed in early 2002, and was modelled on a pre-existing programme run by World Vision in Rajasthan State. Children from the local villages were invited to participate and run for election to leadership positions; a total of twelve children between the ages of 9 and 16 were elected, and the group then chose their own 'prime minister'. The remaining eleven children became the 'cabinet ministers', holding portfolios such as defence, homeland affairs, foreign affairs and education.

The Children's Parliament receives support and encouragement from the local programme manager and other World Vision staff in order to carry out its meetings and areas of responsibility. The children welcomed the idea of the Parliament and have worked consistently and diligently to make it effective.

Irshaad, the former Prime Minister of the Uttranchal Children's Parliament, feels very strongly about child rights, in particular that

> a child should have the freedom to express his views, get education, play and make his own decisions.

The Cabinet Ministers all agree that education is a priority, and that every child should have at least a basic education. They are equally concerned about health and environmental problems, and want to bring about changes to the best of their capacity.

While the Uttranchal Children's Parliament is a small-scale local initiative, the zest and zeal of the Prime Minister and Cabinet Ministers send a positive signal for the future. The effective replication of the model from Rajasthan demonstrates the importance of drawing inspiration from other initiatives and applying their lessons learned. It is hoped that the successful example in Uttranchal will spur others on to promote similar such initiatives in even more communities throughout India and around the world.

Agents of Peace in Colombia

In Colombia, World Vision has employed a very different approach to children's civic engagement. For the past ten years, World Vision Colombia has supported the Gestores de Paz (Agents of Peace) movement, with the aim of contributing to the construction of a culture of peace led by children.

One of World Vision's strategic objectives for Colombia is to prepare community leaders – including children and adolescents – to develop a level of awareness of social issues, along with their responsibilities as actors in the construction of peace in their communities, ultimately resulting in people who are capable of empowering themselves to feel and transform their real conditions. The Gestores de Paz movement is therefore a critical tool through which this objective can be realised. At present, the movement is made up of more than ten thousand boys, girls and adolescents between the ages of 3 and 18, along with some older youths, representing various ethnic groups, religions, and regions of the country.

The movement is implemented in such a way that its activities are identified, designed and promoted by the children themselves and include such things as games, sports, arts (theatre, dance, music, literature), ecology and personal, social and spiritual training (Plate 22.1). The programme aims to develop a process that

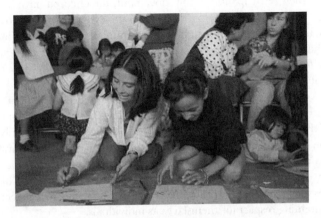

Plate 22.1 Gestores de Paz group meeting. Copyright: World Vision

is sustainable over the long term by promoting a methodology in which children teach other children and thus multiply the impact. The movement also promotes children's participation in the home, moving towards their greater participation in both the community and the municipality.

Gestores de Paz is essentially child led and adult supported. World Vision's Advocacy Coordinator supports a team of children, adolescents and youth (called 'peace promoters') who lead and promote the programme. The peace promoters are a part of a national-level group of young leaders who promote the participation of the children and adolescents and act as the leadership team for the movement. The leaders prepare the plans, including identifying the issues, themes and relevant activities, and then disseminate the plans among all the participants. Within the group of leaders there are children and adolescents who are being trained in different skills such as journalism and public speaking, along with teachers and promoters of children's and adolescents' empowerment and participation. The leaders have small groups of children with whom they develop the curriculum that they have planned in order to be ready to start working with other groups. In this manner, an increasing number of children are involved in the process, thus strengthening the effectiveness and sustainability of the movement.

The participation of children and young people in the movement has contributed in many ways to the participants' developing a stronger sense of belonging, identity and recognition. Belonging, because the formation, execution and evaluation of the plan is the responsibility of the children and adolescents who are leaders and members of the movement; identity, because they named the movement themselves and are responsible for promoting the initiative; and recognition, because the movement has gained notoriety and commendation at both national and global level. World Vision's Gestores de Paz has received three nominations for the Nobel Peace Prize and representatives of the movement have had the opportunity to take part in national and international events on child rights. Most notably, several of the children participated in the United Nations General Assembly Special Session on Children in 2002, when one of the leaders of the movement addressed the UN General Assembly.

Through their participation in the movement, the children have been able to exercise their right to be active participants in the evolution of their own lives as well as the lives of their families and their communities. Their participation originates in their own reality and conception of the world, and it strengthens their dignity, self-awareness and self-esteem, thus contributing to the development of and capacity to realise their citizenship.

The movement has had a significant impact on the lives of thousands of individuals, as well as on the wider Colombian society. On the individual level, the impact of the movement can be seen in the changing attitudes to daily relationships of the children and adolescents with their families, with their community, at school and at church, and with the environment. The children and adolescents are empowered with respect towards their individual background, history and capabilities, their capacity to realise their goals and to belong to a collective cause, while maintaining respect for themselves as individuals.

At the local level, some of the young leaders of the movement have been able to participate in the Youth Municipality Councils, which are legally created bodies that promote the participation of youth in the design of plans for the municipality and for the country. At the national level, recognition of the movement has allowed for active intervention in networks and alliances that design public policies related to children. Furthermore, the movement's capacity to assemble people at the local, regional or nationwide level further strengthens the linkages between the various levels, thus increasing the opportunity for greater impact (Plate 22.2).

While the movement is still young, it has grown significantly in strength and capacity over a short period of time. Some of the factors that have contributed to this positive growth include:

- the creation of alliances with local, regional and national institutions that deal with topics and processes related to childhood, adolescence and youth, with a rights-based approach to peace building;
- the development of a curriculum that was designed through a collaborative process with young people, which serves as a methodological guide for the movement;
- the constant organisation of forums for the preparation of leaders of the movement in different areas, including training on legislative processes;
- the methodology of child-to-child teaching and youth-to-child teaching has also strengthened the process by multiplying knowledge and skills across the country, to benefit a greater number of participants;
- explicit identification of games, art and sports as dynamic and experiential elements in the construction of peace.

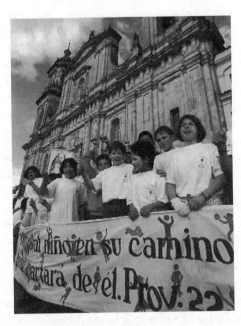

Plate 22.2 Peaceful rally at the parliament building. Copyright: World Vision

As one of Colombia's young advocates has argued:

> We would be fooling ourselves if we tried to deny the problems of our country. But when we focus on the problem, our mind gets blocked, and frustrated; if we focus on what is positive, we multiply this powerful engine we Colombians all have.[1]

The children and youth in the movement are learning to apply this approach in their daily lives, to see their dreams as a reality that is built from the present, and to project it not only towards the future. They are also learning to share their vision, dreams and plans with adults, who may start to see the possibility of a new country through the eyes of a child.

National Children's Congress and Parliament in Bolivia

The participation of children in national-level governance has been a major focus of World Vision's efforts in Bolivia in recent years. World Vision Bolivia is expressly committed to contributing towards the practice of a citizenship culture among the children and adolescents from rural and indigenous communities, so that they can participate actively in their communities and in the political decisions of the country, exercising their right to participate and to express themselves freely regarding issues that interest them.

To accomplish this, World Vision Bolivia facilitates activities directed at forming, strengthening and supporting community-based organisations led by children and adolescents. Such organisations promote the rights and responsibilities of children with families, communities, government organisations and other institutions. Through these activities, both boys and girls become catalysts for the promotion and defence of their own rights in their communities and with the state.

Together with the Social and Political Commission of the Bolivian parliament and a number of other NGOs, World Vision is seeking to facilitate the representation and participation of children in the national Legislative Assembly in two ways. First, through the National Congress of Children and Adolescents, which brings together children and adolescents from different sectors and social groups from the nine regions of Bolivia to discuss issues and produce recommendations to go before the Bolivian parliament. Second, through the Children's and Adolescents' National Parliament, which has provided children with the opportunity to propose draft national laws (see Box 22.1), and to present requests through written reports that will be passed to the Social and Political Commission of the parliament for its response.

The members of the children's parliament are democratically elected by their peers, based on their involvement in children's clubs in their own communities. The parliament itself is composed of a Deputies' Chamber and a Senators' Chamber, with equal representation based on gender, age and geographic distribution.

Through their participation in the parliament, the children are able to identify their own concerns, find potential solutions and suggest proposals for policies and actions that will benefit all of the country's children and adolescents. Additionally,

---

Box 22.1 Legislation drafted by Bolivian Children's and Adolescents' Parliament is passed into law

In 2003 the Bolivian Children's and Adolescents' Parliament presented a draft bill concerning children's right to proper identification/registration, expressing that the Bolivian state should provide birth certificates, free of charge, to all children and adolescents in the country. Based on this proposal, on 18 December 2003 the state of Bolivia passed Law 2616, which establishes the mechanism necessary for the registration of children and adolescents through the National Civil Register.

---

because a number of participants are drawn from rural areas and indigenous communities, particular attention has been given to issues affecting those children who are most marginalised and impoverished.

Participation by children in these processes is supported through workshops where they are taught about the procedures of the Legislative Assembly, the use of formal chamber methods, the election of representatives, and the generation of policy proposals at departmental and national levels.

While the Bolivian children's parliament is still in its infancy, it is evident through the reactions from both the government and the general public that there is interest and commitment from the state and from civil society to begin to listen to children's and adolescents' opinions on issues that concern them, as well as issues of broader national interest. Furthermore, the children's parliament has initiated a process that is leading towards more democratic representation of children in Bolivia, and to consolidating spaces that will allow for the achievement of greater outcomes.

Children's participation in poverty alleviation in the Philippines

In the Philippines, World Vision is working with children to influence government policies and decisions to allocate more resources for children. The Children's Basic Sector Council (CBSC), composed of twenty-five children aged 10 to 17 years, is recognised by the government as an official representation of the children's sector to the Philippines' National Anti-Poverty Commission (NAPC). The task of the NAPC-CBSC is to articulate the needs, demands and positions of the children's sector through dialogue with government agencies. They are also involved in spearheading the monitoring and follow-up of the government's commitments to address the needs of children. The Council consults other children at all levels in formulating a minimum achievable sectoral agenda, with the purpose of soliciting their viewpoints on concerns and policies relevant to children.

For seven years now, the children have campaigned vigorously for the prioritisation of children's concerns in policies and programmes on poverty reduction. For 2005–8, the NAPC-CBSC's agenda is focused on addressing: child abuse, child labour, children in armed conflict, child participation in governance, health and education. On the health agenda, the NAPC-CBSC is campaigning for improved health care and nutrition for mothers and children. This includes advocacy for more resources to fully implement the breastfeeding law, micronutrient supplementation, feeding programmes, food fortification, nutrition training for communities, and other hunger-mitigating interventions. The children are also demanding increased budget allocation to ensure better access to potable water in poor communities, construction of health-care facilities and support for moves towards the reduction of fees for medicines.

In their claim for better access to, and quality of, education, the children passed several resolutions to increase funds for the construction of more classrooms and the provision of mobile schools in remote and poor provinces. They are advocating for an improved student–textbook ratio for public school students (from one book to three students, to one book for each student) and for the improvement of school facilities (renovation of dilapidated classrooms, more libraries, laboratories, toilets etc). The children have urged the Department of Education to improve the situation of teachers by enhancing their competencies and complementing the budget to provide better compensation and benefits for public school teachers, since many are leaving the country to find better alternatives. The children have also asked for the cancellation of miscellaneous fees in public schools.

While some positive developments have been achieved in this area, such as more vigilance in the distribution of textbooks in public schools and increased support for child-friendly schools and for teachers, the children and the organisations supporting them need to continually advocate for changes in policies so as to ensure that children are continually prioritised in the allocation of resources.

Conclusion

In light of the case studies above, it is possible to distil some common themes and lessons learned that contribute to our understanding of children's participation. First, we see the need to ensure that programmes to support children's citizenship are rooted in their own reality. For instance, in the case of Bolivia, the children's parliament served as an important vehicle for them to engage in legislative reform that resulted in free universal birth registration, which was a matter of interest to all children, but particularly to those from indigenous and rural communities. In Colombia, the interests of the children and adolescents drove the promotion of a child-led peace movement, and in the Philippines, concerns about their education gave rise to advocacy for better school facilities and improved access to textbooks.

Second, it is important to recognise children's capacity to make contributions in the present, as well as to equip them for their future contributions as adolescents and in adulthood. In all of the case studies, it is clear that the children gained a greater sense of self and became involved in making important contributions to society, while at the same time they also learned skills and developed a sense of purpose that it is hoped will lead to active civic engagement later in life.

Third, it is critical to ensure that initiatives to support children's civic engagement are linked with local government and civil society organisations. For instance in India, the Philippines and Bolivia, the children's parliaments were not stand-alone entities, but were formally linked with government and civil society structures, so that the children's proposals would gain broader political, legal and social support.

Last, the case studies also point to the importance of building sustainable systems to support children's civic engagement and, where appropriate, to encourage the replication of successful initiatives. Children's citizenship must not be viewed as a one-off project, but must be supported with the appropriate resources and structures to ensure sustainability. Such initiatives must be accessible to new groups of children as the others grow older, and also be flexible enough to adjust to lessons learned and respond to new challenges. For instance, in the case of Colombia, children have been encouraged to take on new roles with greater responsibility as they grow older, and in the case of India, the programme was modelled on and adapted from another successful initiative.

Children must be given the opportunity to participate in democratic systems of governance, so that they can begin to actively engage with the systems and structures that impact their lives, and influence them in a manner that promotes and protects their rights. In doing so, they live out the maxim that when children live with fairness, they learn justice.[2] The result is that their own lives become transformed, and they begin to participate in the transformation of the world around them. The case studies above provide just a few examples of where spaces and structures have been created for this to happen in a sustained and effective manner.

Acknowledgements

Aimyleen Gabriel, Luz Alicra Granada, Philippa Lei, Minnie Portales, Astrid Zacipa, Stefan Germann.

Notes

1. www.yocreoencolombia.com
2. Dorothy Law Nolte, 'Children Learn What They Live', www.empowermentresources.com/info2/childrenlearn-long_version.html.

23 Maintaining the status quo?

Appraising the effectiveness of youth councils in Scotland

Brian McGinley and Ann Grieve

Introduction

In most Western societies youth participation is advocated as part of a discourse on active citizenship, with increased youth participation being equated with the inclusion of young people (Bessant 2004). However, there is a paradox whereby young people continue to be viewed as 'part citizen and part villain' (McCulloch 2007) by adults simultaneously seeking their involvement while still regarding them as a threat.

There is recognition that young people are thus socially excluded, due to both age and reputation (MacDonald 1997; Barry 2005). The formation and support of youth councils across Britain has been one of the most popular mechanisms for government and voluntary agencies to promote the participation of young people (Matthews 2001; BYC 2007). The aim of youth councils is to provide a forum to enable the expression of opinions and encourage young people's active involvement in community decision making. However, these mechanisms created by adults have not been demanded by young people, and their purpose and organisation have been questioned over the past 10 years (Fitzpatrick and Kintrea 2000; Matthews 2001; Smith et al. 2005).

This chapter will discuss the effectiveness of youth council structures in enabling the participation of young people in Scotland. It considers three perspectives: the ways young people are involved, how well the voice of young people is facilitated by youth councils, and to what extent they lead to improvements in the lives of young people. In addition, the chapter provides both a rationale and an action plan for developing a more inclusive participatory process based on human rights. This discussion is important, because the demand for increased participation is inexorably linked to the concept of citizenship which has become an 'indispensable component of modern social theory as a perspective on social rights, welfare issues, political membership and social identity' (Shotter 1993: ix).

Locating participation in the Scottish context

The extent and purpose of participation for children and young people in Scotland has many different meanings. For example, it is a concept used to determine involvement in leisure programmes, as a form of social conditioning to change behaviour (Scottish Executive 2004) and as a way of working in child welfare programmes (Murray and Hallett 2000). In addition, it denotes involvement rates in Post-Compulsory Education and Training (Raffe et al. 2001) and the contribution of individuals and peers in specialist programmes (Coburn et al. 2007). However, participation also holds the promise of overcoming the alleged democratic deficit of young people, addressing exclusion and promoting active citizenship, through involvement in decision making.

In Scotland the approaches deemed most appropriate for increasing youth participation and enhancing active citizenship are through the establishment and support of youth councils (BYC 2007). Historically, youth councils have been developed as structural responses to government policy directives (Scottish Executive 2007). Thus, the meaning and context for participation is strongly influenced by this political discourse, and ultimately politicians have the power to create or remove rights for ordinary citizens. As Prior, Stewart and Walsh (1995: 8) remind us, 'the status of citizens in Britain is founded on no more than an act of faith in the reasonableness of their elected representatives.'

In Scotland, the promotion of youth councils is founded on the assumption that participation is the best way to release human potential and inculcate cultural capacity (Scottish Parliament 2002) through a 'bottom-up' approach which focuses on the natural assets of a given locality (Rondinelli 1993). However, in reality, there are contradictions in policies affecting young people. On the one hand, positive developments have emerged from policy through the creation of a Children's Rights Commissioner and a legislative requirement on community planning partners to consult with young people. At the same time, policy simultaneously advocates the control and containment of young people through increased surveillance and Anti-Social Behaviour Orders, the use of which may contribute to, rather than reduce, the criminalisation of young people (Davies and McMahon 2007). Thus, it could be argued that these contrary messages have perpetuated ambiguity in the social status of young people. This ambiguity in policy stances raises questions about the effectiveness of youth councils as a way of engaging young people.

Youth councils: facilitating the youth voice?

The following discussion draws on two recent studies undertaken with 76 young people aged 12 to 18 years in six youth councils across Scotland, which explored the effectiveness of youth councils according to three key areas of debate (Reynolds 2007; McGinley 2006). These are: the extent to which youth voice is facilitated; a critique of the level of youth involvement in local decision making; and the reported improvements and benefits in the lives of young people.

The studies suggested that those chosen to participate in youth councils were hand-picked by adults and known to be potentially interested. This finding is exemplified by comments from John, who intimated that 'it was the youth worker who asked me if I wanted to come along to the youth council meetings to see if I was interested in joining'. Young people's perception of the recruitment process is that it does not encourage the voice of 'outsider' youth to be heard.

It's the good ones who get to go to speak to the council about stuff … it's for the geeks who think they know everything.

Findings from the research suggest that significant numbers of young people continue to be socially excluded and disadvantaged through lack of participatory opportunities. Two categories of 'outsider' youth were identified. The first are those who are not involved in any club or organisation and who therefore have no way of knowing that participatory opportunities exist. The second category are those who are involved in youth projects but are not picked to represent their club or forum, due to both the validity that they attach to this involvement and their strained relationships with powerful local adults. Checkoway and Gutierrez (2006) suggest that there should be more examination of issues of 'relative power, privilege and position' (p. 114) of those involved in youth councils, as well as of their adult 'allies'.

The studies also found that being included as member of the local youth council is a route into a whole host of other participatory structures both locally and nationally. Participants can be self-nominated or elected by peers, but there is a prerequisite that they are successfully involved, to some extent, prior to selection.

In spite of the rationale for youth councils of empowering young people, those involved reported feeling a lack of personal power. They recognised that their voices were regarded as a common voice which was dependent on being a member of the group. The balance of promoting the individual within the group context is a complex and interesting area for those working with young people. In essence, three aspects need to be nurtured when seeking to enhance the participation of young people: the individual, the group and the community.

Involvement in local decision making

Most significantly, youth councils are seen as being key to providing opportunities for young people to get involved in local, regional and national decision making. Dialogue Youth is a major youth initiative working with 12- to 18-year-olds to improve youth councils and encourage participation. Interestingly, the evaluation report (Scottish Executive 2005) identified a range of successful developments, but also found that there was a small core group of truly engaged young people providing information for the less engaged (Scottish Executive Social Research 2005). However, the Scottish Executive is clear that the problem does not lie with the policy or structure, and that, through the spaces provided by these structures, opportunities for enhancing the participation of young people across the community can be realised.

Of course, there are general opportunities for young people to get involved. For example, they have the right to be consulted and involved in the community planning process in Scotland, which is a partnership arrangement between public bodies as part of the modernising agenda. There are a number of successful partnerships, for example, Argyll and Bute Young Scot Dialogue Youth Unit, Sauchie Community Green Map (Scottish Executive 2006). However, the extent to which these have successfully engaged young people is open to question. Barber and Naulty (2005: 49) make a range of observations and recommendations to improve this process. They report that 'not all young people – nor local authority workers and community planning partners are ready to engage in this type of dialogue'. This is in spite of a statutory requirement imposed through the Local Government Scotland (2003) Act.

However, it is clear that if a young person wants and is able to get involved, then a fuller range of participatory opportunities can open up, such as the Young People's Fund (National Lottery), the Prince's Trust and a number of voluntary uniformed organisations. In addition, they can become a member of the Scottish Youth Parliament, which was launched in 1999. The vast majority of members represent a youth forum, while others represent youth organisations or are individually nominated. Conversely, the vast majority of young people in Scotland do not participate in these types of structures. Youth Bank (www.youthbank.org.uk), a successful youth participation model, itself recognises the difficulties in recruiting young people who are harder to reach. It argues the need for specific strategies to encourage participation by this group if reproduction of the inequalities inherent in the representative democratic structures already in place is to be avoided.

Youth councils: changing the lives of young people?

A key measure of the effectiveness of youth councils is the extent to which they bring about change in the lives of young people. Youth councils across Scotland report changes being effected by young people's participation. For example, in Dumfries and Galloway a Youth Strategy Executive Group was formed to work in partnership with other young people, to voice young people's opinions, to be noticed and heard and to deal with Youth Bank funding. Another example, Fife Youth Forum, states it has made impacts through countering negative stereotypes of young people and helping the community. However, it is harder to find evidence to substantiate these claims. It appears that youth councils are being seen by the wider political community as effecting limited change, but perhaps only within a restricted political agenda.

Young people themselves believe that youth councils promote involvement in organised activities, can promote the views of young people and encourage awareness of the channels available to air those views, be it through surveys, local pages or other means (Scottish Executive Social Research 2005).

Most significantly, youth council participation is seen by those young people involved as having personal benefits. These include:

- increased confidence in presenting their ideas to others
- new skills acquired
- making new contacts and developing friendships
- increased motivation to work with others
- broader perspective on their life
- increased interest in their environment.

While young people perceive personal benefits from participation in youth councils, the impact of participation in youth councils in bringing about change in young people's lives more generally is a contentious issue. Evidence suggests that youth councils do indeed give rise to outcomes for young people, but these tend to concern 'safe' issues which do not significantly challenge the power or agenda of adults.

Youth councils may be perceived to be successful, depending on the agenda and understandings of stakeholders. They appear to work well as an apprentice-ship for a small cohort of young people who wish to continue their involvement in politics. However, when viewed as a structure for empowering a majority of young people and redefining the structures for their participation, youth councils arguably have less impact (Matthews et al. 1999).

Signposting a way forward: a rights-based approach?

Evidence from these studies points to a continuing lack of local participatory opportunities for many, the validation of those already capable of being involved, the continuing discrimination against those who could potentially benefit most from this structure and the lack of rigorous evaluation of youth councils as an effective medium for bringing about change. If we are to address and rectify these problems, then we must recognise the complex nature of participation and devise a systematic way of involving people and inculcating participation as a core feature of our relationship with young people and children (Sinclair 2004).

To improve the status quo, there is a need to develop 'a rights-based approach' to working with young people, based on the UN Convention on the Rights of the Child. To date, Scottish administrations have failed to fully recognise the rights of children and young people in law, policy and practice (Matthews and Limb 2003). Thus, we need to find new ways to promote involvement which improves the experiences of Scottish young people in line with those of other Europeans (Margo et al. 2006).

Part of the answer may be to move from a representative approach, symbolised by youth councils, to create a participatory culture which encourages the claiming of rights and promotes social justice, with full active citizenship within everyday social practices. This will affect every aspect of the child's life and will have conse-quences for adult–child relations (Cockburn 2007). The legislative basis for this is clear and acknowledges that all under-18s have the right to be heard and involved in a respectful way. Moving forward in this way involves creating a nurturing rela-tionship which encourages active listening and moves into purposeful conversa-tions and meaningful dialogue. This approach has the potential to lead to mutual critical consciousness and praxis (Freire 1972), which is a prerequisite for engaging with the current hegemonic forces that demonise young people. It is through this developing sense of critical consciousness that the rights of young people can be established and their citizenship role indubitably recognised.

In order for this to happen, political actions are needed to increase resources, improve spaces and structures and share power through meaningful engagement with young people. The following five-point action plan (Box 23.1) could provide a

Box 23.1 Five-point action plan

1 Provide a national charter which enshrines the rights of children and young people as being protected, promoted and enacted in every subsequent piece of legislation.
2 Set substantial levels of dedicated resources at national and local levels to ensure that children and young people have ways of being involved which are jointly identified, flexible, developmental and reviewed at regular intervals.
3 Ensure that children and young people's voices are recognised and that decision-making processes reflect the exercise of political power, including the creation of a vibrant youth workforce to act as a dedicated 'civil service' which holds the young person as its primary client.
4 Ensure that children and young people are actively involved in equal partnerships with adults to develop policies which reflect their identified concerns, understandings and aspirations.
5 Establish monitoring and development mechanisms for children and young people to claim their equal rights as the basis for negotiation with other power brokers.

starting point for a rights-based approach and is based on identifying the relevant legislative processes, resource implications, decision-making mechanisms, policy development and procedures for evaluation.

If enacted in a consistent manner, then these actions can lead to improved structures and spaces for enhancing the participation of children and young people. This would support the development of a rights-based approach which focuses on both processes and outcomes and moves the young person centre-stage as an actor in, rather than a recipient of, policy. It is a practice which challenges those who hide behind culture to undermine rights and integrity, while actively listening to the voices of young people (Braeken and Cardinal 2006).

This is not a deficit model that seeks to build capacity and resolve social problems. Rather, it recognises and celebrates current capacities and encourages levels of involvement that are meaningful and aspirational. The starting point for this is to recognise the significant obstacles that young people currently experience when trying to participate socially, economically and politically through currently accepted societal routes. Thus, new structures and environments must be grounded in a reality that starts where young people are at, reflect their experiences and is created in tune with their views of the world.

This action plan demands a commitment to democratic practice that is well planned, resourced and evaluated to ensure that it delivers the intended opportunities in an equitable and just manner. It also requires a cultural change both conceptually and operationally where official youth participation policies actively champion, listen and act upon the voices of young people. Perhaps in this way an innovative, empowering joint agenda will be created that strengthens the active social commitment and growth of both young people and adults alike.

Conclusion

Participation in youth councils is perceived by 'insider' youth and adults as beneficial in giving young people a voice, yet the voices of many young people are not heard. Youth councils allow limited involvement in decision making, usually at the level of consultation rather than of encouraging young people to drive their own agenda. There is limited evidence of impact on the lives of young people generally, although those involved reported personal benefits. Given this situation, a case is made for an alternative 'rights-based' discourse to evolve new forms of youth participation rooted in the everyday lives and relationships of young people. This proposal is within our reach and can be achieved by building on good practice and the commitment that already exists at all levels. Inspirational examples of good practice do exist, but it is only through renewed and continuous commitment and the realisation of the principles of justice, rights, equality, democracy and participation that our children and young people will feel secure and valued on their life journey.

Opportunities for involvement should be based on an increasing confidence nurtured from an early age, with an appreciation of the significance and benefits of contributing to society. However, this will only be achieved when we tackle the inconsistencies and discrimination inherent in top-down, adult-dominated policies. If we have the courage to truly situate children and young people at the heart of social processes then the status quo will be challenged.

References

Barber, T. and Naulty, M. (2005) *Your Place or Mine? A research study exploring young people's participation in community planning*, Dundee: University of Dundee.

Barry, M. (2005) *Youth Policy and Social Inclusion: Critical debates with young people*, London and New York: Routledge.

Bessant, J. (2004) 'Mixed messages: Youth participation and democratic practice', *Australian Journal of Political Science* 39(2): 387–404.

Braeken, D. and Cardinal, M. (2006) 'Sexuality education', paper presented at the International Expert Consultation on Promotion of Sexual Health, World Association for Sexual Health, Oaxaca City, 1–2 May 2006.

BYC (British Youth Council) (2007) 'Getting it right for every child: Draft Children's Services (Scotland) Bill consultation: British Council Submission', London: British Youth Council, available at www.byc.org.uk/asset_store/documents/draft_children's_ services__scotland__bill.pdf.

Checkoway, B. and Gutierrez, L. (2006) *Youth Participation and Community Change*, London: Routledge.

Coburn, A., McGinley, B. and McNally, C. (2007) 'Peer education: Individual learning or service delivery?', *Youth and Policy* 94(1): 19–33.

Cockburn, T. (2007) 'Partners in power: A radically pluralistic form of participative democracy for children and young people', *Children & Society* 21(6) 446–57.

Davies, Z. and McMahon, W. (eds) (2007) *Debating youth justice: From punishment to problem solving*, London: Centre for Crime and Justice Studies.

Fitzpatrick, S. A. and Kintrea, K. (2000) 'Youth involvement in urban regeneration: Hard lessons – future directions', *Policy and Politics* 28(4): 493–509.

Freire, P. (1972) *Pedagogy of the Oppressed*, Harmondsworth: Penguin.

Smith, N., Lister, R., Middleton, S. and Cox, L. (2005) 'Young people as real citizens: Towards an inclusionary understanding of citizenship', *Journal of Youth Studies* 8(4): 425–43.

McCulloch, K. (2007) 'Democratic participation or surveillance? Structures and practices for young people's decision making', *Scottish Youth Issues Journal* 9(1): 9–22.

MacDonald, R. (1997) 'Dangerous youth and the dangerous class', in R. MacDonald (ed.) *Youth, the Underclass and Social Exclusion* London: Routledge, pp. 1–26.

McGinley, B. (2006) 'Seeking change or same? An insight into the workings of youth councils in Scotland', unpublished research, Strathclyde: University of Strathclyde.

Margo, J., Dixon, M., Pearce, N. and Reed, H. (2006) *Freedom's Orphans: Raising youth in a changing world*, London: IPPR Publications.

Matthews, H. (2001) 'Citizenship, youth councils and young people's participation', *Journal of Youth Studies* 4(3): 299–318.

Matthews, H. and Limb, M. (2003) 'Another white elephant? Youth councils as democratic structures', *Space and Polity* 7(2): 173–92.

Matthews, H., Limb, M. and Taylor, M. (1999) 'Young people's participation and representation in society', *Geoforum* 30: 135–44.

Murray, C. and Hallett, C. (2000) 'Young people's participation in decisions affecting their welfare', *Childhood* 7(1): 11–25.

Prior, D., Stewart, J., and Walsh, K. (1995) *Citizenship: Rights, community and participation*, London: Pitman.

Raffe, D., Brannen, K., Fairgrieve, J. and Martin, C. (2001) 'Participation, inclusiveness, academic drift and parity of esteem: A comparison of post-compulsory education and training in England, Wales, Scotland and Northern Ireland', *Oxford Review of Education* 27(2): 173–203.

Reynolds, A. (2007) 'The recruitment and selection for youth councils: Are outsider youths socially excluded from youth participatory structures in their local area?', unpublished thesis, Strathclyde: University of Strathclyde.

Rondinelli, D. (1993) *Development Projects as Policy Experiments: An adaptive approach to development administration*, London: Routledge.

Scottish Executive (2004) 'A literature review of the evidence base for culture, the arts and sports policy', Edinburgh: Scottish Executive, available at www.scotland.gov.uk/Publications/2004/08/19784/41507, accessed 23 January 2008.

Scottish Executive (2005) *Evaluation of the Dialogue Youth Programme*, Edinburgh: Scottish Executive, www.scotland.gov.uk/Publications/2006/03/08144046/0.

Scottish Executive (2006) 'Engaging children and young people in community planning', accessible at www.scotland.gov.uk/Resource/Doc/154089/0041433.pdf.

Scottish Executive (2007) *Moving Forward: A strategy for improving young people's chances through youth work*, Edinburgh: Scottish Executive.

Scottish Executive Social Research (2005) *Local Government Evaluation of the Dialogue Youth Programme*, Edinburgh: Scottish Executive.

Scottish Parliament (2002) *Youth Participation*, Edinburgh: Scottish Executive.

Shotter, J. (1993) 'Psychology and citizenship: Identity and belonging', in B. Turner (ed.) *Citizenship and Social Theory*, London: Sage.

Sinclair, R. (2004) 'Participation in practice: Making it meaningful, effective and sustainable', *Children & Society* 18(2): 106–18.

Smith, N., Lister, R., Middleton, S. and Cox, L. (2005) 'Young people as real citizens: Towards an inclusionary understanding of citizenship', *Journal of Youth Studies* 8(4): 425–43.

24 More than crumbs from the table

A critique of youth parliaments as models of representation for marginalised young people

Alan Turkie

Introduction

This paper addresses issues of inclusion and exclusion, not between young people and adults, but between included and excluded young people. By exploring and challenging commonly held assumptions about youth democracy and participation it also questions whether inclusion is aided or hindered by the pursuit of a representative democracy model. The paper draws primarily on the experience of the UK Youth Parliament (UKYP) and the views of young people involved.[1]

Context

In broad terms, the UKYP operates a model of representation similar to that of the Westminster parliament. Members of the Youth Parliament (MYPs) are elected by 11- to 18-year-olds within prescribed geographic areas, on the basis of one MYP per 25,000 young people. For example, in England these are based on local authority areas, with the largest electing seven MYPs and the smallest one MYP. Young people in Northern Ireland, with a population of approximately one-twentieth that of England, can elect 16 young people, while England has a total of 308.

Data on intake to the UKYP over the two years 2006 and 2007 (Table 24.1) appears to suggest a healthy spread in terms of gender and ethnicity. However, similar data on social class, potentially equally revealing, is not readily available. More detailed analysis in fact shows that only 1 per cent of young people in 2007 were of African Caribbean origin, as compared to 6 per cent of Indian origin, which mirrors very directly young people's experience of, and success in, formal education.

Factors affecting the inclusion of socially excluded or vulnerable young people

A number of factors militate against the involvement of socially excluded young people in youth parliaments and other representative bodies. In particular, barriers to inclusion may be influenced by a number of assumptions.

Table 24.1 Percentages of young people elected to Youth Parliament, 2006 and 2007

Elected as MYPs	2006 (%)	2007 (%)
Girls and young women	53	54
Black and minority ethnic young people	21	21
Disabled young people	2	5
Young gypsies and travellers	0.3	0.3
Young people in care	1	3
Homeless young people	1	3

Assumption 1: Young people who put themselves forward are highly motivated, artic-ulate and ambitious young people, who have striven to get elected on merit by their peers. They are not necessarily generously disposed to the extra efforts youth workers make to involve vulnerable or marginalised young people

There are, of course, many views on this, but overwhelmingly, MYPs and depu-ties argue that, as fair-minded people, they are elected to represent the views of all young people. The following represent a range of views:

> If we want to be effective we need young people with get up and go who are prepared to represent everyone. I don't like the idea of bringing people in because of labels. To label is to disable. We can't afford to waste time on pointless rubbish … UKYP shouldn't change to accommodate this … workers should work to our existing procedures.
>
> (MYP, Scotland)

> If there is someone who didn't feel comfortable with certain aspects of UKYP, then we should change to accommodate them … As long as it does not affect the way in which UKYP runs in terms of successes and aims. It depends on the individual situation.
>
> (Deputy MYP, West Midlands)

> If there is a need for a specific voice for young gypsies, homeless people and so on then there needs to be a separate group established for that purpose. It should not be lumped in with a group that is in place to represent all young people.
>
> (Ex-MYP, South West Region)

In fact, the diversity of any cohort of MYPs depends less on the determination and motivation of individual young people than on factors such as the resources devoted to the election process locally and the commitment and attitudes of youth workers and their senior officers. For example, in 2007 the turnout of voters was 28,804 in one local authority and 83 in another! A third authority delivered a plebiscite of over 50 per cent of all young people aged between 11 and 18. One area had two candidates with cerebral palsy, while a young gypsy was elected as MYP in another. Others are experimenting with proportional voting systems, which give more opportunity to young people attending special schools with only fifty pupils; otherwise, pupils attending large comprehensives tend to benefit greatly from a first-past-the-post system. In one local authority the candidates themselves argued strongly for a first-past-the-post process while gay, lesbian and bisexual young people and Black and minority ethnic young people argued for a proportional voting procedure. Some youth workers put most of their energy into supporting young people who may not initially feel confident to stand for election, while others focus on ensuring that the process of election is watertight.

What does this tell us? First, that elected MYPs are by no means a homogeneous group and statistical data does not take account of young people's complex or multilayered identities: musician, sportsperson, gay *and* autistic; potholer, environmentalist *and* homeless; feminist, scientist *and* asylum-seeker. Some are concerned to 'get up and go' on behalf of others, while some want to ensure that *others* have a seat at the table. Second, youth workers are also not a homogeneous group. Ideology informs their practice and the models of representation they will push for. Third, the chosen structures will determine the outcome of elections and are usually not determined by young people.

Assumption 2: It is too time consuming/expensive/inappropriate to involve vulnerable or marginalised young people

There are a number of common rationalisations for not making efforts to enlist young people from excluded groups:

- Vulnerable young people are hounded to become active citizens by endless professionals; this puts more demands on these young people's already difficult or complex lives.
- Disabled young people are vulnerable or have 'evolving capacities' which may make involvement too difficult.
- Gypsies and traveller children, or homeless young people, lead lifestyles which are too chaotic for active citizenship.
- Disaffected young people do not want to become involved.
- Young carers are too tied to their domestic commitments.
- Refugee and asylum-seeking young people or young people in care are too burdened by day-to-day survival to become involved.

These arguments can easily be self-fulfilling, and so serve to maintain the confinement of marginalised young people to the edges of society. Although some of the obstacles to involving young people in these groups are real, with creativity and persistence they can be overcome, as the following examples show.

For disabled young people, while barriers to involvement are perhaps greater in national structures, best-practice local initiatives (for example City Equals in Sunderland, the Disability Youth Forum in Calderdale, Speaking Out in Cambridge) are showing the ways forward as young people with disabilities break new ground in developing inclusive participative structures. But limited under-standing, skills and awareness mean that there is still a long way to go; recent research indicates that:

- participation only happens for very few disabled young people, and especially not among those with complex needs or communication impairments;
- a clearer understanding about the meaning of participation is needed on the part of professionals, especially the need for activity which is undertaken at levels appropriate to young people's abilities or capacities for involvement;
- preparing children and young people to express their views takes time and an individual approach.

(Franklin and Sloper 2007)

Gypsy and traveller young people face multiple barriers, as recent work under-taken by the Ormiston Children and Families Trust indicates. Racism, the need to hide their identity in order to avoid conflict, misunderstanding and lack of posi-tive representation of their culture are all additional reasons why young people from this most excluded community are reluctant to become involved in civic life (Warrington 2006). With the employment of a specialist worker over the past two years, the UKYP aims in the future to properly involve young gypsies and travel-lers, and high-quality democracy work in Kent has already resulted in one young gypsy being elected as an MYP for the county.

While refugee and asylum-seeking young people frequently face overwhelming pressures, extensive research conducted by the Centre for Multicultural Youth Issues (2006) indicates that young refugees tend to be particularly independent, resilient, strong-minded and more than capable of making their own decisions. To argue that a preoccupation with day-to-day survival should disenfranchise people is therefore spurious.

While public policy and professional practice are, with varying levels of success, encouraging the involvement of looked-after children in the planning and delivery of services that directly affect them (see Children in Scotland 2006), they remain largely excluded from influence and involvement in wider decisions. Pursuing the argument posited previously about multilayered identities, it stands to reason that while some young people in care, or previously in care, will want to develop their skills as musicians or scientists, others may want the opportunity to engage with campaigning organisations, such as youth councils or youth parliaments.

Mapping of children and young people's participation in England (Oldfield and Fowler 2004) indicates that statutory and voluntary agencies are less successful in involving young travellers, lesbian, gay or bisexual young people, young refugees and asylum seekers, and disaffected or disengaged young people. In this context, the UKYP appears successful in many respects. It has consistently high involve-ment from Black and minority ethnic young people. Gay young men are a promi-nent force, although lesbian young women are less visible. There is increasing involvement from disabled young people, homeless young people and young people who are or have been in care. On the other hand, refugee and asylum-seeking young people and gypsies and travellers remain under-represented.

While targeted work with disabled young people and with gypsy and traveller young people is being undertaken within the Youth Parliament, embedding new processes will take time, as this also requires cultural change. For instance, for many young people attending the four-day Annual Sitting, at which almost 400 young people develop their campaign strategies, it can be a confusing experience at best, and for some a very challenging one. In such an environment success can be viewed – by the young people themselves – as the capacity to speak with self-assurance to a large group, to quickly research complex information or to facilitate groups, tasks which many experienced adult workers would find challenging. The views of two young people with disabilities reinforce this point:

> With 60 young people in my group the event was too noisy, and I frequently had to leave the room. I was too ambitious and have bitten off more than I can chew.
>
> (Letter of resignation from MYP, South West England)

> The other MYPs don't need sleep breaks. We use and need so much more energy to function. If everyone had more free time we could have just sloped off … and there's been a problem about where responsibility lies. I'm not allowed to do anything without a youth worker so I've had to fit into their schedule. It makes me a bit useless.
>
> (MYP, Yorkshire and Humberside)

Ethnographic research undertaken on behalf of the UKYP by a young person with a learning disability (Clancy 2008), with support from Mencap and the Open University, found that, while her experience of the UKYP at a local level was entirely positive, this was not the case at regional or national events. The young researcher's recommendations included the use of small groups; only one person speaking at one time; no jargon; use of pictures and symbols; the availability of support workers; plenty of breaks; fun and games; time to think; time to speak; and a friendly and helpful atmosphere. It is reasonable to argue that these 'top tips' are in fact good-practice guidelines which should be applied universally. Not to do so could in fact exclude the majority of young people, as the following quotation illustrates:

> When the government ministers were here yesterday I thought it was amazing having young people challenge them. But rather than making this accessible maybe we need to look at better ways of feeding in the views of other young people. Not just disabled young people. The vast majority of young people are excluded from this process … it doesn't suit most young people. Without a lot of support and training it excludes most young people.
>
> (Inclusion development worker, Calderdale Council, attending the 2007 UKYP Annual Sitting in Glasgow)

The experiences of young people with disabilities within the Youth Parliament bring us back to the question of whether genuine inclusion is viable in complex national organisations such as the UKYP. Perhaps parallel structures feeding into larger national ones can provide a way forward, but perhaps also young people need not be bound by representative traditions which, many would argue, have not delivered for disadvantaged or minority voices in national democracies. Hill et al. (2004: 85) speak directly to this point:

> There are many adults who are not empowered by the operation of the representative democratic process ... and it would be surprising if this did not apply equally to children and young people.

Reflective evaluation of our practice points to the need for deeper cultural change within the organisation if vulnerable and socially excluded young people are to feel that the Youth Parliament offers an equal opportunity for election by their peers and, once elected, a level playing field on which to operate. In responding to this second assumption, yes, it is expensive and time consuming, but not inappropriate.

Assumption 3: Quotas ensuring the involvement of marginalised young people are unworkable, tokenistic or patronising

It is interesting that Members of the Scottish Youth Parliament (MSYPs), who already operate within a quota system, mainly responded in the affirmative to the question 'Do you think a specific number of seats should be allocated to young people from marginalised or excluded groups', while most UK Youth Parliament MYPs, who do not have a quota system, argued against:

> I believe it is both reasonable and realistic to involve a diverse range of people. The easiest way would be to partner with more organisations. For example the Scottish Youth Parliament allows national bodies to put forward two youth representatives, who work alongside the constituency MSYPs. This enables varied groups to get involved but also ensures that the representation isn't tokenistic. So young people representing a marginalised group have the support of a national organisation behind them.
>
> (MSYP)

> I think it's a good idea to allocate some seats to excluded groups within society. This will help in getting a wide range of ideas, and also help them in getting their voices heard.
>
> (MSYP)

> I do not think that a specific number of seats should be allocated to marginalised or excluded groups as I believe this is almost positive discrimination. But if any group is left feeling unrepresented (be they marginalised or not) the system must be failing and needs to be rectified. The most effective way is to work with such groups across the country finding out the best ways to get them involved in the Youth Parliament.
>
> (Young trustee of UKYP and ex-MYP)

As mentioned previously, UKYP functions as a representative democracy, with areas, regions and devolved nations allocated numbers of seats based strictly on the population of 11- to 18-year-olds within each 'constituency'. This results in an inbuilt Anglo-centric bias, with, for instance, issues of national identity being raised frequently but regularly sidelined by the majority. While the Scottish Youth Parliament and Funky Dragon, the youth representative body for Wales, have both adopted approaches which guarantee the involvement of at least some targeted groups of young people, population size as the single determining factor for representation within the UKYP makes marginal voices hard to hear. Notwithstanding that, there is much creative work going on at present within the UKYP, as mentioned above, including imaginative approaches to the election process, targeted work with gypsies and travellers, work with Muslim young people, partnership work with disability organisations and planned targeted work with looked-after young people and refugee and asylum-seeking young people. Youth service practitioners in one local authority speak for many others who contribute to the increasingly mature youth participation debate, which attempts to function at both universal and targeted levels:

> We start by creating safe environments which enable inclusion. This opens the door to integration, but if, for instance, disabled young people or lesbian and gay young people do not feel safe in a mainstream provision, they still have opportunities to feed into and engage with the mainstream.
>
> (Local authority youth participation manager)

Conclusion

Whether the UK Youth Parliament, and other youth participation organisations, need to choose between supporting young people to achieve change by taking the quickest or straightest route, or challenging the very structures on which adult decision making is based, is a question for debate. I would argue that change cannot be achieved without challenging the structures. More specifically, if socially excluded groups of people do not have a chair at the table, or are forced to compete for a place at that table, they are only ever likely to get the crumbs. Experience over the two years 2006 and 2007 reinforces this argument. For instance, concerns about tackling racism, sexism or homophobia have not been raised as campaign choices within the UKYP, in spite of strong representation by Black young people, young women and young gay men. Similarly, disabled young people have to date campaigned on global issues rather than on disability-specific ones; more detailed research might show that this has more to do with the culture of the organisation rather than the unencumbered choices made by young people.

Mimicking flawed adult structures is not the only way forward for young people, who need not be constrained by tradition. Letting election processes, however democratic, simply take their course without thinking through what makes participation possible will not deliver the equal involvement of socially excluded young people. Once involved in large national structures, many young people will continue to feel excluded unless minority voices and access requirements are put centre-stage. A participative approach (Hill et al. 2004) or a participatory democracy style of engagement, similar to the well-respected Investing in Children Durham model (Cairns 2006: 217–34), might provide more opportunities for young people to decide for themselves how and when they wish to engage.

Specific, considered measures are needed, based on the first-hand views and experiences of marginalised young people. Commitment, knowledge, skills, awareness, money and open, not predetermined, approaches are all needed in order to remove barriers to participation, but the benefits to both included and excluded young people are considerable. As Lloyd (2002: 83) points out,

> In the process of becoming marginalised a group becomes dehumanised and people within it become treated like objects … objects of the actions of others, a statistic to be achieved.

That process dehumanises us all, and we all must work together to prevent it.

Notes

1. Interviews conducted by Alice Clancy at the UKYP Annual Sitting in Glasgow in July 2007 and by Alan Turkie in January/February 2008.

References

Cairns, L. (2006) 'Participation with purpose', in E. K. M. Tisdall, J. Davis, M. Hill, and A. Prout (eds) *Children, Young People and Social Inclusion: Participation for what?* Bristol: The Policy Press.

Centre for Multicultural Youth Issues (2006) *What is Good Youth Settlement? Exploring what it means for refugee young people to settle well in Australia*, Melbourne: Centre for Multicultural Youth Issues.

Children in Scotland (2006) *My Turn to Talk? The participation of looked after and accommodated children in decision-making about their own care*, Edinburgh: Children in Scotland.

Clancy, A. (2008) 'What it is like for me to take part in UK Youth Parliament' (unpublished).

Franklin, A. and Sloper, P. (2007) *Supporting the Participation of Disabled Children and Young People in Decision Making*, York: Social Policy Research Unit, University of York.

Hill, M., Davis, J., Prout, A. and Tisdall, E. (2004) 'Moving the participation agenda forward', *Children & Society*, 18(2): 77–96.

Lloyd, M. (2002) *The Invisible Table: Perspectives on youth and youth work in New Zealand*, Wellington: Dunmore Press.

Oldfield, C. and Fowler, C. (2004) *Mapping Children and Young People's Participation in England*, London: Department for Education and Skills.

Warrington, C. (2006) *Children's Voices: Changing futures. The views and experiences of young gypsies and travellers*, Ipswich: Ormiston Children and Families Trust.

25 *Nil desperandum* **as long as you** *carpe diem*

Jack Lewars

Introduction

In a publication with so many eminent contributors, it is perhaps worth starting with an introduction and an explanation of my interest in Student Voice. I am a 19-year-old student heading to university after around five years in the field of participation. After various Student Voice activities at school, I have worked for a year as the Student Support Officer of the English Secondary Students' Association (ESSA). ESSA is a representative organisation for young people in secondary education in England, i.e. people between 11 and 19 years of age. The association operates much like a union, gathering the views of its members and representing them to government, the media, academics and any other interested bodies. ESSA also delivers a large amount of training in schools to enable students to express themselves most efficiently and effectively, and in the last year has branched more into political lobbying and contracted consultation work. At the time of writing the organisation (established in 2005) is three years old and continues to expand its membership base and the breadth of its activities. In line with its ethos, ESSA is run at a strategic level by a National Council of elected students, two from each government region. These young people drive the organisation forward and make all the key decisions associated with its operation. The Student Support Officer, nearly always a student on a gap year between school and university, coordinates ESSA's activities, with a focus on enabling the association's members to get involved in ESSA's work as fully as possible. My interest in Student Voice is, therefore, both personal and professional, and I hope to bring a 'youthful' perspective to the debate to balance my relative inexperience in the field.

The title of this chapter reflects, inevitably, my interest in classical languages. I say 'inevitably' because I believe that your whole life is shaped by your experiences at school, be they academic, social or political. The importance of active participation in education cannot therefore be underestimated, as it has the potential to dramatically alter the course of a student's life. This can be through new skills acquired through Student Voice activities; through an individual's new-found belief that his or her views actually matter, and that they can change things by acting on them; or even through the broader horizons and interests of a student who is actively involved in the decisions concerning every facet of his or her education. In this chapter I intend to examine first the current state of participation (*nil desperandum*) and then the key challenges for driving this work forward (how to *carpe diem*).

Student Voice in England

As things stand, Student Voice in England occupies a strange position with regard to how far we can consider it 'official'. There is now significant guidance encouraging Student Voice, some of it even coming from the government's Department for Children, Schools and Families. Every teaching union recognises the value of participation, at least in part. Perhaps most significantly in terms of its practical effects, the school inspection body, Ofsted, is now actively seeking evidence of consultation with students when it visits schools. All this means that the 'virgin Student Voice school' or the 'school with absolutely no participation at all' is now almost entirely hypothetical, and research shows that 97 per cent of schools have a school council (Whitty and Wisby 2007). However, if we broaden the definition of our 'virgin school' to one without any *effective* Student Voice, the landscape changes somewhat. There is already a danger in England that, with the Ofsted stipulation mentioned above, schools are indulging in box-ticking exercises with their school councils. Making a concept such as Student Voice statutory is filled with potential pitfalls, as the situation in Wales shows. Welsh legislation already exists requiring schools to have a student council. Although the status of school councils has been strengthened by the regulations, research shows that they have very rarely led to broader Student Voice work; that school councils deal largely with 'decisions about practical arrangements, in most schools'; and that the policy has only really formalised existing practice (Estyn 2008). Despite the fact that the Welsh legislation could be considered overly prescriptive, it is certainly interesting that the regulations have in reality *narrowed* the remit of Student Voice, rather than extending it. It is not difficult to imagine the relief of a teacher who is seriously against student involvement in decision making, as they can simply set up a 'puppet' school council to decide on the colour of the uniform, or other trivialities.

   This example flags up two of the biggest weaknesses in, and biggest dangers to, Student Voice in England. First, there is tokenism. The consequences of tokenistic Student Voice are well documented – disaffected, cynical students; ineffectual processes; and a genuine lack of many of the potential benefits of successful participation. However, second, there is another, equally unfortunate situation, which is much less dwelt upon – *limited but effective* Student Voice. Many schools, senior staff and, *in particular*, students unintentionally limit the scope of participation in their schools, thus missing out on countless opportunities to reap the rewards of full-scale, widespread Student Voice, even though what they are doing is done well. This is frequently because they are unaware of the full canon of participatory practice; and the need for better information sharing is slowly attracting more attention within Student Voice. Many staff and students simply do not think of the more unusual mechanisms for participation: student interview panels for staff; students writing part of their school development plan; and even students designing and delivering lessons. The real problem here is that, even if teachers and students do think of such concepts, they are unable to get in touch with those who have already tried them, so as to get advice and explore any caveats. The value of a database of such case-study material cannot be overstated, and it is hoped that the Movement for Active Participation[1] will soon address this quite critical requirement.

Despite the above, however, *nil desperandum*! Student Voice is undoubtedly growing, and gathering momentum in England. Indeed, the various pressures and incentives mentioned above mean that, in the majority of schools, Student Voice is in the process of introduction. It is interesting to consider the advantages and disadvantages of the various ways in which Student Voice is being introduced.

Approaches to developing Student Voice: evolution or revolution?

First, there is the gradual approach. This is the most common route, involving a phased introduction of various participatory structures (school councils, working groups, students as researchers etc.). This is commonly twinned with a keenly interested member of staff to mentor and oversee Student Voice, and often involves some sort of 'kick-start': an off-timetable Student Voice day, or some formal training. The advantages of this gradual introduction are considerable. With a gradual approach, there tends to be a lack of serious opposition from staff, who feel less threatened by a series of small concessions; there is more control over the initiation of potentially controversial processes, reducing the danger of misused or inappropriate activities; and the students are less likely to feel out of their depth. However, it is very easy for this gradual approach to stagnate, especially if a key member of staff moves on. Equally, there is a danger that the ultimate extent of Student Voice will be inevitably limited, as the initial aspirations of the concept were themselves constrained and moderate.

The other route is not one I have encountered thus far, but is an exciting one nonetheless. This is a full-scale Student Voice 'revolution', where radical changes are made to existing structures and relationships – students are taken straight to the heart of school decision making, with input into school development plans, students as associate governors, meetings with the senior management team and a fully operational, budgeted school council that is included in all areas of teaching, learning and the school environment. This approach relies on placing considerable trust in the student body, and would no doubt be met with opposition by more conservative elements within the staff room (and quite possibly the student body as well). However, if staff and students can overcome the initial culture shock, it has the potential to extend Student Voice well beyond the mundane, tokenistic boundaries that exist in many of the more cautious school environments. It also has the distinct advantage of allowing the students to see that they really *are* being listened to, and really *are* making decisions key to the running of their education.

Much as I would love to reach a firm conclusion as to which is the better of the above approaches, I feel unable to do so without further research, especially as I don't know of an example of the second approach. I do feel, however, that a large number of schools in England are falling short of the more radical possibilities for Student Voice. During my time at ESSA, I encountered disappointing examples of practice more frequently than encouraging ones. In particular, I found that students or teachers were often blinkered by their local context. Unaware of the wider possibilities presented by participation, they were stuck somewhere between rungs four and six on Hart's famous 'Ladder of Participation' (Figure 25.1). If this were only a stage in the gradual progression towards rung eight, it might be a cause for cautious optimism. Too often, however, I found that staff and students were perfectly content to remain at that level – classic examples of the stagnation that I mentioned above. When you also consider the natural conservatism in education in England as a whole, realised in the limited extent of our pupil participation, this is not especially surprising.

How, then, can we truly *carpe diem* and realise the more exciting possibilities of Student Voice? There is no easy answer to this question, but I think there are three main challenges that education in England needs to address if it is to drive participation on to a more meaningful, more inclusive and more radical level.

Challenges to Student Voice

Becoming more inclusive

First, Student Voice needs to become more inclusive. The traditional school council, the most common and the 'safest' of participation mechanisms, involves

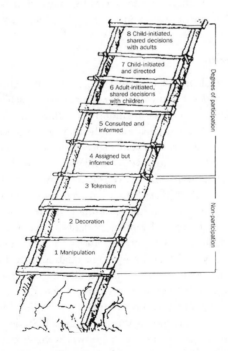

Figure 25.1 Hart's 'Ladder of Participation'
Source: www.hort.cornell.edu/gbl/greenervoices/images/ladder.pdf

elected students meeting after school to debate an agenda. This model is entirely geared towards articulate, confident students with flexible arrangements for getting home. Frequently, these students come from a small section of the student demographic, and this automatically creates disengagement in the majority of students. Widening involvement to every student is one of the biggest challenges for Student Voice, especially if it is to be considered democratic and truly inclusive. For the best ideas on doing this within the confines of a school council structure, the School Councils UK guidance is invaluable.[2] However, I believe that even the most carefully constructed school council still revolves around a central concept – that of oral debate – which is inaccessible to many students. This is why I believe that alternative mechanisms are necessary in order to get as many students as possible involved in participatory processes such as:

- writing research reports;
- using art, photography and drama to contribute;
- being given their own time and space to consider their opinions, however they choose to express them.

The latter is particularly important, given the current drive to use participation as a method of encouraging those who are not in education, employment or training back into some form of formal learning. ESSA's work in the borough of Waltham Forest clearly demonstrates that students in this situation contribute best when allowed to use their own methods (in the case of that particular borough, through music and rap) and when encouraged and supervised by their own trained peers.

Changing relationships

Second, there is the challenge of changing the traditional school relationships, between teachers and students and within the student body itself. A lot of Student Voice does not dramatically alter the relationships within school. This is perhaps related to the fact that student participation in the majority of schools is dominated by a certain type of student – academically successful, well behaved and usually middle class. These students tend to have good relationships with staff already, and so no noticeable improvements take place in terms of behaviour and teacher–student interaction. However, as the *Inspiring Schools* research shows (Davies et al. 2006), Student Voice has the potential to result in dramatic improvements in both these areas, and also to decrease bullying. By giving students a greater sense of ownership over their education, encouraging teachers and students to work together outside the classroom and fostering better student-to-student relationships through buddying and peer mentoring, participation can completely alter the classroom dynamic of a school. However, if this is to happen it is necessary for the students who previously struggled in these areas (i.e. those with previously poor relationships with staff and other students) to be included in Student Voice processes. If Student Voice is limited to narrow, exclusive mechanisms, these changes will never take place. The challenge of altering the relationships within a school or college is therefore intrinsically linked to the challenge of broadening the demographic of Student Voice.

Widening the scope: impacting all aspects of school life

Third, there is a need to widen the scope of participation so that it impacts on all aspects of school life, including teaching and learning. At the heart of Student Voice is a desire to improve education as a whole. There is now considerable research to show that the benefits of effective participation are almost unlimited, from more skilled students to better school organisation, from more active citizenship to more effective teaching and learning (Davies et al. 2006: 3). It therefore follows that the only things that stop Student Voice being the most powerful mechanism for positive change in education are the constraints that individuals and individual institutions place upon it. When Student Voice is no longer an add-on or an adornment, but is an integral part of the school ethos, its true potential will be realised. That is why I believe it needs to permeate and underlie every aspect of school life, from staff appointments to curriculum, from school environments to the very process of learning and information exchange within the classroom.

Conclusion

In conclusion, there are a number of challenges that must be addressed so that Student Voice can be driven forward. First, tokenism and limited participation are both dangerous concepts – they need to be eradicated. They produce cynical, disengaged students; confrontational situations and relationships between staff and students and within the student body; and they often represent an opportunity missed in terms of the potential improvements that can be initiated via pupil participation. An effective mechanism for sharing the wealth of information and case studies in Student Voice would help this immeasurably, if only by opening the minds of those involved at a grassroots level to the less common, sometimes more extreme manifestations of Student Voice work. Second, legislating Student Voice is a dangerous game, although it can lead to significant advantages if successfully done. The gain in status for school councils in Wales is a good example, although this legislation is an equally good example of the box ticking that prescriptive regulations can engender. The key here is to allow schools and students the freedom to experiment with different mechanisms and structures, in order that they can find the system that works best for them. The reservations attached to prescriptive regulations, and the limited success of the Welsh policy, do not exclude the possibility of a flexible legislative grounding for Student Voice, however, and these should not be considered as impassable barriers. Third, it is important to remember the potential of participation, and what is required to unleash it. If the full benefits of shared decision making are to be felt, the opportunity to engage with the concept must be extended to all students and must be backed up by an ethos that values Student Voice in all areas of a school. This ethos must also be shared between all students and all staff, most especially those from each body who lead on the various aspects of participatory work. Finally, it strikes me that that the success of ESSA is crucial to the success of Student Voice in this country. As the only organisation which actively promotes student participation in all its forms via individual *and* affiliated representation, ESSA has a unique role. It is the only organisation which aims to cover *all* aspects of student involvement, consistently promoting the rights of the less articulate and the voice of minority groups. It is, and must remain, a constant reminder to government, teachers and students not to despair, because they can always seize the day.

Notes

1. www.participationforschools.org.uk.
2. www.schoolcouncils.org.

References

Davies, L., Williams, C. and Yamashita, H. with Man-Hing, K. O. (2006) *Inspiring Schools: Impact and outcomes: Taking up the challenge of pupil participation*, London: Carnegie UK Trust.
Estyn (HM Inspectorate for Education and Training in Wales) (2008) *Having Your Say – Young people, participation and school councils*, Cardiff: Estyn, available at www.estyn.gov.uk/publications/Having_your_say_young_people_participation_and_school_councils.pdf.
Whitty, G. and Wisby, E. (2007) *Real Decision Making? School councils in action*, London: Institute of Education, p. 37, available at www.dcsf.gov.uk/research/data/uploadfiles/DCSF-RR001.pdf.

26 In search of agency

Participation in a youth organisation in Turkey

Fahriye Hazer Sancar and Yucel Can Severcan

Since the mid-1990s, in part due to the accession talks to join the European Union, there are a myriad of activities and projects focused on participatory governance and youth participation in Turkey. These are happening across the nation in a variety of institutional, community and/or informal settings, supported by all kinds of national and international public, private and non-governmental entities. This chapter is based on research that sought to identify and study cases where children/youth are able to exercise agency. We define *agency* as 'having the power to make decisions that impact on self and others and to act on them'; and consider participation as a precondition for agency. We are particularly interested in agency directed towards and/or grounded in *place*.

In our search we reviewed internet sites and wrote to and interviewed a number of informants to identify ongoing activism or organisations established and led by disadvantaged youth aged 18 or younger. Here we tell the story of the Young Volunteers, the only organisation that we found that met our criteria, its formation, membership, relationship with other organisations and with the government (central and local), its programmatic activities, accomplishments and challenges. We use the case to illustrate how the governance and administrative structures, attitudes and norms, political conjunction and cultural factors affect this form of youth participation as well as its sphere of influence. The description is based on interviews with the elected leader and another founding member of the organisation, project reports and media coverage, and workshops with neighbourhood children who are involved in various capacities.

Background: context and issues

In Turkey, where (according to the 2007 census) 44 per cent of the population are 24 years of age or younger, youth are perceived as the major resource for the development and prosperity of the country, as well as guardians of the Republic, a role ascribed to them since the formation of the Republic. The official rhetoric of the state acknowledges the well-being of Turkish youth as a requirement of economic and social development, although reality on the ground belies the sincerity of such statements. The majority of the youth population is composed of economically disadvantaged individuals, and youth unemployment is a serious problem. A leading cause of youth poverty is widespread, continuous migration from rural to urban areas and from east to west, resulting in large families living in poverty in big cities and the rural hinterland.

The social and economic development of the nation clearly depends on the realisation of the full potential of a young population to become productive members of society. The participation of youth in decisions that affect them is an essential aspect of this process. Youth advocates hypothesise that participation benefits individual youth, their communities and the wider society in both the short and the long term. International agencies and various non-governmental organisations in Turkey and elsewhere endorse youth participation in planning, and principles and techniques to guide practice on the ground are widely available. Despite such progress, youth involvement in governance and planning is rare, indicating that there are significant barriers in practice (Checkoway, Pothukuchi, and Finn 1995; Adams and Ingham 1998; Hart 1997). In Turkey, having a majority of youth in poverty is a major impediment in this regard. Due to both lack of money and separation from places that incorporate adequate functions, disadvantaged young people lack access to the means for encouraging their participatory actions, visions and sense of community (Fitzpatrick et al. 1998). Moreover, in low-income communities parents generally view their children as generators of income (Kagitcibasi 1986), leaving them with no time to devote to other types of activity. As a result, there are very few youth-initiated associations across the nation. Most are in central and western Anatolia, especially in communities where income and education levels are high. Almost all the associations target only university students, which constitute no more than 4 per cent of the total youth population of Turkey. Furthermore, few remain active over time. A study of Istanbul youth organisations found that only a small percentage of children and youth participate in civic associations. Almost all of these bodies are composed of university students (ages 17 to 25). A majority of members are boys, and most are from economically wealthy and educated classes (Yenturk et al. 2006).

Cultural attitudes and norms also affect the level and type of youth participation in civil society. As guardians of the republic, youth have been assigned the duty of putting the country back on course, should governments go astray on the road to a just, prosperous and scientifically and technologically modern nation or when national unity is under threat. Ironically this mission empowers youth as an oppositional force, one that Turkish youth has historically fulfilled time and again, but not as members of civil society with equal rights for participation in day-to-day decision making. Parental permission is required by law if a child applies for membership in a registered association. Moreover, today, parents who experienced oppression due to their political affiliations during the military coups (1970s–80s), do not want their children to get involved in any activity that may be perceived as social activism. These attitudes also affect the programmes of youth organisations, especially those supported by international or government agencies. These organisations, rather than focusing on transformative activities that will enable youth to have more control over their immediate environments, engage in one-off events and project-specific initiatives that often target non-controversial issues and concerns that are somewhat removed from young people's immediate localities.

A youth organisation in Ayazaga, Istanbul: Young Volunteers

Young Volunteers is a rare example of a youth organisation established by disadvantaged youth, in 2004. The headquarters of the organisation is located in Ayazaga, a squatter neighbourhood in Sisli, one of the most prestigious municipalities of Istanbul (Plate 26.1). The neighbourhood is surrounded by middle- and high-class residential communities and is adjacent to a forested area and a small private university campus.

Despite the locational advantages, unemployment and illiteracy levels remain high. Most of the residents are third-generation immigrants from the Black Sea coast who are still in touch with their rural roots. They are highly conservative, and tied to their traditional values.

Young Volunteers was founded in 2004 by a 16-year-old high school student, Eyup Coskun (Plate 26.2). During his high school years, Eyup belonged to an environmental club and was involved in periodic neighbourhood clean-up and tree planting activities. He started questioning adult-initiated, tokenistic activities and decided to form his own organisation where youth would become the engine of community change towards self-governance, and help to solve significant problems. In 2003, with a group of around ten high school and university students, all from Ayazaga, Eyup went to the mayor of Sisli and asked for help. Their bold initiatives and the potential for funding from European Union grants impressed the mayor, who agreed to provide space and pay for utilities in an apartment building in downtown Ayazaga. The executive board of Young Volunteers, whose ages vary between 16 and 35, elected Eyup as the president and the organisation embarked on a wide range of activities, including setting up branches in a number of cities beyond Istanbul and forming a membership in Ankara, the capital, to enable easier communication and follow-up with regard to project proposals at the seat of the central government.

One of the first and most highly profiled activities of the organisation was to establish the 'People's Assembly of Ayazaga', attended by 550 people from the

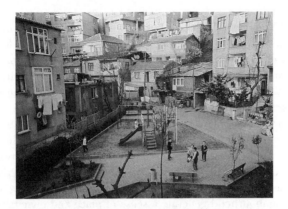

Plate 26.1 Ayazaga. Copyright: the authors and children of Ayazaga

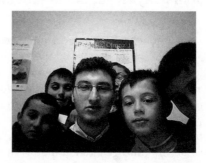

Plate 26.2   Eyup Coskun and children of Ayazaga. Copyright: Fahriye Hazer Sancar

neighbourhood and where they discussed neighbourhood issues and problems and formed a dozen committees to work on them.

It is unclear whether these committees achieved tangible results on the ground. Nevertheless this initiative must have played an important role in the neighbourhood's embracing the youth organisation as its own. In the following years, Young Volunteers focused on a variety of projects that were national, regional and local in scope. Another highly profiled project that was funded by the European Union focused on alleviating hit-and-run gangs and drug abuse among youth in Istanbul. In these projects the organisation solicited the participation of adults, experts from university faculties, representatives from relevant government agencies and elected officials. In a related project it successfully organised a retreat (on the Black Sea coast), with a series of workshops and panel discussions with participation of youth offenders and volunteer youth from Turkey and European countries. A particular category of activities involved school restoration and library projects in their parents' and grandparents' home towns in the Black Sea region. At the national level, Young Volunteers developed links with international youth to learn from each other's experiences and to contribute to multicultural understanding. Again, whether any of these activities are sustainable in the long term, or how lasting or broad their impacts are, remains to be seen.

Activities of Young Volunteers at the local level have been the most enduring, with tangible impacts. They established free preparatory courses for high school and university entrance exams for children and youth who cannot afford to pay for private courses. The after-school and weekend programme, where the volunteers help Ayazaga children with their academic work, has close to 200 registered students, more than 50 per cent of whom are girls. Seasonal environmental programmes are also part of the after-school activities. According to a media report, these educational programmes helped to improve Ayazaga children's academic performance (Salman 2006). We observed that a core of fifteen to twenty children (ages 8 to 12) come to the 'association place' daily to help out with the chores and take care of the space. This type of dedication shows that ongoing activities with and for the neighbourhood generate a sense of place and ownership. Similarly, in a participatory photography study with the children who use the facilities, we found that they are highly perceptive and knowledgeable about physical, social and economic problems in their own neighbourhoods, sensitive to issues of children in other parts of the city and capable of finding solutions to these problems. They were enthusiastic about the prospects of improving their environments and confident of their own abilities (Plate 26.3).

The organisation recruits volunteers from the private university in Ayazaga, thus helping to integrate the otherwise insular campus into the neighbourhood. A recent project to tackle land tenure and property ownership in Ayazaga was scheduled to take place on campus facilities but was thwarted at the last minute by 'the authorities'. As we will discuss in the next section, local activities that arguably have the most impact have turned out to be the most controversial, to the point of threatening the organisation's very existence.

Drivers of and challenges to success

In reviewing the activities and impacts of the organisation, we observed that the Young Volunteers Association is unique in several aspects when compared to other youth organisations in Turkey. First, it was initiated and is governed by youth. Second, it represents disadvantaged youth from low-income families. Third, it is based in a low-income *gecekondu* (squatter) neighbourhood. Fourth, its activities include provision of services for the neighbourhood children, and other place-based initiatives meaningful to the residents. In our interviews we asked Eyup Coskun, the founding leader of the organisation, and Kerem Ates, a founding member, to articulate the reasons for the successes and describe the main challenges they face.

Kerem Ates (currently the leader of a national environmental youth organisation) noted that other youth organisations do not function properly because leadership positions are often distributed arbitrarily. Only those young individuals, such as Eyup, who know local issues well and who have developed strong attachments to their neighbourhoods and cities can be successful as leaders. He added that developing competence by doing issue-specific projects is a helpful strategy. For instance, Eyup, who had worked previously on the issue of youth crime, initiated and directed projects that were related to alleviating hit-and-run youth gangs and

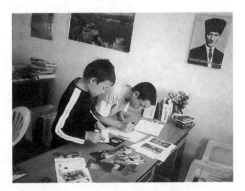

Plate 26.3   Children annotating place pictures. Copyright: the archives of Young Volunteers

drug abuse among youth in Istanbul. First-hand knowledge of the local environment, building on previous experiences, enthusiasm for changing the condition of disadvantaged youth, and the learning and practice environment offered by the organisation have led to the success of the Young Volunteers' activities.

Eyup Coskun explained that one of the most important principles of practice they had adopted was to be politically and ideologically neutral in guiding their members, and instead to aim only to develop their skills. He stressed that the organisation has been especially careful to be inclusive in its membership and provision of services:

> Everybody is welcome, regardless of their political views or ethnic backgrounds, but has to respect others. No one can use the organisation as a platform to advance some political agenda. People come here to fulfil their social responsibility.

Thus, because of its distant stance towards political parties, equal attitude towards children from different ethnic, age and gender backgrounds, proficient knowledge of local issues, and intent to improve and shape the neighbourhood, the Young Volunteers established a strong relationship of trust with the local residents. Another strategy for success was intergenerational collaboration (Plate 26.4). Some of the executive members of the organisation are adults who have experience with social development projects. These people did not take on leadership functions, but helped Eyup and his young colleagues with project proposals, grant applications and networking.

Referring to the formative years of the association, Kerem Ates stated that:

> Although there were some adults in the executive board, all of the leading actors and the event planners and organisers were youth. Adults were there only for guiding the youth. Almost everything was done by the young members.

All these factors enhanced the effectiveness of project interventions at the local level.

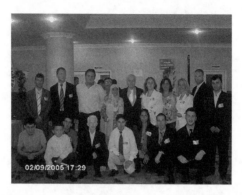

Plate 26.4 Intergenerational collaboration. Copyright: the authors

Maintaining good relationships with the municipal government and the mayor was another key factor in helping young activists to move forward. During the formative phases, the mayor supported the organisation by providing space in a central location adjacent to other community facilities such as community courses for women, a computer-literacy training room and community day care. Local officials participated in some of the projects, such as the people's assembly project. However, the organisation's policy of staying away from local politics became a sore point in its relationship with the mayor, whose party had received slightly less than 50 per cent of the votes in Ayazaga precinct during the last local elections. When we visited the organisation in 2006, unlike the year before, communication with the mayor had reached breaking point and Young Volunteers was asked to leave the premises. It all started when the mayor fixed a signboard to the entrance of the apartment with the name of the organisation, followed by the name of the municipality. This was read by neighbourhood residents who had voted for the competing party as representing allegiance to the mayor's political party; they also expected the organisation to provide services regardless of the availability of space or resources, since they now perceived it to be part of the municipality. Youth leaders took the sign down and the mayor retaliated by asking them to leave the building. Opposing factions in the neighbourhood tried to take advantage of the conflict and to buy off the organisation by offering new space, but fortunately the municipality had the foresight to back down, and the organisation continued to operate in its original location as an independent entity. This experience demonstrates the inherent tension between elected officials and youth organisations that operate at the local level in contexts where local elections are dominated by party politics, as they are in Turkey.

Engaging in local issues, while essential for youth organisations, can also be a source of conflict, especially when the discussion threatens powerful interests. This was apparently the case when the Young Volunteers decided to organise a day-long panel workshop about land tenure and property ownership. The issue of secure tenure is arguably the most important and sensitive issue in Ayazaga, a squatter neighbourhood surrounded by high-value property and destined to become the next large swathe of urban redevelopment. This initiative was thwarted by closing off the venue (the auditorium of the university) at the last minute, allegedly because an of electrical power cut.

Finally, all youth organisations are faced with the challenge of filling leadership positions, since their leaders are obliged to pass on the torch when they grow up. The terms of office for these organisations are much shorter than for any other public service. This is even more challenging in Turkey, where military service is compulsory for all aged 18 years or older, unless deferred by enrolment in higher education. Youth often define their attachment to an organisation in terms of their relationship with a caring, experienced leader (Pittman 1992). When a leader transfers his/her position to another member of the organisation, the relationships formed over time between the leader, the youth and the local residents are lost, leading to frustration and a loss of confidence among the members (Matthews 2001). When Eyup left the organisation in 2006 (only two years after its establishment) to perform his military service, he did leave other members in his place and the organisation survived his absence, even though it was less active during that year.

Conclusion: place as a central concept for youth organising

During our interview, Eyup Coskun told the story of how the organisation found its place:

> They offered us space in a nice building located in central Nisantasi. We did not accept it. We said, 'What kind of problems do the wealthy folks in Nisantasi have? Maybe traffic congestion?' Let them solve it on their own. In other words, we wanted to begin a movement for development here in our own backyard. We can instigate our projects from this place and reach out. And that is how we began. If we can solve problems here, we can do the same anywhere. This is our context where we can learn.

When we review the experiences of the Young Volunteers we find that *place* emerges as a central concept. When a youth organisation is clearly bound to a particular place, its membership, leaders, activities and choice of projects are local and specific to that place but may represent a broad range of socio-economic and environmental issues rather than narrowly defined interests or problems. Being place-focused compels the organisation to establish and rely on local resources and develop social capital. Intergenerational collaboration is a natural driving force *and* an outcome. Youth servicing the children of the neighbourhood is an obvious strategy that creates a multitude of positive outcomes, including establishing trust and nurturing future youth leaders. The physical environment becomes salient and significant when an organisation is place-based. Activities and projects begin to have explicit spatial components. Heightened sensitivity towards the immediate environment, in turn, enhances sense of place, desire for care and improvement, and intensifies attachment to place (Plate 26.5).

Developing place-specific competence often translates into understanding and effective participation elsewhere and begins to transcend the narrow confines of particular locales. Having a place to originate from facilitates branching out, both

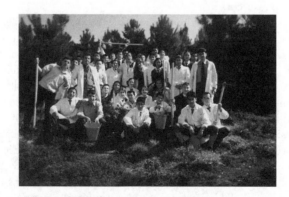

Plate 26.5   The environmental club: taking care of local places. Copyright: the authors

in the sense of establishing links or sub-units and in crafting approaches to deal with national or global issues and problems.

On the other hand, being place-bound creates tensions and a host of challenges. Unless the organisation can deal with these effectively, instead of realising the benefits, the process may result in failure or marginalisation of the organisation. A politically neutral stance and assuring ethnic and value diversity are essential for establishing relationships based on trust with the non-political actors. However, this is likely to disappoint local elected officials, especially if party politics (and patronage) is strong in municipal elections. Since place-bound youth organisations are likely to depend on allocation of resources by local government, they run the risk of losing financial support when they engage sensitive issues. The experiences of Volunteer Youth in Ayazaga underscore the complexities of youth involvement in urban planning. Current efforts largely focus on capturing the youth voice and, in so doing, help them become active and engaged citizens (Race and Torma 1998). More ambitious initiatives aim at establishing youth councils within the municipal government. We are doubtful that such a strategy would be in the best interests of youth or the public if adopted in a place such as Ayazaga, where there is a real danger of co-optation. Perhaps the strategy of building trust, serving local needs and maintaining neutrality, if practised consistently and for a significant period of time by a youth organisation, may establish it as an independent voice that the planning agencies do not dare to ignore.

Acknowledgement

The authors acknowledge the contributions of Eyup Coskun, Kerem Ates and children of Ayazaga in the writing of this chapter.

References

Adams, E. and Ingham, S. (1998) *Changing Places: Children's participation in environmental planning*, London: The Children's Society.

Checkoway, B., Pothukuchi, K., and Finn, J. (1995) 'Youth participation in community planning: What are the benefits?', *Journal of Planning Education and Research* 14: 134–9.

Fitzpatrick, S., Hastings, A., and Kintrea, K. (1998) *Including Young People in Urban Regeneration*, Bristol: The Policy Press.

Hart, R. A. (1997) *Children's Participation: The theory and practice of involving young citizens in community development and environmental care*, London: Earthscan.

Kagitcibasi, C. (1986) 'Status of women in Turkey: Cross-cultural perspectives', *International Journal of Middle East Studies* 18(4): 485–99.

Matthews, H. (2001) 'Citizenship, youth councils and young people's participation', *Journal of Youth Studies* 4(3): 299–318.

Pittman, K. (1992) *Defining the Fourth R: Promoting youth development through building relationships*, Washington, DC: Academy for Educational Development, Center for Youth Development and Policy Research.

Race, B. and Torma, C. (1998) *Youth Planning Charrettes: A manual for planners, teachers and youth advocates*, Chicago: American Planning Association.

Salman, U. A. (2006) 'Her derde deva gencler' (Youth as the panacea), *Radical* (7 February) (newspaper article).

Yenturk, N., Kurtaran, Y., Uran, S., Yurttaguler, L., Akyuz, A. and Nemutlu, G. (2006) 'Istanbul gencligi – STK uyeligi bir fark yaratiyor mu?' (Istanbul youth – Does being a member of a civic organisation make a difference?), research report, Children's Studies Center (February), available at http://genclik.bilgi.edu.tr/docs/istanbulstkuyeligigen-clik.pdf.

Commentary 6

Spaces and structures
Looking from the outside

Colin Williams, Jessica Edlin and Fiona Beals

Coming from the mighty 'down under' (that's Aotearoa/New Zealand, not Australia), the three of us represent different aspects of the youth voice in New Zealand. In Aotearoa/New Zealand, we have a phrase *'tino rangatiratanga'*. It is one of the foundational cornerstones to the Treaty of Waitangi – the document that established Aotearoa/New Zealand as we know it today. A short definition of this phrase is the ability to make choices and decisions in one's own life about issues relevant to oneself – it's about striving for self-determination in one's own life. So, basically, it is about agency. When we look at the chapters in this section, we can see that effective youth participation is about *tino rangatiratanga* – giving young people the space to have a choice and to exercise some agency when it comes to making decisions about their own lives.

As reflected throughout the chapters, young people now make a significant portion of the world's population – both in the majority world (those countries that have once been considered 'developing,' but which make up a significant portion of the world's population) and the minority world (those countries often referred to as 'developed' or Western). It is because of this fact that we need to recognise the need for youth involvement, voice and agency. Young people have valuable ideas and perspectives that can enrich decision making at local, national and international levels. As Austin eloquently points out – the significant proportion of young people in our society simply gives adults more of an opportunity to embrace the moment, listen to them and include them in decisions rather than feed a fear that young people simply present problems to society.

It seems that in the minority world, there is an assumption that young people do not have the capacity or ability to participate effectively without adult intervention or control. In the three chapters that talk about examples from the United Kingdom it seems that adults are not letting go of the process; decision making by young people is not about *tino rangatiratanga*, but about simply endorsing what adults want to be said. Whereas in the examples given from the majority world, there is a sense of trust in young people on the part of adults; adults understand and know that youth can make informed decisions and changes in the community. This is because these examples recognise the importance of both the adult voice and the youth voice in addressing local and national issues. Furthermore, initiatives such as the examples given by Austin and Sancar and Severcan, recognise the maturity of youth; they understand that young people can lead organisations and have valuable opinions. In the minority world, people tend to think that youth don't have the capacity to think for themselves; adults in the minority world think that young people might just 'screw it up' if they are given the responsibility.

The majority world examples also show adults prepared to take a risk with youth by giving power and opportunity for young people to make real decisions. For example, in both Austin's and Sancar and Severcan's chapters there are clear moments in which, to a certain extent, adults let go of the process and allow young people space and opportunity to lead and make significant decisions which impact locally and nationally. In comparison, the examples by Lewars, Turkie, and McGinley and Grieve all show some aversion on the part of adults to giving young people complete control. For example, Lewars challenges us to take the risk of giving power to young people. He points out that it takes time to establish enough trust, if ever, because effective trust requires the acceptance of new ideas, ideas that may contradict and counter the original opinions of adults.

One of the key stumbling blocks to effective participation noted throughout Lewars's, Turkie's, and McGinley and Grieve's chapters is the need for diverse representation. This seems to be a real problem in the minority world, where communities tend to be fragmented across a variety of interest groups who all have different needs. It did not come through as an issue so much for Austin and Sancar and Severcan, possibly due to the homogeneous structure of the communities described. The United Kingdom examples advocate for representation from a broad selection of society; but even in these examples there are limited moments of success. One possible reason comes from our own experiences in Aotearoa/New Zealand. We are aware of instances in which selection is all about diversity – to fill spaces – rather than the inclusion of the skill set needed for a project or initiative. Our experience in New Zealand is that diversity is important, but participation is about asset building – building on the skills that young people bring and equipping them with the resources they need to be successful.

In the United Kingdom examples, the authors note that it is important for youth participation initiatives to move beyond just including young people who have already experienced success in places such as school. These authors note that valuable ideas don't always come from 'successful' young people and that in places like the United Kingdom it is important to look beyond the social strata of society. Despite this, McGinley and Grieve also note that it is often difficult to achieve full participation and representation – you may have a diverse group of young people, but often some included young people feel excluded in discussions. This is a challenge that any youth participation initiative wanting to be effective and representative faces. For example, in New Zealand, participation initiatives are often not advertised, rather, able young people are selected, mainly by teachers and sometimes youth workers. In other words, you have to be 'in the know' and identified.

Another important lesson we can take from these chapters is that we need to start youth participation initiatives in the community before expanding to a regional, national or international level. Furthermore, we need to develop initiatives slowly to make use of available resources. When we do this we can address problems such as representation and trust. Starting small also means that we can get behind and support youth participation initiatives; we are able (both as young people and as adults) to build success upon success. If we look at the chapters presented in this section, we can find clear evidence of both the successfulness of projects that start small and the problematic nature of projects that begin at a national level. For example, the volunteer programme that Sancar and Severcan describe in Turkey was initiated by young people at a community level. This way they were able to build trust between adults in the community and themselves, which enabled them to act at a local level. This later progressed to impacting on decisions made at regional and national levels.

In contrast, the United Kingdom examples tended to be nationally driven and have led to several key problems regarding youth voice and participation. The first problem is that regions and communities need to buy into the initiative in order for it to be successful and there seems to be variable buy-in across regions, with some fully behind the initiatives and others just paying tokenistic lip-service to them. Another problem is that you need to have more support than if you start local. If you start at a national level, then you rely heavily on adult support for guidance and risk adult ideas and agendas permeating the original intention of the initiative or programme.

It is impressive and interesting that many of these initiatives mimic adult-based governance systems. However, it is important that to some extent they reflect the types of initiatives talked about by Austin, where there are key moments of *tino rangatiratanga*, moments when young people are actively making decisions and actively working with adults in 'power'. Our experience in New Zealand is that often practices that give young people an experience of adult governance structures do not result in effective participation. Instead, they are merely a day, or a week, in parliament for the more intelligent and able students. The United Kingdom initiatives try to address the limitations of tokenistic parliaments, but still face the problem of adult buy-in and support.

One interesting point in Sancar and Severcan's chapter is the political neutrality of the initiative. It seems that they reflected all the strengths of youth participation by being unattached to political agendas. It enabled them to address the needs of a wide group of young people without risking taking sides. If they took a side they would not have reflected the wishes of the community in which they were based and they would have had to take a side which would possibly exclude some young people. Also, taking a political side would have meant that they would have had to wait for an adult stance or opinion to be stated before progressing through to the community level. That is, if you are on a political side you will be dependent upon what the adults say at a governmental level to drive your own initiatives. You couldn't have a mission statement driven by youth, but rather would have an ever-changing political stance given by adults in power.

Reading these five chapters provided moments of learning for all of us. Before we read the chapters we assumed that the majority world would not have an interest in youth participation. After all, we thought, they have bigger problems, like poverty and inequality. However, as we read, we realised that it is precisely because of these 'problems' that youth participation is so needed and so effective. It is about time that we listened to young people in other countries and communities.

The lessons that we will learn will help to inform our own practices in Aotearoa/ New Zealand and beyond.

The authors

Colin Williams has been involved since he was 12 years of age in Urge/ Whakamanawa – a health and resource service for young people which has transformed itself from being controlled by adults into a youth-led initiative, and has been recognised in New Zealand as an exemplar.

Jessica Edlin has been a member of a school youth council which she found somewhat tokenistic, and is now in a youth leadership group at the local community church, advising the youth pastor and taking part in decisions about the direction of youth ministry.

Fiona Beals works at the New Zealand non-governmental organisation Global Education as a resource writer and adviser. She recently completed her doctoral study on the ways in which young people and youth crime have been written about in New Zealand.

PART III

New theoretical perspectives

27 Children's participation as a struggle over recognition

Exploring the promise of dialogue

Robyn Fitzgerald, Anne Graham, Anne Smith and Nicola Taylor

(with contributions from young people who are part of the Centre for Children and Young People's Youth Advisory Committee, 'Young People, Big Voice')

Introduction

A number of the earlier chapters in this Handbook have signalled the possibilities for children's participation to contribute positively to children's lives, while at the same time acknowledging the unresolved tensions, ambiguities and social power relations that undermine its emancipatory potential.[1] In this chapter, we approach children's participation as a *struggle over recognition* so as to further explore its increasingly complex and contested nature (Honneth 1995; Taylor 1995; Tully 2004). Such a conceptualisation enables us to reflect on the politico-historical conditions that have shaped the theory and practice of participation, including where and how children have been located within emerging discourses. Conceptualising participation as a struggle *over* recognition is also useful because it focuses on participation as a negotiated space that is dialogical rather than monological in nature, which, in turn, more adequately captures the mutual and inter-connected layering of children's participation. We conclude by exploring some of the possibilities and implications for both theory and practice when participation is conceptualised as a struggle over recognition.

Setting the context

Since the late 1980s there has been increasing interest in New Zealand and Australia in the possibilities that participatory practices might hold for enabling the inclusion of children in social and political life. A diverse range of organisations now seek to represent and promote the interests of children in the development and implementation of law, policy and services. In New Zealand, the national plan Agenda for Children aims to 'promote the place of children and young people in society and make the country a better place for them' (Agenda for Children Project Team 2002: 6). One of the key action areas involves increasing children's participation, and this has subsequently been associated with some innovative policy developments across many settings of children's lives, including early childhood education, schools, family law, out-of-home care and local government decision making. In Australia, demands for the voice of the child to be heard in decision making can be seen in plans to establish a National Commissioner for Children and Young People to promote the interests of children, and the development and implementation of a national plan for consultation with and inclusion of children (ALP 2007).

A number of powerful influences, including the United Nations Convention on the Rights of the Child (UNCRC)[2] and the broad field of childhood studies, have challenged the very nature and meaning of participation itself, prompting a fundamental shift in thinking about children's status and capacity to participate in social and political life. From this substantial body of work we know that children's participation offers important and far-reaching benefits for children, their families and wider communities. Consequently, children's participation is now legitimated as 'something that contributes to children's positive development of individual identity, competence and sense of responsibility' (Kjørholt 2002: 76). Children themselves cite participation across any number of contexts, whether in planning and policy evaluation or in relation to their own lives, as helping them to develop a sense of belonging, to gain new skills and experiences, to meet new people and friends and to build a sense of their own agency (Greene and Hill 2006; Smart 2002; 2006; Smith 2002; 2007). Research shows that children attribute a great deal of importance to being recognised and acknowledged as individuals with opinions and feelings of their own and as agents capable of contributing to decisions made in their everyday lives (Graham, 2004; Parkinson, Cashmore and Single 2007; Smart 2002; Taylor 2006). This view contrasts with previous conceptions of children as 'non-citizens', 'not-full citizens' or 'citizens in the making', unable to know their own best interests, or as dependants in need of protection (Taylor, Tapp and Henaghan 2007).

Yet, while in many countries children may have become increasingly important to contemporary social and political agendas, their views and perspectives have not been as central (Hill et al. 2004). Many observers are voicing concerns as to the extent to which children are taken seriously as participants, even in those policy and project initiatives intended to promote their participation (Davis and Hill 2006). An increasing number of critiques point to a widening gap between the rationale for participation and documented evidence evaluating the impact and outcomes of children's participation, what difference it makes, and for whom (Davis, Farrier and Whiting 2006; Kirby with Bryson 2002; Partridge 2005). James (2007) captures this emerging disjuncture between policy claims about participation and practices that facilitate children's participation:

> Despite such representations of the 'voices of children' children themselves may, nonetheless, continue to find their voices silenced, suppressed, or ignored in their everyday lives. Children may not be asked their views and opinions, and even if they are consulted, their views may be dismissed.

(James 2007: 261)

James's concerns are echoed across a variety of settings. Despite the enthusiasm among children for getting involved in innovations such as school councils, youth parliaments, local community governance and planning, as well as family law and care proceedings, their involvement is often undemocratic and fails to fulfil its original aims (Davis and Hill 2006; Percy-Smith 2005; Thomas 2007). Importantly, children report that even when they are involved in participatory opportunities, they receive little feedback regarding the value of their contribution and observe little evidence in the actions or decisions taken that their views are responded to (Kirby with Bryson 2002; Morgan 2005).

Similar concerns were raised by members of a youth consultative committee[3] that we consulted at a 2008 forum for their views on the nature, purpose, benefits and challenges of participation. They defined participation in terms of purpose, change and action:

Participation is when you are actively involved in something.

Not just saying you are going to do it, but doing it.

Presenting an idea and following through with it.

Being involved in things you choose to be involved in ... having a choice.

Participation is about making a difference.

I think it's about contributing to society.

When the international researchers came we were given the opportunity to contribute to how youth are portrayed ... so that's making a difference.

Nevertheless, the young people identified limited opportunities for participation and were strongly of the view their 'participation' is experienced as superficial and constrained:

About the only thing the SRC [Student Representative Council] did was raise money for Daffodil Day.

SRCs are ... a popularity contest ... it's not necessarily who'll do the best job.

There is a fear about letting students have a voice ... giving them power ... but most kids would contribute something positive.

The people who have to go through a school don't really have a say in whether and what should change.

This gap between the principle and the practice of participation is not the only area of uncertainty in the study of children's participation. Children often express caution or ambivalence about the nature and value of their participation. Even when they are at the centre of participatory initiatives, they are not always prepared to readily accept the mantle of 'child participant'. Children do not necessarily always want to participate, or they may, simultaneously, want and not want to participate – an experience that is not too dissimilar to that of many adults (Thomas 2007; Wyness, Harrison and Buchanan 2004).

In addition, there is a growing realisation that, while listening to the voices of children represents an important start in addressing the issues arising from the social inclusion of children, actually to do the listening and responding authentically is challenging. When asked about participation, for example, children sometimes tell a story that does not necessarily fit with that of the agentic-participant child, that is, of wanting to participate in activities that are important to them, or of having 'message like thoughts that can be exchanged, and intentions that match situations defined by adults' (Komulainen 2007: 25). In our work with children from families whose parents have separated, many children 'to and fro' between accounts of vulnerability, hurt and sadness arising from the experience of their parents' separation and of wanting to be heard (Graham and Fitzgerald 2006; Smith, Taylor and Tapp 2003).

In order to further clarify the 'problem' of children's participation, an overview of the conceptual conditions that have privileged certain interpretations is required. Central to such an analysis is how we have come to recognise both the status and the voice of children.

Participation as a site of struggle

Until now, debates about children's participation have been located primarily in discourses of childhood. However, the focus on children's participation also reflects a more widespread movement in Western society towards acknowledging participation as central to the way we understand democracy (Arnott 2006; Taylor and Smith, 2009). Approached from this perspective, children's participation can be said to have emerged in response to a 'concatenation of factors', including some that have challenged the very nature and meaning of democracy itself (Christensen and Prout 2005: 53). Such developments have increasingly challenged the democratic norms that govern the inclusion of individuals and groups as they struggle for recognition of their ethnicity, race, class, gender and, more recently, age, in order to be able to participate as citizens (Christensen and Prout 2005; Kulynych 2001). Arnott (2006) suggests that we are witnessing an increasingly complex governance and policy environment where government's key role is to 'co-ordinate and steer the diverse range of policy actors' (p. 5). This is evident in the changing relations between government, civil society and the individual, as governments seek to respond to calls for recognition of the voice and status of groups otherwise positioned in the margins of society, including children.

It is important, then, to analyse closely the procedural enactment of participation. To this end, we propose three key 'moments' in the recent history of participation. Such moments attempt to capture the ways in which individuals and groups have been recognised within particular political and democratic cultures, and hence how their participation has been shaped and acted upon. Consequently, we suggest that the serious inclusion of children is both enabled and constrained by a struggle around recognition – at philosophical, theoretical and practical levels. In attempting to situate children's participation in this way, we suggest it is useful to do so through the construct of historical 'moments', only insofar as these continue to inform and challenge how we have come to 'know' participation. We do not, then, intend that our analysis locate or confine particular understandings of participation to a time and place in history; rather, that it is possible to identify 'genuine ruptures in the fabrics of our histories, precise or fuzzy points at which we are irrevocably changed' (Lincoln and Denzin 2005: 1116) and thus to signal the appearance of new sensibilities that potentially shape how we see and do participation in the contemporary social context.

While the following discussion focuses primarily on the procedural enactment of participation, our thinking is grounded in wider debates about the politics of recognition. For this reason, it is useful to briefly clarify what we mean by 'recognition', given that there is little agreement about the term and how it should be approached (Fraser 2000). The *Concise Oxford Dictionary* (1964; 2008) defines recognition in terms of acknowledgement of someone's or something's existence, validity or legality; according notice or consideration to; discovering or realising the nature of; to treat as, acknowledge, realise or admit that; and to know again or identify as known before. Building upon such definitional understandings, a number of philosophers, such as Charles Taylor (1995) and Axel Honneth (2004), propose that recognition is facilitated or negotiated through dialogue with others. This dialogical relationship is said to be crucial for the development of an individual's identity and takes place through a process of *mutual* recognition. Furthermore, the converse is said to hold true – misrecognition is constituted in the depreciation of the identity of the group or individual by the dominant culture. Such misrecognition has the potential to inflict harm, and to be a form of oppression that can potentially imprison individuals within a 'false, distorted, and reduced mode of being' (Taylor 1995: 225).

Other philosophers, including Nancy Fraser (2000), have argued that recognition is a question not so much of identity, but rather of social status. Accordingly, misrecognition should be taken to mean social subordination, rather than the depreciation and deformation of group identity (Fraser 2000). From this perspective, redressing injustice requires a politics aimed at overcoming subordination by positioning the misrecognised person (or group) as a 'full member of society, capable of participating on par with the rest' (Fraser 2000: 4). Such debates attest to the potential of recognition as an appropriate lens through which to examine and conceptualise participation, because it allows for a focus on identity (children's understanding of who they are) as well as on status (the ways in which they are able to fully participate in society).

With this rationale in mind, we now describe three moments that have shaped the emergence of participation. These moments frame participation in terms of an emphasis on equality, difference and dialogue and underline a struggle that is inextricably linked to recognition.

The first moment: the claim for participation based on equality (the 1960s and 1970s)

The first 'moment' can be seen in the early struggles for recognition of cultural, ethnic and religious minorities in the 1960s and 1970s, whereby dominant approaches to participation embedded within juridical theories, rules and policies were based on a framework of citizenship and strongly aligned with the right of every (adult) citizen to equal participation in political life. With the move to equality came a politics of universalism, emphasising the equal dignity of all citizens, and the emergence of the right and entitlement to participation (Taylor 1995).

Tully (2004) argues that the most obvious evidence of struggles for recognition in this first moment lies in the legal rules used to work out a definitive and final solution to claims. He suggests that the preconditions of participation are first, that participation is limited to those who possess legal status to assert a claim; second, that a claim must be made out; third, that individuals are deemed to accept the fundamental terms of their association, and so must frame their claim so that it can be heard within a legal forum; fourth, that decision makers are assumed to be neutral with respect to such claims; and fifth, that solutions to conflicts are handed down from on high. In this way, the process of participation is characterised as imposing a definitive solution capable of neutral translation and handed down to individual members from 'on high', that is, by theorists, courts and policy makers. Tully (2004: 85) has described this approach as proceeding from a 'monological' perspective.

Consequently, while the strength of the rights formulation lies in its recognition of children as humans equally worthy of respect, its limitation stems from its reliance on a monological interpretation of autonomy that privileges self-determination in order to initiate a claim for recognition. Within this conceptualisation, children lack the 'entrance requirements' necessary to participate (Arneil 2002: 70), that is, they are not, and cannot be, assigned the status of the subject and so cannot possess the right to participate. Even if children were to be assigned legal status, the exclusionary nature of participatory processes, which has been so strongly asserted in the first moment, precludes their participation.

In response to the expanding field of claims for participation rights, many theorists and policy makers sought to enrich the principles of freedom and equality by working out theories and policies addressing minority and cultural rights that might acknowledge the legitimacy of minority rights to equal participation. In other words, the emphasis was shifting to the recognition of difference (Fraser 2000; Taylor 1995; Tully 2004).

The second moment: the claim for participation based on difference (the 1980s and 1990s)

With its early origins in the US civil rights movement, the rise of a politics of difference was accompanied by a shift in the exclusive focus on participation as a political right towards a more inclusively understood concept of participation as an activity that could also be realised in social and cultural spheres (Benhabib 1992). The second moment thus witnessed the rallying of individuals and groups to express their political agency and to participate in social and political life, underpinned by the pursuit of a more inclusive interpretation of participation that might better accommodate diversity (Fraser 2000).

Although relative latecomers to the participatory sphere, children were acknowledged during the second moment as participants, with their rights to participation taken seriously for the first time. Prompted by a new discourse of children as social actors and, importantly, by the UNCRC, the 'invited space' of participation in the second moment reveals a rethinking of the possibilities around 'children's rights', central to which is the idea of recognising and respecting children's agency.

Yet, as we have already signalled, such recognition has not necessarily resulted in what might be described as deeply authentic participation whereby young people are involved in their communities as 'co-constitutors of change ... in addressing social problems and as agents in their own lives' (Percy-Smith and Weil 2003: 84). Instead, children's participation has continued to be characterised by a gap between expectations for their participation and their lived experiences of participation across the many settings of their lives. In this way, while there has been a shift towards acknowledging the voices of children, their status as participants remains largely untouched by the possibilities that arise out of a politics of difference. The second moment can therefore be said to have enabled, to a far greater degree, the symbolic inclusion of children, but at the same time has struggled to address an underlying resistance to political and social agency embedded in monological approaches to participation.

For Tully (2004), this is not surprising, as he argues that the discursive framing of participation in the first moment as a monological process remained largely unchanged in the second. Since the focus in the second moment has primarily been on the *claim* for recognition, rather than on the *conditions* that must be in place, the net result has been the positioning of children outside the discursive space of participation altogether. Thus, in the second moment, even though children were recognised as holding rights to participate, they continued to be indirectly excluded from the 'invited space' of participation because, in essence, they were unable to assert or to claim these rights. Understood in this way, children's participation reveals a paradox: while contemporary calls for children to 'have a say' and for adults to listen to the 'voices of children' have gained prominence as a result of the politics of universalism and difference, the framing of the procedural terms of participation continues to ensure that few children are able to assert the claim for recognition of that right.

We suggest, however, that a further development in the way we think about participation is now under way. Rather than approaching participation from a monological perspective, theorists, courts and policy makers are seeking to reconcile tensions over recognition by means of dialogue, that is, by listening to the people engaged in the struggle to be recognised as participants in social and political life (Tully 2004).

The third moment: the turn to dialogue

As the concept of participation has been shaped by growing calls for recognition of the diversity of 'voices', so too have demands for new forms of engagement and inclusion between individuals and the state. Gaventa (2007) argues that implicit in such calls are challenges to the notion of democracy as a set of rules, procedures and institutional design, and a widespread movement is now building on participatory claims for equality and difference, but which is focused on the practice and process of participation. A burgeoning array of decision-making practices is emerging which are designed to ensure that individuals are able to enter into dialogue with those who govern and who have a duty to listen and to respond, so as to ensure that there is openness to review, evaluation and possible renegotiation if required (Tully 2004). From this perspective, participation is increasingly being seen as 'a process through which citizens exercise ever-deepening control over decisions which affect their lives through a number of forums and in a variety of arenas' (Gaventa 2007: xii).

A dialogical approach is further revealed in sociocultural frameworks for studying childhood which emphasise that relationships and interactions are a key component in enhancing children's participation (Smith 2002). In order for children to understand and participate meaningfully, sociocultural theory emphasises the importance of children's engagement in the shared experience of relevant scripts, events and objects. In this way, adults' awareness of children's understanding and experience in their daily lives is a prerequisite for meaningful engagement with children. Close relationships between adult and child are necessary to establish intersubjectivity (a shared focus of understanding and purpose), which is essential for a dialogic approach to participation. Burman (2008) notes that sociocultural models provide models of learning in context and communities of practice, which are replacing individualistic units of analysis and which focus on dialogue as informing broader theoretical approaches to understanding and knowledge production.

This dialogical shift implies that children's participation is not tied to the efforts of an individual child asserting a claim, but rather emerges within a mutual interdependence, recognition and respect for children and their views and experiences. Significantly, the young people we consulted emphasised the importance of dialogue with adults for affirming, challenging and developing them as people. Supporting young people for dialogue was considered important, with schools in particular needing to examine the value they place on engaging in dialogue with students:

> As teenagers get older we want to discuss things ... the sooner that's introduced to youth it means they mature ... they learn how to interpret their thoughts better ... so discussion is a really good thing. When students start to talk more they mature ... gain confidence ... that's why I like participating in as many things as possible. There's too much for kids to live up to, but not enough discussion about what matters to kids.

Embedded in this shift from a monological to a dialogical approach is a strengthening conceptualisation of participation as a 'struggle over recognition', where the word *over* begs emphasis. Monological approaches to participation focus primarily on claims that can best be conceptualised as a struggle *for* recognition, which is advanced by an agent and evaluated in abstraction from the field in which it is raised. In approaching children's participation as a struggle *over* recognition, attention is drawn to the relational and mutual nature of participation and to the dialogical space within which norms of recognition and intersubjectivity are constituted and negotiated.

In the following discussion we suggest that several challenges remain for researchers and practitioners if we are to endeavour to respond to the inherent emphasis within a dialogical approach, that being the central role of authentic dialogue in recognising both the status and voice of children.

The turn to dialogue: new possibilities and challenges for children's participation

A dialogical approach begs for more critical awareness of the ways in which children have remained excluded by the monological understandings of participation implicit in the first and second moments. Merely granting children rights or proclaiming that they are capable participants does not, in and of itself, create, effect or transform participation. In other words, children's participation depends principally on the invitation offered through dialogue to be acknowledged and to negotiate the terms of their recognition (Kulynych 2001; Percy-Smith and Weil 2003).

While at first glance the significance of dialogue with children seems very self-evident, we need to ensure that it is not simply adopted as a new orthodoxy, such that we fail to understand the implications of the underlying structure of dialogue and the dangers inherent in its uncritical appropriation. It would be both idealistic and naive to approach dialogue as if it were devoid of power, or to assume that deeply embedded practices of power and authority can be readily untangled from the ways we listen to, interpret and act upon what children have to say.

So what are the conditions for a dialogical approach? First, as indicated above, it requires us to focus attention on the workings of power, that is, the *struggle* over recognition. By its very nature, children's participation is imbued with power relations which simultaneously constrain and enable any emancipatory possibilities that may emerge from this. Thus, while inviting children into dialogue is the first step, the accounts that they share cannot be heard outside of, or free from, the political, legal, social and cultural discourses that potentially enable, inhibit and resist what they have to say (Kögler 1999). This requires that we question precisely how all of those involved in participatory initiatives are exercising power, in much the same way as Michael Gallagher suggests here:

> What are the strategies and tactics of participation? Is power being exercised through tactics of coaxing, persuasion, refusal, persistence or evasion? Is it being exercised through the medium of space, bodies, objects, hearing,

vision or words? Is it being exercised through economic resources, sanctions, punishments, rewards?

(2006: 8)

Second, it is not enough simply to assert that addressing the workings and exercise of power will create the conditions for dialogue. Just as important is the analysis of how children's knowledge about participation is organised and sustained, that is, how they think about, interpret and articulate what it is they are struggling for. To speak of children's participation as a struggle over *recognition* suggests that we must commit to a deeper consciousness of just what it is we seek through their participation and be prepared to recognise and act on it when we invite them into a participatory space. In doing so, we commit to a perspective and process that strives to understand, and to trust, how children themselves make sense of the world – in others words, a commitment to the self-understanding and reflexivity of children.

Third, approaching children's participation in terms of struggles *over* recognition denotes a shift towards accepting its mutual and interconnected nature, and hence its conceptualisation as a negotiated space. Adopting a dialogical approach challenges understandings of the *ways in which children are recognised*, which, in turn, adds impetus to the acknowledgement of their rights and their capacity to participate. When the interpretive process of participation is guided by an orientation towards dialogue with children, the self-understanding and individual agency of children (their competence, dependency and vulnerability) does not determine their inclusion or exclusion from the participatory processes, but rather informs the conditions in which their participation occurs. Such an approach thus acknowledges children's dialogue with important adults in their lives (parents, case workers, professionals, lawyers) as deeply implicated in creating and sustaining their identities, in both positive and negative ways.

There is, then, a need to focus on the ways in which we invite, engage and interpret dialogue with children. This includes the systematic, critical explication of the act of dialogue itself so as to position the listener/interpreter for participatory practices that generate a deeper recognition of children. Such recognition is likely to be accompanied by empathy towards, and intersubjectivity with, children, positioning them to formulate their own views and engage in reciprocal interaction and shared responsibility with others. Assigning *dialogue* to a central role in the conceptualisation and practice of participation is a challenge for researchers and practitioners. It is important that they understand and communicate with a range of different children who have complex, diverging life experiences. Dialogue (and the ways in which we communicate more generally) has different rules in different cultures and contexts, and the task of sharing meaning in genuine dialogue requires more than transitory listening, when there are experiential gaps to fill. Generalised assumptions about children do not help us to understand children of different cultures, those from new-immigrant families, children who have disabilities, are chronically ill, or in other ways have experiences many have not shared. Inviting authentic participation from, and dialogue with, children requires a new set of skills from parents and professionals, requiring them to work alongside children, familiarising themselves with the child's context, orienting themselves to 'read' and understand the child's point of view, and providing respectful but non-intrusive support for their engagement in dialogue. This is difficult and challenging work, but worthwhile and rewarding.

Conclusion

Our purpose in this chapter has been to posit a conceptualisation of participation that locates recognition as its *raison d'être*. In doing so, we set out on a path that acknowledges the complex and contested nature of children's participation, which may work to undermine its potential unless we give further attention to the conditions which enable and constrain the elevation of both status and voice. By conceptualising participation as a 'struggle over recognition' we have suggested the need for a shift from a monological to a dialogical approach that opens up new possibilities for children's participation. Far from oversimplifying the conditions which shape our interactions with children, we argue that at the heart of a dialogical approach remains a recursive challenge: how do we engage in dialogue with children and young people about the issues that matter to them? What do we do with their sometimes uninterested or contradictory accounts? How do we respectfully hear and act upon what children tell us is important to them? It is only through pursuing and refining our responses to such questions that we fully acknowledge the complex interplay between agency and power and, in so doing, gently but resolutely hold the voice and status of children at the forefront of our endeavours.

Notes

1. For ease of reading, the term 'children' is used to refer to both children and young people.
2. Ratified in 1990 by Australia and in 1993 by New Zealand.
3. These young people, aged 13 to 20 years, are members of the 'Young People, Big Voice' consultative group who are actively involved with the Centre for Children and Young People at Southern Cross University.

References

Agenda for Children Project Team (2002) '"Listen to us and take us seriously": Young people's responses to the Government's Agenda for Children consultation', *Childrenz Issues*, 6(1): 6–10.

ALP (Australian Labor Party) (2007) *National Platform and Constitution*, www.alp.org.au/download/now/2007_national_platform.pdf (accessed 30 April 2009).

Arneil, B. (2002) 'Becoming versus being: A critical analysis of the child in Liberal Theory', in D. MacLeod (ed.) *The Moral and Political Status of the Child*, Oxford: Oxford University Press, pp. 70–96.

Arnott, M. (2006) 'Democratic renewal and civil society: A perspective from political science', paper presented at the Conference on Theorising Children's Participation: International and Interdisciplinary Perspectives, 4–6 September, University of Edinburgh.

Benhabib, S. (1992) *Situating the Self*, Cambridge: Polity Press.

Burman, E. (2008) *Deconstructing Developmental Psychology* (2nd edn), London: Routledge.

Christensen, P. and Prout, A. (2005) 'Anthropological and sociological perspectives on the study of children', in S. Greene and D. Hogan (eds) *Researching Children's Experiences: Approaches and methods*, London: Sage, pp. 42–60.

Davis, J. and Hill, M. (2006) 'Introduction', in E. K. M. Tisdall, J. Davis, M. Hill, and A. Prout (eds) *Children, Young People and Social Inclusion: Participation for what?* Bristol: The Policy Press, pp. 1–22.

Davis, J. M., Farrier, S. and Whiting, C. (2006) 'Literature review: Participation', paper presented at the Conference on Theorising Children's Participation: International and Interdisciplinary Perspectives, 4–6 September, University of Edinburgh.

Fraser, N. (2000) 'Rethinking recognition', *New Left Review* 3: 107–20.

Gallagher, M. (2006) 'Foucault, power and participation', paper presented at the Conference on Theorising Children's Participation: International and Interdisciplinary Perspectives, 4–6 September, University of Edinburgh.

Gaventa, G. (2007) 'Foreword', in A. Cornwall and V. Coelho (eds) *Spaces for Change?*, London: Zed Books, pp. x–xviii.

Graham, A. (2004) 'Life is like the seasons: Responding to change, loss, and grief through a peer-based education programme', *Childhood Education* 80(6): 317–21.

Graham, A. and Fitzgerald, R. (2006) 'Taking account of the "to and fro" of children's experiences in family law', *Children Australia* 31(2): 30–36.

Greene, S. and Hill, M. (2006) 'Researching children's experience: Methods and methodological issues', in S. Greene and D. Hogan (eds) *Researching Children's Experiences: Approaches and methods*, London: Sage, pp. 1–21.

Hill, M., Davis, J., Prout, A. and Tisdall, K. (2004) 'Moving the participation agenda forward', *Children & Society* 18: 77–96.

Honneth, A. (1995) *The Struggle for Recognition*, trans. J. Anderson, Cambridge: Polity Press.

Honneth, A. (2004) 'Recognition and respect', *Acta Sociologica* 47(4): 351–64.

James, A. (2007) 'Giving voice to children's voices: Practices and problems, pitfalls and potentials', *American Anthropologist* 109(2): 261–72.

Kirby, P. with Bryson, S. (2002) *Measuring the Magic? Evaluating and researching young people's participation in public decision making*, London: Carnegie Young People Initiative.

Kjørholt, A. (2002) 'Small is powerful', *Childhood* 9(1): 63–82.

Kögler, H. (1999) *The Power of Dialogue: Critical hermeneutics after Gadamer and Foucault*, London: MIT Press.

Komulainen, S. (2007) 'The ambiguity of the child's "voice" in social research', *Childhood* 14(1): 11–28.

Kulynych, J. (2001) 'No playing in the public sphere: Democratic theory and the exclusion of children', *Social Theory and Practice* 27(2): 231–64.

Lincoln, Y. and Denzin, N. (2005) 'The eighth and ninth moments – Qualitative research in/and the fractured future', in N. Denzin and Y. Lincoln (eds) *Handbook of Qualitative Research*, Thousand Oaks: Sage, pp. 1116–26.

Morgan, R. (2005) 'Finding what children say they want: Messages from children', *Representing Children* 17(3): 180–9.

Parkinson, P., Cashmore, J. and Single, J. (2007) 'Parents' and children's views on talking to judges in parenting disputes in Australia', *International Journal of Law, Policy and the Family* 21(1): 84–107.

Partridge, A. (2005) 'Children and young people's inclusion in public decision-making', *Support for Learning* 20(4): 181–9.

Percy-Smith, B. (2005) '"I've had my say and nothing's changed!": Where to now? Critical reflections on children's participation', paper presented at Emerging Issues in the Geographies of Children and Youth Conference, 23–24 June, Brunel University.

Percy-Smith, B. and Weil, S. (2003) 'Practice-based research as development: Innovation and empowerment in youth intervention initiatives using collaborative action inquiry', in A. Bennett, M. Cieslik and S. Miles (eds) *Researching Youth*, London: Palgrave Macmillan, pp. 66–84.

Smart, C. (2002) 'From children's shoes to children's voices', *Family Court Review* 40(3): 307–19.

Smart, C. (2006) 'Children's narratives of post-divorce family life: From individual experience to an ethical disposition', *The Sociological Review* 54(1): 155–70.

Smith, A. B. (2002) 'Interpreting and supporting participation rights: Contributions from sociocultural theory', *International Journal of Children's Rights* 10: 73–88.

Smith, A. B. (2007) 'Children and young people's participation rights in education', *International Journal of Children's Rights* 15: 147–64.

Smith, A. B., Taylor, N. J. and Tapp, P. (2003) 'Rethinking children's involvement in decision-making after parental separation', *Childhood* 10(2): 201–16.

Taylor, C. (1995) *Philosophical Arguments*, London: Harvard University Press.

Taylor, N. J. (2006) 'What do we know about involving children and young people in family law decision making? A research update', *Australian Journal of Family Law* 20(2): 154–78.

Taylor, N. J. and Smith, A. B. (eds) (2009) *Children as Citizens? International voices*, Dunedin: University of Otago Press.

Taylor, N. J., Tapp, P. and Henaghan, R. M. (2007) 'Respecting children's participation in family law proceedings', *The International Journal of Children's Rights* 15(1): 61–82.

Thomas, N. (2007) 'Towards a theory of children's participation', *International Journal of Children's Rights* 15(2): 199–218.

Tully, J. (2004) 'Recognition and dialogue: The emergence of a new field', *Critical Review of International, Social and Political Philosophy* 7(3): 84–106.

Wyness, M., Harrison, L. and Buchanan, I. (2004) 'Childhood, politics and ambiguity: Towards an agenda for children's political inclusion', *Sociology* 38(1): 81–99.

28 Children and deliberative democracy in England

Tom Cockburn

Although democracy manifests itself in many forms (see Held 1987), three broad types have been debated in the literature around children and young people's participation. First, 'representational democracy' involves the model of a large number of people voting for someone to represent their views from a menu of candidates. By way of contrast, 'participatory democracy' emphasises the greater involvement of everyone in decision making. This involves the democratisation of everyday life beyond assemblies, parliaments and councils. Third, 'deliberative democracy' lies somewhere in between these forms and involves a selection (possibly randomly chosen, using a structured sample design, not necessarily 'elected') to represent the make-up of a population. In the forum, participants hear evidence, then question the evidence and discuss it among themselves, i.e. they deliberate.

There are a number of themes in children's general participation that have involved a great deal of academic debate; including the role of adults, the struggle to find appropriate forms of participation to develop meaningful practice; problems of theory and implementation (Crimmens and West 2004). While recognising that children may need help through participatory practice in developing their social and cultural capital (Pinkney 2006), research raises significant questions about the extent to which participation promotes inclusion. Further questions concern how to bridge the gap between children's interest in local issues and wider political debates, from which they feel distanced, with older children showing most cynicism about politicians and citizenship (Buckingham 2000).

Furthermore, there are ambiguities within deliberative participatory structures in the developed world, such as in England, where enthusiasm for citizenship is weak, based on an undemocratic education system, a short-term 'consumerist' notion of participation and an emphasis on 'partnership' rather than an expression and contestation of difference. The analysis in this chapter and others in this volume contrasts the spaces for participation 'from above', that is, the spaces that are instigated and defined by policy makers and practitioners, and those 'from below' that have arisen out of community networks. However, the spaces of policy and deliberation to date have not been able to adapt themselves to the worlds of children and young people.

This chapter explores children's engagement with deliberative democratic mechanisms and discusses the potential and limitations of this approach in including the voices of children and young people. Recent reforms in the UK have potentially opened up spaces for citizen participation in decision making. This includes innovations in children and young people participating in 'deliberative' mechanisms. Such initiatives must be broadly welcomed, as any opportunity that potentially opens up the possibility of dialogue with young citizens can only be beneficial. However, there are some important pitfalls to bear in mind.

Participation of children and young people

Children's participation operates in the context of an increasingly complex and differentiated nature of both global and local power relations (Stoker 2000). These wider processes have been operating amid a parallel pull of involving children and young people in state decision making. In particular, the 2003 publication of the *Every Child Matters* green paper (DfES, 2003) has directed service providers to involve children and young people in the delivery of services. In 2005 the DfES Children and Youth Board aimed to support children and young people's involvement in 'the heart of government'. Yet there is little evidence of children and young people making an impact at a central government level in England. Children and young people's views are invited at the 'consultation' stage and examples of children's views are cited in government reports, but there are no significant examples of children initiating a policy *change* at the heart of government.

Perhaps a greater opportunity needs to present itself for children's citizenship to have an impact at a local government level? After all, the 2007 Local Government Act enables local authorities to be 'freed' from central government in their development of local solutions to meet the needs of core groups, including children and young people. It aims to put more decision making into the hands of communities. This 'freeing' of local government from the centre reflects the limits of central government in the global market and the difficulties in shaping interpersonal, inter-organisational and inter-systemic coordination in such a complicated and rapidly changing governance context (Jessop 2000). Governments in the UK have attempted to open up spaces at a local level for citizens to participate in deliberative mechanisms of decision making. This was established in 1999 under the New Deal for Communities, outlined in the Strategy for Neighbourhood Renewal in 2001 and in the establishment of Local Strategic Partnerships in 'deprived areas'. Local authorities have responded to these initiatives and have attempted to link in with local communities in a broad spectrum of methods characterised by Stoker (2004) from the 'consumerist' methods of satisfaction surveys to the 'deliberative mechanisms' such as citizens juries, visioning exercises and community planning schemes. The recent Lyons Inquiry found that there was a need for local government to see itself not merely as a site for service delivery but as 'a place of debate, discussion and collective decision-making' (Lyons Inquiry into Local Government 2007).

Despite the greater opportunities for, and access of local authorities to, young people, considerable barriers persist, as fewer than 4 per cent of local councillors are under 30 years old and local engagements with young people tend to be 'one-off initiatives' (Councillors Commission 2007). In 2007 the Councillors Commission declared concern about:

the lack of faith in existing methods of participation; perceptions that local government is not interested in the views of young people ... of particular importance perhaps is the fact that young people perceive local government to be disinterested [*sic*] in their views. Even when young people acknowledge that there are opportunities to participate they sometimes abstain, assuming that their views will either be given little status or simply ignored.

(Councillors Commission 2007: 81)

Interestingly, the Councillors Commission advocate a reduction in the voting age to 16 and strive to involve young people in more deliberative and participative 'experiments' in democratic engagement. These concerns are reflected in the wider political community through debates around the 'democratic deficit' of young people. Participation in deliberative mechanisms is frequently advocated as a means of increasing young people's involvement in democracy and policy making and 'educating' young people in the benefits of political participation. Oona King (2007), for instance, has suggested that children and young people's engagement with politics can be improved by:

- publication of youth manifestos by election candidates, aimed at young people, to be distributed to schools and youth groups;
- lowering the voting age to 16;
- strengthening youth mayors, school councils, local youth funds and youth parliaments;
- budgets for youth mayors;
- new laws requiring local and national government to consult young people.

Deliberative mechanisms and children and young people

Policy makers see deliberative institutions and practices as having potential through young people for the democratic renewal of the country. There are a number of ways in which people can 'participate', ranging from filling in a questionnaire, to a deliberative forum where dialogue takes place and decisions are made. Local authorities, for instance, have used focus groups, community planning exercises, visioning exercises and user management programmes (see Birch 2002). In England there are district-level youth councils, assemblies, forums, youth parliaments and young mayors through which young people are consulted about services in their area. Within these forums, deliberations occur where ideas are presented, argued for and against, alternatives considered and agreement is arrived at, possibly through compromises.

Middleton (2006) has counted that there are over 500 youth forumss or school councils nationally, of varying shapes and sizes. Deliberative mechanisms have also been encouraged in schools as illustrations of good practice, although to date they are not compulsory. Participation in pupil forums in school is believed to improve the performance, commitment and attitude of students (DfES, 2003). As Yamashita and Davies in this volume acknowledge, if properly done, such participation leads to real school improvement and student development.

'Youth parliaments' have been established across the country, including a national UK Youth Parliament, but have been criticised for replicating adult political structures. They have been proved to be characterised by high disaffection rates among 18- to 24-year-olds and to reinforce the lack of involvement by marginalised young people (Green and Sender 2005; Turkie this volume). However, a different study of youth parliaments explored how far young people adopt the accepted norms of representative democracy (for symbolic/legitimacy/efficacy reasons) and has shown how far they challenge these norms in order to foreground youth priorities and agendas (O'Toole and Gale 2006). The language and practices of politics and policy making tend to be alienating for children, and children's preferred ways of expressing opinions need to be better understood and translated for policy processes. Such understandings are important, as partial or poorly executed attempts to foster participation can have strong negative effects, leading to disaffection and social exclusion, and can compound young people's disadvantage (Matthews 2003).

In 2005 the *Youth Matters* Green Paper instigated the development of the Youth Opportunity Fund (YOF) and the Youth Capital Fund (YCF). Under these funding streams, young people were to be actively involved with the local authority in administering the ring-fenced £115 million awards to develop facilities and 'positive activities' in their area. The guidance stipulated the involvement of young people aged 13 to 19, especially young people from disadvantaged backgrounds and hard-to-reach groups.[1] Participants engaged in training provided by the National Youth Agency, YouthBank and government offices. An evaluation of the YOF/YCF identified 'educational' benefits from young people's involvement in the fund, as it would lead to 'further insights into what young people need, to identify gaps in provision, to engage with new groups of young people and to develop their confidence in combining empowering young people with finance' (O'Donnell, et al. 2007: iv). Interestingly, the most efficient local authorities (that is, those who had allocated or spent all the money within the financial year) had 'all taken a youth-driven approach from the outset, had used gatekeepers to access hard-to-reach young people and young people applied to join the panel, as distinct from being elected by peers' (O'Donnell et al. 2007: 15). Participatory budgeting (PB) is in its infancy in England, but in Brazil and other South American countries it has been used since at least the 1980s; in Porto Allegre, for instance, between 15 and 25 per cent of the city's budget is allocated through PB, where 30,000 people vote each year.

There are, however, a number of constraining factors to 'devolving decisions'. First, there is often the difficulty of localities being run by 'self-styled community leaders', who may restrict funding to their own pet projects. Second, participatory budgeting could foster community competition at the expense of community cohesion.

Third, participatory budgeting processes, despite their best efforts, can still be lacking in inclusion. All socially excluded children and young people still find it very hard to participate, despite the government's attempts to include 'hard-to-reach' groups. How participants are selected or not selected is an important issue, and research shows how easy it is for disadvantaged groups to become marginalised. Feminists show how women can be sidelined from decisions (Abrar 2000).

Similarly, research has shown how ethnic minorities are infrequently included in deliberative mechanisms, especially in important decision-making processes (Spicer and Evans 2006). This is especially so for some communities, such as Chinese or new-immigrant communities. In terms of the YOF/YCF, tensions and resentment may occur if projects are not successful in their applications. Unsuccessful projects may be tempted to appeal directly to the Department for Children, Families and Schools (DCFS), thus undermining the decisions of local children and young people.

Last, young people don't have the time or confidence to run services themselves or to deliberate and mull over issues. Children generally have increasing demands on their time, through school commitments around the National Curriculum. Children and young people need support when they engage in adult institutions. The British Youth Council (2005) noted that only 16 per cent of youth councils have some form of staff support. They need resources and support, or they will end up feeling isolated and bored (Hipskind and Poremski 2005). Mentorship and support by adults happen in a variety of ways. They can show support, engage at practical and strategic levels and also, controversially, '*translate*' children and young people's 'voices' (Lauwers and Vanderstede 2005).

Further assessment of the impact (or otherwise) of deliberative projects involving children and young people is very hard to achieve and is rarely done in a system-atic way (see Halsey et al. 2006). The best precondition is for those establishing deliberative projects to be clear about what kind of *decision* participants are able to make. They need to be aware of why they are offering participation; are the deliberative processes there for bureaucrats to learn and make better policies? Is it for the young people to take part and monitor policies? Or is it to make bureau-crats become more accountable? It is well accepted that participation in anything, especially in deliberative mechanisms, needs to be followed through with tangible 'results' that can be seen by young people. This usually involves further spending, so it is important to link initiatives with further funding sources. This may, of course, be limited in the context of the public sector. However, further funds do exist and the new Youth Opportunities Fund does offer some scope.

Moving to children and young people's spaces

The above discussion perhaps refers to a 'technical' means of optimising delibera-tive mechanisms. However, other research shows that it is necessary for partici-pation in public and formal decision making to be entwined with children and young people's everyday lives and personal and family decision making (Hill et al. 2004). In this sense, the limited nature of citizenship that relies on 'individuals' rather than on interdependencies can be discerned (Cockburn 1998). There is also a tension in young people's participation in mechanisms that on the one hand reside in the culture of public policy and service delivery and on the other hand in the lifeworlds of children and young people (Clark and Percy-Smith 2006). This has significant implications for establishing and embedding ongoing relation-ships through which adults and organisations relate to children, rather than simply focusing on one-off participatory events or isolated structures (Sinclair 2004).

Tisdall and Davis (2004) question whether 'adult-led promotional groups', such as those deliberative mechanisms outlined above, are more effective than representational groups of children, as representative groups have more political skills and are less likely to be dismissed by policy makers as 'unrepresentative'.

However, representational models of democracy also have severe problems. First, once someone becomes a 'representative' there is not necessarily any explicit means of accountability and feedback to those 'represented', the voice becomes an individual opinion (Cairns 2006). Second, creaming off 'representatives' may exacerbate divisions, as investment in the training of individuals to take part in adult structures may lead to limiting the number of children and young people who feel able to take part (Hill et al. 2004). Third, representational means do not encourage involvement across the spectrum of organisations and society. Instead, reflecting a participative democratic approach, recognising the impact of many young people being involved at different levels and in different ways facilitates collaborative working and shared decisions (Badham and Davies 2007).

Theda Skocpol perhaps had this in mind when she developed the notion of 'diminished democracy', where small numbers of representative individuals encourage an 'advocate universe that magnifies polarised voices and encourages class-biased policy outcomes' as the result of 'participation by small groups of activists with intense commitments to (often) extreme causes, coupled with obstacles to routine participation by ambivalent citizens with everyday concerns' (cited in Edwards 2004: 78).

There is an underlying belief in the assumption that children and young people will be willing and able to share their wishes, beliefs and views with bureaucrats if they are provided with specific structures and spaces to do this. However, it is important to pay attention to the specific spaces where children and young people are invited in, and questions need to be asked about whose terms are defining these spaces (Cornwall and Coelho 2007). Hickey and Mohan (2004) have noted the importance of the spatial now entering into political theory. They argue that there are three ways in which spaces are an important component of analysis. First, participation and associational life are *situated in practice*. Often in policy, 'practice spaces' are romanticised and homogenised through self-evident evocations of 'the local community'. Who forms this local community and who 'speaks for' the community is a complex process that is simplified through representational and deliberative structures. Instead, local communities consist of complicated social worlds where social identities are shaped by local dynamics, constructions of space/place, as well as being shaped by wider social forces. In this sense, children and young people can be silenced in social constructions of 'the local community' and often local young people are constructed as problems by the 'voice' of local communities.

Second, places are shaped by market forces and material well-being. This has implications for how a geographical space is shaped in relation to other adjoining spaces that may be richer and poorer.

Third, it is important to focus analytic attention onto how participatory or associational spaces are presented. For instance, 'provided' spaces, such as council meetings noted above, are often disempowering to local people. Those subject to discrimination and exclusion entering these spaces can find them intimidating. How young people talk and what they talk about may be seen as incoherent, irrelevant or even disruptive. Marian Barnes (2007) has described how young people were coached by youth workers to present versions of their concerns that were seen to be 'acceptable', rather than being expressed in their own language. The ownership of these spaces is therefore a crucial element. Moss and Petrie's (2002) analysis of children's participative spaces draws our attention to how space is constructed through 'place', that is, how children and childhood are placed within broader social relations.

Children and young people in 'offered' deliberative spaces

So what does deliberative democracy offer for the citizenship of children and young people? At first sight there are enormous obstacles to deliberative democracy's being successful in England. First, there is the distinct lack of interest in politics in Britain, and this reluctance is not limited to children and young people. By way of contrast to England, where enthusiasm for citizenship is weak, the developing world experiences situations such as the collapse of the economy or conflict, which pull individuals out of the social languor that characterises political lives. We have also seen children and young people becoming stirred up about things, but professionals often dismiss these as trivial or unimportant. Furthermore, a citizenship 'bored' of politics is characteristic of a centralised and bureaucratic party structure in England, in contrast to the decentralised mass of local associations and personal relationships that constitute the basis of party politics in Latin America (Rodgers 2007).

Second, children and young people's citizenship is shaped by an undemocratic education system (Lockyer 2003). Alderson (1999) has noted that the introduction of student councils in schools has deflected attention away from children's real participation in school by focusing on peripheral issues. Indeed, such experiences of 'tokenistic' deliberative mechanisms reinforce the general apathy and cynicism towards participation in general. Further analysis of school councils within governance spaces is presented by Tisdall in the next chapter.

Third, citizenship is based on a short-term 'consumerist' notion of participation. One of the most damaging critiques of children and young people's participation has been the charge of the 'consumerist' tendency by which they are presented with a 'choice' of services or how they might feel about them. The shift from welfare to monetarism has allowed the state to disengage itself from the economy and from political accountability in challenging inequalities. This consumerist element is harmful for children and young people in that they are already economically marginalised and do not have a strong consumerist hand to play. Such shallow consumerism does not encourage political participation, as young people are encouraged into an apolitical form of participation where they are able to display only a rather limited amount of agency. Thus, children and young people are portrayed as self-interested and politically uninformed citizens only capable of commenting on a very narrow aspect of their own lives (Mizen 2004).

Fourth, concepts of deliberative citizenship in the UK have an emphasis on 'partnership' rather than on an expression and contestation of difference. As noted above, those from marginalised groups feel intimidated by 'provided' spaces. Deliberative structures are framed by those who have created them and they are thus instilled with power relations and the practices of interactions that people bring with them from other spaces. There is an assumption that participation will assuage heterogeneous relationships to the state (see Acharya et al. 2004). Deliberative mechanisms exist within this competitive terrain, and such spaces facilitate 'reasonable' actions and define others as 'unreasonable', 'immature' and so on. It is erroneous to suggest that people can form associations and engage in deliberative activity on an equal basis, as associations between adults and young people are structured by vertical dependencies, routine exclusion, patronising attitudes and non-democratic forms of authority. For instance, professionals bring in 'expertise' and are reluctant to listen to alternative knowledge or even to recognise it. Young people's culture is more often than not portrayed as chaotic, disruptive and unproductive, and in stark contrast to the rationalised world of professionals. Furthermore, those from some socially excluded backgrounds will be familiar with their parents' politics which is more confrontational and partisan than the consensus-seeking and 'rational' modes of argumentation and delibera-tion. Despite all the innovation and build-up of technical knowledge, delibera-tive participatory structures in the UK continue to exclude the poorer and more marginalised citizen.

Inclusive deliberative citizenship?

How, therefore, can these obstacles be overcome in developing deliberative mech-anisms? Most importantly, it is necessary to develop deliberative mechanisms into spaces where all children, including the most marginalised, feel most comfortable. As noted above, much of the development of children and young people in delib-erative democracy to date has been undertaken by formal, adult-led organisations. There has been a focus on procedures, policies, processes, practices and techniques of improving children's participation in formal processes. However, researchers and practitioners are beginning to realise the importance of 'the informal sector', of peers, parents, friends and less formal networks. For instance, Yuen et al. (2005) note the importance of leisure activities in providing a foundation for the devel-opment of shared meanings through the familiarisation of participants in leisure into social learning that leads to the emergence of social capital. Allender et al. (2006) have made similar points about engagement in sport. Helen Haste and Amy Hogan (2006) have helpfully extended the analytic focus of 'civic engage-ment' from the narrow confines of voting to include helping (in a broad sense) and struggling to make one's voice heard.

Young people are spending an increasing amount of time with peers, rather than in family situations (Dixon et al. 2006). It is therefore important to focus on this aspect of their lives. It is vital to notice the importance children and young people attach to their peer networks, and policy needs to focus on supporting these networks. If children and young people are happy with their peers, we find that they are indeed capable of critical thinking, responsibility and learning. By way of contrast to adult-initiated structures, they can at the same time be places of curiosity, fun and negotiation. William Corsaro (1999) has written much about the way children adapt ideas from the adult world to address their own concerns. They therefore do deliberate already, it is just that the structures of these spaces are not recognised, recorded, taken seriously and certainly do not feed into social policy. Nancy Rosenblum (1998), in her discussion of civil society, argued that it is necessary to include a wider group of structures not included by other political theorists. She includes not only identity-based groups but also street gangs, and points out that within these spaces young people gain deliberative skills such as taking turns in talking, leadership and learning reciprocity.

The opening up of deliberative mechanisms to children needs to be understood in the context of changes in citizenship ideas. Recent debates on citizenship in England have been concerned with notions of 'active citizenship', of which the various political campaigns against 'voter apathy' and 'welfare dependency' are the issues most covered by the media. Central to the 'active citizenship' campaign are the encouragement of greater participation in civil society organisations, 'volunteering' and involvement in structures such as deliberative mechanisms. This promotion of active citizenship has occurred at the same time as the attack on many aspects of 'social citizenship' that in T. H. Marshall's (1950) classic conception included the 'evolution of social rights to welfare, housing, education, etc. A key concern for government has been the movement of those 'dependent' on social rights into the labour market. Recent examples in England include lone parents and those receiving Disability Living Allowance. Most children (under 16), of course, are the exception to this, as they are expected to be dependent upon other householders and are full-time beneficiaries of the social right to education.

In the Latin American context there is an enormous enthusiasm for participating in deliberative mechanisms, as the establishment of social rights (and in some cases civil and political rights) is an aspiration and goal to be achieved. It is thus easier to generate energy and enthusiasm if people can clearly see that they will get something out of participating. By way of contrast, there is more ambiguity towards the social rights that are under attack in England; social rights are seen as an entitlement and people tend to be less interested in the processes by which they receive them, than in that they so receive them.

Some activists of course can see the threat to their social rights, and this is manifested in England in a number of 'user groups'. In this sense, 'user groups' are an example of a deliberative forum, and a lot of children and young people's deliberative forums, such as schools councils, local authority initiatives and to some extent youth parliaments are examples of 'user groups'. As such, the young people attempt to involve themselves in their struggle for social rights, as they struggle to be listened to, argue for adequate facilities, for more resources or for help in 'more efficient' delivery of services.

Deliberative mechanisms are about capturing the 'voice' of children and young people. Yet expressing voice, having your voice heard, and dialogue with those in public forums are extremely difficult for young people. A recent study (Cockburn and Cleaver 2008) I was involved in looked at children and young people's involvement in a range of civil society settings and found the enormous difficulty they had in having their 'voices' heard. Included in our study were a highly skilled group of young people involved in a local youth parliament. My colleague referred to these young people as 'super participators', as they were involved not only in the youth parliament but also in a large range of political, social and religious organisations, yet these confident and experienced young people still required support from professionals. They felt the importance of their ties with parents, friends, peers and the other young people they represented. However, they felt a tension and a disconnection in their roles as youth parliamentarians and their 'other lives' of family, friends and social lives. Thus, advancing a children and young person's voice was a tremendous struggle.

Conclusion

Taylor and Percy-Smith (2008) cite the key findings of a symposium of academics and practitioners in Oslo in 2000 on 'the importance of recognising different forms of participation in both formal and informal settings; building on existing cultural norms and practices of children in their everyday settings; engaging children according to issues which are meaningful' (p. 379). These observations reflect the above arguments about deliberative democracy in England, and the lack of movement in these issues over the years since then is cause for some pessimism.

However, some progress has been made in making deliberative spaces less alienating. Alan Turkie's contribution to this volume recognises some advances (as well as the persistent problems) in capturing the voices of marginalised groups in youth parliaments. Furthermore, as the contributions in this volume by Greg Mannion and Kay Tisdall make clear, more analytical attention is rightly being focused on the *spaces* of deliberations and the way adult–child relationships may 'co-evolve' with shared deliberations. Children and young people's own resourcefulness of course must not be underestimated, and some young people achieve effectiveness despite the obstacles and difficulties discussed here. The next step is for there to be a leap of faith as well as to mobilise resources and, rather than expecting young people to come to democracy, for democracy to go to children and young people.

Notes

1. Including young disabled people, young care leavers, looked-after young people, young offenders, young carers, young refugees, young lesbian women and gay men, young Black and minority ethnic people, travellers and those in rural areas.

References

Abrar, S. (2000) 'Feminist intervention and local domestic violence policy', in G. Stoker (ed.) *The New Politics of British Local Governance*, Basingstoke: Macmillan, pp. 249–67.

Acharya, A. et al. (2004) 'Civil society representation in the participatory budget and deliberative councils of Sao Paulo, Brazil', *IDS Bulletin* 35(2): 40–8.

Alderson, P. (1999) 'Human rights and democracy in school', *International Journal of Children's Rights* 7: 195–205.

Allender, S., Cowburn, G. and Foster, C. (2006) 'Understanding participation in sport and physical activity among children and adults: A review of qualitative studies', *Health Education Research* 21(6): 826–35.

Badham, B. and Davies, T. (2007) 'The active involvement of young people', in R. Harrison et al. (eds) *Leading Work with Young People*, London: Sage.

Barnes, M. (2007) 'Whose spaces?' in A. Cornwall and V. S. Coelho (eds) *Spaces for Change*, London: Zed Books.

Birch, A. (2002) *Public Participation in Local Government: A survey of local authorities*, London: ODPM.

British Youth Council (2005) *The Youth White Paper: Strong local voices*, London: British Youth Council.

Buckingham, D. (2000) *The Making of Citizens: Young people, news and politics*, London: Routledge.

Cairns, L. (2006) 'Participation with purpose', in E. K. M. Tisdall, J. Davis, M. Hill, and A. Prout (eds) *Children, Young People and Social Inclusion: Participation for what?* Bristol: The Policy Press.

Clark, A. and Percy-Smith, B. (2006) 'Beyond consultation: Participatory practices in everyday spaces', *Children, Youth and Environments* 16(2): 1–9.

Cockburn, T. (1998) 'Children and citizenship in Britain: A case for a socially interdependent model of citizenship', *Childhood: A Global Journal of Child Research* 5(1): 99–117.

Cockburn, T. and Cleaver, F. (2008) 'How children and young people win friends and influence people: children and young people's association, their opportunities, strategies and obstacles', unpublished report to Carnegie UK

Cornwall, A. and Schattan Coelho, V. (2007) *Spaces for Change*, London: Zed Books.

Corsaro, W. (1999) *The Sociology of Childhood*, London: Sage.

Councillors Commission (2007) *Representing the Future*, Department for Communities and Local Government.

Crimmens, D. and West, A. (2004) *Having Their Say. Young people and participation: European experiences*, Lyme Regis: Russell House Publishing.

DfES (2003) *Every Child Matters*, London: Department of Health.

Dixon, M. et al. (2006) *Freedom's Orphans: Raising youth in a changing world*, London: IPPR.

Edwards, M. (2004) *Civil Society*, Cambridge: Polity Press.

Green, R. and Sender, H. (2005) 'Marginal inclusion: What is the future for the UK Youth Parliament?' *Youth and Policy* 82: 1–14.

Halsey, K. et al. (2006) *The Voice of Young People: An engine for improvement? Scoping the evidence: Literature Review*, Reading: CfBT Education Trust.

Haste, H. and Hogan, A. (2006) 'Beyond conventional civic participation, beyond the moral-political divide: Young people and contemporary debates around citizenship', *Journal of Moral Education* 35(4): 473–93.

Held, D. (1987) *Models of Democracy*, Cambridge: Polity Press.

Hickey, S. and Mohan, G. (2004) *Participation: From tyranny to transformation?*, London: Zed Books.

Hill, M. et al. (2004) 'Moving the participation agenda forward', *Children & Society* 18(2): 77–96.

Hipskind, A. and Poremski, C. (2005) 'Youth governance: Supports and resources are critical components for youth success', *Children, Youth and Environments* 15(2): 245–53.

Jessop, B. (2000) 'Governance failure', in G. Stoker (ed.) *The New Politics of British Local Governance*, Basingstoke: Macmillan, pp. 11–32.

King, Oona (2007) *The Battle to Engage*, 4Children: www.4children.org.uk/information/show/ref/1077.

Lauwers, H. and Vanderstede, W. (2005) 'Spatial planning and opportunities for children's participation: A local governance network analysis', *Children, Youth and Environments* 15(2): 278–89.

Lockyer, A. (2003) 'The political status of children and young people' in A. Lockyer, B. Crick and J. Annette (eds) *Education for Democratic Citizenship: Issues of theory and practice*, Aldershot: Ashgate, pp. 120–38.

Lyons Inquiry into Local Government (2007) *Place Shaping: A shared ambition for the future of local government*, London: The Stationery Office.

Marshall, T. H. (1950) *Citizenship and Social Class*, Cambridge: Cambridge University Press.

Matthews, H. (2003) 'Children and regeneration: Setting an agenda for community participation and integration', *Children & Society* 17: 264–76.

Middleton, E. (2006) 'proYouth Participation in the UK', *Children, Youth and Environments* 16(2): 180–90.

Mizen, P. (2004) *The Changing State of Youth*, Basingstoke: Palgrave Macmillan.

Moss, P. and Petrie, P. (2002) *From Children's Services to Children's Spaces*, London: Routledge.

O'Donnell, L. et al. (2007) *Youth Opportunity Fund and Youth Capital Fund: Evaluation findings from initial case study visits*, London: DCFS.

O'Toole, T. and Gale, R. (2006) 'Participative governance and youth inclusion: The case of youth parliaments', paper presented at the Conference on Theorising Children's Participation: International and Interdisciplinary Perspectives, 4–6 September, University of Edinburgh.

Pinkney, S. (2006) 'Response to Nigel Thomas, Joy Moncrieffe and Michael Gallagher', paper presented at the Conference on Theorising Children's Participation: International and Interdisciplinary Perspectives, 4–6 September, University of Edinburgh.

Rodgers, D. (2007) 'Subverting the spaces of invitation? Local politics and participatory budgeting in post-crisis Buenos Aires', in A. Cornwall and V. Coelho (eds) *Spaces for Change: The politics of participation in new democratic arenas*, London: Zed Books.

Rosenblum, N. (1998) *Membership and Morals*, Princeton, NJ: Princeton University Press.

Sinclair, R. (2004) 'Participation in Practice: making it meaningful, effective and sustainable', *Children & Society* 18: 106–18.

Spicer, N. and Evans, R. (2006) 'Developing children and young people's participation in strategic processes: The experience of the Children's Fund initiative', *Social Policy and Society* 5(2): 177–88

Stoker, G. (ed.) (2000) *The New Politics of British Local Governance*, London: Macmillan.

Stoker, G. (2004) *Transforming Local Governance: From Thatcherism to New Labour*, Basingstoke: Palgrave Macmillan.

Taylor, M. and Percy-Smith, B. (2008) 'Children's participation: Learning from and for community development', *International Journal of Children's Rights* 16(3): 379–94.

Tisdall, K. and Davis, J. (2004) 'Making a difference? Bringing children's and young people's views into policy making', *Children & Society* 18: 131–42.

Yuen, F., Pedlar, A. and Mannell, R. (2005) 'Building community and social capital through children's leisure in the context of an international camp', *Journal of Leisure Research* 37(4): 494–518.

29 Governance and participation

E. Kay M. Tisdall

Theorisations of children and young people's[1] participation in collective decision making have been largely inward looking in recent decades. Typologies – such as Hart's ladder (1992), Treseder's subsequent circle (1997) and Shier's step-wise progression (2001) – have been immensely useful to challenge policy and practice, as they have been powerful tools to highlight the *lack* of children's participation and to advocate for change. And there has been substantial change: participation activities involving children and young people have blossomed over recent years, in the UK and also internationally (see, for example, special issues of *Children, Youth and Environments* (2006, 2007 and 2008); Tisdall et al. 2006; Hinton 2008). With this growth, it has become apparent that the typologies are insufficient to address current tensions in children and young people's participation and assist in moving such participation forward. It is time for theorisations of children and young people's participation to look more widely.

A potentially fruitful area lies within political science and public policy ideas, with their recent obsession with governance. This chapter first reviews such ideas, highlighting those of potential use for children and young people's participation in collective decision making. It then considers schools as a site for governance, and school (or pupil) councils, in particular, as especially testing for children and young people's participation. On the one hand, the right to education features strongly for children across international human rights instruments, from the Universal Declaration of Human Rights, to the UNCRC, to the recent UN Convention on the Rights of Persons with Disabilities. With the international agenda of *Education for All*, the goal is for primary schooling to be universal. Schooling is thus becoming a central frame for childhoods in the global South, just as it already frames Northern childhoods. On the other hand, schools (at least in the UK) have been accused of typically being poor in recognising and promoting children and young people's rights generally, and specifically their participation (e.g. Alderson 2000; Jeffs 2002; Fielding 2007; UK Children's Commissioners 2008). Schooling is compulsory, and thus at their heart schools are not voluntary associations for children and young people (see Cockburn's chapter in this volume). What can we learn if we consider schools as sites of governance and (potential) associational spaces?

Governance

Interest in governance – as a concept, as a descriptive device, as a normative value – exploded within public policy and political theory in the mid 1990s. Almost inevitably, therefore, definitions are diverse and diffuse.

As a starting point, Richards and Smith (2002: 2) describe the perceived shift from top-down government to more horizontal relationships of 'governance':

> 'Governance' is a descriptive label that is used to highlight the changing nature of the policy process in recent decades. In particular, it sensitizes us to the ever-increasing variety of terrains and actors involved in the making of public policy. Thus, it demands that we consider all the actors and locations beyond the 'core executive' involved in the policy-making process.

Certain definitions of governance explicitly link to participation. One of the most optimistic is expressed by Lovan and colleagues:

> Governance, in short, is a process of participation which depends on networks of engagement, which attempts to embrace diversity in contemporary society; which promotes greater responsiveness to service users and, in so doing, seeks to reshape accountability relationships.
>
> (2004: 7–8)

Participation will improve both the quality and the legitimacy of government decisions (Barnes et al. 2007). A consensus is growing, writes Gaventa, in both the North and South, that 'a more active and engaged citizenry' is needed *and* a 'more responsive and effective state' (2004: 6).

This consensus is part of and parallels the 'deliberative turn' (Cornwall and Coelho 2007). Rather than relying on passive voting, people are brought together to deliberate, to discuss, to work together in exploring and taking forward policy solutions. This participatory approach, it is argued, is the way to engage people and truly create democratic renewal. But it has potential pitfalls, as Cockburn and Cleaver point out, as 'attention needs to be paid not just to the "select few" who are involved in these deliberations but to extending participation to the majority' (2008: 11). To avoid these and other problems, Cornwall and Coelho (2007: 8–10) set out five requirements for participatory institutions to be inclusive and effect change:

1   People need more than invitations to participate: they need to recognise themselves as citizens, rather than as beneficiaries or clients.
2   Representative claims must be considered critically and mechanisms to be representative must be in place.
3   Structures are not enough. The motives of those who participate – including state actors – can be competing and are in constant negotiation.
4   Three factors are essential for change: involvement by a 'wide spectrum of popular movements and civil associations, committed bureaucrats and inclusive institutional designs' (9).

5   Participation is a process over time and must be situated alongside other polit-
     ical institutions and within its own social, cultural and historical context.

How does children and young people's participation in schools – and particularly
through school councils – marry up to these requirements? Below, examples and
empirical evidence from England and Scotland are used to explore this question.

Schools as participative institutions?

1 Children and young people as citizens

Cornwall and Coelho's first requirement is problematic for children and young
people generally and for schooling in particular. There are resurgent academic
claims for children as citizens (e.g. Invernizzi and Milne 2005; Jans 2004; Liebel
2008), but debates continue about whether children are semi- or partial citizens
or whether they can claim citizenship on the basis of a restricted cluster of rights
(Lister 2007; Stalford 2000; see Tisdall 2008 for discussion).

Education policies in the UK have only recently recognised children as the
consumers of schooling, as education legislation has traditionally been structured
around parents' responsibilities to ensure that their children are educated and
the state's responsibility to provide. The 2000 Standards in Scotland's Schools
etc. Act in the UK was the first to recognise children's own right to schooling
(s.1, although the legal enforceability of this provision is questionable). Further,
rights to participate have now been included, in various ways, in most devolved
educational legislation (see Tisdall 2007). School inspection regimes now inquire
about pupil participation and involve pupil views in their assessments. Children's
participation is now on the educational policy agenda.

Citizenship education, re-emphasised from the mid 1990s, is another (potential)
lever to promote children and young people's participation. Its implementation in
England has been roundly and frequently criticised for focusing on *teaching* children and young people about and to be citizens (e.g. see Faulks 2006) – with far
less recognition that children and young people are citizens in the present and that
their school participation is vital to their current and future engagement in citizenship. Other nations in the UK have taken a different approach to England's.
For example, in Scotland citizenship was set as one of the national priorities of
education but its implementation was across the curriculum and throughout the
school – 'there is no intention of specifying rigid age- and stage-related outcomes
for education for citizenship here' (LTS 2002: 22). 'Citizenship through experience' was advocated in pupil participation (LTS 2002: 19), harking back to the
provisions in the 2000 Standards in Scotland's Schools etc. Act. But the new
curriculum, the Curriculum for Excellence, prioritises children recognising their
responsibilities, relating to a 'responsibilisation' discourse where rights are condi-
tional rather than inalienable (Lewis 2003).

If rights are a fundamental building block of citizenship (e.g. T. H. Marshall's
(1963) seminal paper on citizenship), then children's lack of awareness of their
rights limits their ability to recognise their citizenship. Only 44 per cent of children

in Scotland have heard of the UNCRC, with even lower numbers in England (13 per cent) and Wales (8 per cent) (survey results reported in UK Children's Commissioners (2008)).[3] Overall, the UK Children's Commissioners reflect that there has been only 'limited progress in children's participation in education' and 'there remains resistance to allowing children to exercise their right to participate in decisions that affect them at school' (2008: 13).

In short, recognition of children and young people as citizens is not assured by theorists, educational policies or organisations, let alone by children and young people themselves. Yet there are new openings and opportunities and an enthusiasm about innovative practice.

2 Representation

A popular response to the demands for 'pupil voice' has been the growth in school councils throughout the UK. From around 50 per cent of schools having councils in the mid 1990s, surveys report around 85 to 90 per cent of schools having such councils in England and Scotland (Whitty and Wisby 2007; Tisdall 2007). The Welsh Assembly required all primary, secondary and special schools to have a school council by November 2006.

Despite their popularity, school councils are a contentious mechanism for children and young people's participation. On the one hand, Alderson (2000: 124) notes the powerful position of school councils:

> School councils are a key practical and symbolic indicator of respect for children's rights. There are other useful methods for pupils to contribute to school policy ... Yet only councils provide a formal, democratic, transparent, accountable, whole-school policy forum.

But her research team also found that, if children and young people perceived their school council as tokenistic and ineffective, they were more disappointed and disengaged than if there were no school council at all. Criticisms of school councils go further, with attacks on their replication of a failed adult structure of representative politics (Cairns 2006). They are seen to privilege a small, articulate elite and exclude others from involvement (for this potential, see Yamashita and Davies' chapter in this book) – the select few that Cockburn and Cleaver (2008) warn us about.

We have new evidence on school councils, confirming some of these criticisms – but also pointing to more positive potential. Recent surveys have been taken of secondary school pupils in England and Wales (reported in Whitty and Wisby 2007) and in Scotland (Tisdall 2007), providing results from a statistically representative sample of such pupils. The surveys do show that a minority of pupils are school council members at any one time: 8 per cent in Scotland, with a higher result of 12 per cent in England and Wales. But the Scottish survey also asked respondents about past experience of being school council members, finding that one-third had such experience – mostly from primary schools. With the growing numbers of school councils in primary schools, there may be upward pressures on secondary schools to be more participative (Whitty and Wisby 2007): certainly, the Scottish survey found respondents in lower grades considerably more positive about school councils than those in higher grades.

In short, school councils can potentially meet Cornwall and Coelho's second requirement, with mechanisms to be representative in place. They have been contentious for repeating failed models of democracy and enhancing participation for the few. Deeper consideration of representativeness claims and mechanisms could combine the flexibility of associational democracy with accountability.

3 Beyond structures

Cornwall and Coelho conclude that much depends on the motivations of those who enter participatory institutions and on what 'participation' means to them. This chimes with Fielding's highly critical analysis (2006: 306) of the 'the high performance learning' school, which has a broad range of formal and informal pupil participation but where participation is put to largely instrumental use, for particular adult purposes:

> It is often technologically and emotionally sophisticated, seemingly interested in young people's points of view, and attentive to suggestions that may enhance the school's effectiveness and reputation. It is, however, ultimately totalitarian and often dissembling in its dispositions and its operation: here student voice only has significance and is only legitimate insofar as it enhances organisational ends.

With this analysis, Fielding unsurprisingly prefers the second type, the 'person-centred learning community', where 'student voice is essentially dialogic and, in its most exploratory mode, challenging of boundaries and demarcations, preferring instead the intimations of a radical collegiality' (2006: 300). To achieve this, Fielding writes that leadership must support an inclusive, value-driven approach, provide commitment over time, be willing to transcend traditional hierarchy and demarcations, and intend to create dialogic public spaces.

A number of motivations have been suggested for children and young people's participation, which can be divided into four types: appeals to moral and legal rights; consumerism and service user involvement; addressing democratic engagement; and enhancing children's well-being and development (see Department for Education and Skills 2004). The influence of these can be tracked through teachers' responses to an English and Welsh survey, reported by Whitty and Wisby (2007), which asked about purposes (rather than motivations) (Table 29.1).

How can we interpret these results, in light of the various motivations promoting children and young people's participation? Purposes G (as a response to the UNCRC) and I (to meet Ofsted's requirements) align to moral or legal rights, but only 2 per cent and 1 per cent of teachers, respectively, identified these as the top purpose for pupil consultation. A rights-based, legalistic approach has the advantages of a 'trump' card (Dworkin 1978), raising the status of children and young people's participation to an imperative. But pupil participation rights in UK legislation remain legally weak, with little enforcement potential. Clearly, more legalistic motivations were not perceived by teachers as being foremost.

Table 29.1 Teachers' views on the purposes of school councils or other forms of pupil consultation

Purpose	Which of the following, if any, best describes the purpose of your school's form of pupil consultation? (%)	And to what extent, if at all, has the introduction of the school council achieved the purpose? Respondents answering 'a great deal or a fair amount' (%)
A To improve the school's environment and facilities	27	87
B To develop pupils' social and emotional skills	21	88
C To enhance our citizenship provision	17	–
D To help the school respond to the personalisation agenda	10	–
E To improve teaching and learning	7	78
F To raise pupil attainment	2	83
G As a response to the UNCRC	2	–
H To improve pupil behaviour	2	85
I To meet Ofsted's requirements	1	–
J Other	4	–
K Can't say – a combination of these things	3	–
L Don't know	2	–

Source: Ipsos Mori, reported in Whitty and Wisby (2007: 118, 199).

Instead, purposes aligned with consumerism or service user involvement predominated. A large number of the teachers' responses could come under this category (e.g. A, C, D, E, F, H) and these were some of the top-scoring responses for the primary purpose of pupil consultation *and* positively scored as a result of the consultation.[2] As consumerism discourses have been so strong in UK policy, bringing children and young people into them has been a successful ploy. While seemingly persuasive, consumerism has well-rehearsed disadvantages (see Prior et al. 1995; Barnes et al. 2007; Cockburn's chapter in this book). For example, market ideas of supply and demand do not necessarily work well with public goods and quasi-markets. A consumer's ultimate power is that of exit, which hardly applies for many children and young people in compulsory education (and those who do exercise the power of exit are penalised as truants). Consumerism can focus on narrow agendas of service improvement rather than on more radical options; it tends towards more superficial involvement, such as consultation, rather than deeper engagement.

It is possible that purpose C, 'to enhance our citizenship provision', could be aligned instead with motivations to address the democratic crisis. Certainly, this concern influenced the revised focus on citizenship education (see Crick Report 1998), with its advantages and disadvantages discussed above.

Finally, the appeals to children's well-being and development have been persuasive – most clearly linked with purpose B and one of the highest scoring purposes to both questions. Given education's focus on children and young people's development, this purpose may feel particularly comfortable to teachers. Children and young people do report their appreciation of the skills and self-esteem they gain from their participation (e.g. Kirby with Bryson 2002). But research also finds their frustration if their participation is tokenistic or ineffective, with no impact or results (Alderson 2000; Dorrian et al. 1999). A focus on well-being and development can concentrate solely on process and fail to consider outcomes as well.

While motivations are important to Cornwall and Coelho (2007), they do not expect unanimity among participants. Instead, they recognise potential diversity of expectations and how expectations can be in constant negotiation. But some expectations and motivations sit compatibly with each other, while others can clash: for example, a rights-based approach is interested in both process and outcomes, while one based on well-being and development may only emphasise the former. The survey asked solely about teachers' perceptions of the school participation's purpose; forthcoming research will report further on the perceptions of children and young people (see Having A Say at School, www.havingasay-atschool.org.uk/).

4 Effectiveness – a tripartite approach

Cornwall and Coelho (2007) write of the need to connect with wider popular movements and civil associations. The disconnection between children and young people's participation in school, with adult associational or governance structures either within or outside schools, is a considerable weakness in the UK. For example, in England children and young people were stopped from being school governors in 1986. Only since 2003 have young representatives been allowed back on school governing bodies, as associate (but not full) members. The 2006 Scottish Schools (Parental Involvement) Act abolished school boards. Instead, new, flexible and hopefully more inclusive structures were put in place to encourage parental involvement in schools. But the Scottish Executive and the Scottish Parliament refused to legislate for parental and pupil involvement together, to create a coherent and constructive institutional framework for school governance. Joint, intergenerational frameworks for school governance are not required. Children and young people's participation is largely isolated from other forms of school governance, civil associations and movements, cutting off opportunities for dialogue and change.

Cornwall and Coelho (2007) expand on the requirements for inclusive institutional designs, writing of limiting deliberations to implementation rather than rethinking policies, and trade-offs of legitimacy, justice and effectiveness. These limitations can be found in research on school councils. For example, qualitative school council research has been critical of councils' limited power, restricted to decisions on school facilities and environments (e.g. school meals, toilets and after-school activities) and kept from core issues of teaching and learning, staff appointments and other strategic activities (see Wyse 2001; Cotmore 2003; Wyness 2005; Fielding 2006; Yamashita and Davis's chapter and Lewars's chapter in this book). The 2007 survey of secondary school pupils in Scotland found them only moderately positive about school councils in practice. In Scotland, a minority of secondary school respondents agreed or strongly agreed (21 per cent) with the statement 'The council has given me a say on how my school is run', while 40 per cent disagreed or strongly disagreed. Only 29 per cent strongly agreed or agreed with the statement 'The council has improved things at my school', while 28 per cent disagreed or strongly disagreed.

Yet pupils were considerably more positive about school councils in principle, with 44 per cent of the Scottish secondary pupils strongly agreeing or agreeing with the statement 'I think school councils are a good way of listening to pupils'. In the English survey, a small majority of secondary school pupils think 'every school should be required to have a school council': 26 per cent strongly agreed and 29 per cent tended to agree. The experience of Wales with its mandatory school councils will be telling. Do the majority of children and young people approve of school councils' legitimacy as a form of participation, but question their effectiveness?

5 Participation as a process

If anything is unique about children and young people's participation, it may be that children and young people 'grow out' of that identity with considerable speed. Participation focused around schools must deal with the particular groupings of children by age/stage, the ebb and flow of the school year, and the changing populations of teachers and pupils. Whitty and Wisby (2007) note the fragility of school councils, where even some of their case study schools required 'revitalisation' after one or two years and were highly dependent on certain teachers' enthusiasm. How to create hand-over from one academic year to the next, to have useful institutional memory and continuity for children and young people who have gained skills and experience in influencing change to share these with other children and young people, are particular challenges for school-based participation.

But these difficulties arise in part because of the isolation of children and young people's participation from other (adult) groups, which could provide an ongoing trajectory for children and young people themselves, and also the associational continuity to celebrate and encourage people having differential involvement at various points in their lives. Here, movements from other countries which involve all generations may provide illumination on alternatives to age-based isolation of children and young people's participation (e.g. see Smith 2007, Mexico; Butler 2008, Brazil).

New perspectives?

Bringing together the UK and international discussions of governance with children and young people's participation encourages new perspectives. For example, considering schools as sites of governance illuminates their emancipatory and controlling reality – and their potential. Most children spend a great deal of their waking lives in schools, and this will only extend internationally should *Education for All* be successful in extending compulsory primary schooling worldwide. If the hopefulness of Lovan and colleagues' definition of governance were realised, schools could provide networks of engagement, embracing diversity among children and young people. They could allow education (as well as other services) to be more responsive to children and young people and to reshape accountability relationships.

School councils tend to follow a representative model, as underlined by the definition used by School Councils UK (2008):

> An elected body of pupils whose purpose is to represent their classes and to be a forum for active and constructive pupil input into the daily life of the school community.

Some school councils are structured to enhance the capacity of school council members to be representative: designing selection methods that are seen as fair for all children and young people; ensuring feedback mechanisms to and from those who are represented and their representatives. Some schools are experimenting with alternative models, involving open meetings and multiple channels, closer to Hirst's (1994) promotion of participative or associational democracy (see Whitty and Wisby 2007 for survey results from teachers and pupils; HMIE (2006) for Scottish examples). Schools may choose to have class councils, working at a smaller scale, either alongside or instead of school councils. School councils need not follow one model and, indeed, arguably are more inclusive when they take advantage of the possibilities of governance rather than seeking to replicate adult forms of formal democratic representativeness and procedural deliberation. These may be particularly inappropriate, given the transitory nature of school councils, which typically must be renewed every academic year, and as children and young people progress into and out of schools annually. Time, as well as space, needs to be considered for participatory institutions.

Considering governance illuminates the greatest weakness of current trends in UK school participation. Why are school councils, as well as so many of children and young people's participation activities, so isolated from other associative activities? Schools are centrally situated within other partnership and network arrangements, increasingly asked to fulfil a key role in improving communities as well as children and young people's well-being. If schools met Lovan and colleagues' participative agenda, then they could be a central node in broader networks of community participation. Indeed, this appears to be the central rationale for Whitty and Wisby (2007) in recommending that school councils become mandatory in schools; broader structures of youth participation can tap into secondary school councils for representatives.

Governance is not a panacea. The move from government to governance has blurred accountability, with the risk that articulate voices prevail and those who are excluded by conventional politics and systems only become more excluded (O'Toole and Gale 2008). Governance can control and channel dissent, leashing it while creating a mirage of legitimacy and limiting a more substantial critique (Bragg 2007). Thus, for example, children and young people may have more opportunities for participation, but this is only allowed on certain terms: e.g. when children and young people engage in anti-war protests (Cunningham and

Lavalette 2004) they are considered truants rather than citizens expressing their views. School councils may proliferate but, unless their decisions actually impact on decisions and unless they are networked into governance structures, their potential is limited (see Lewars's chapter for a young person's perspective on the scope of student voice activities). Children and young people's participation is kept officially apolitical, fitting more nicely into the governance ideals of partnership and shoring up legitimacy, but potentially missing the more radical potential and demands of a political framing. It highlights that, despite the potential of the civil rights encapsulated in the UNCRC (see Theis's chapter in this book), Article 12 is in fact a very qualified right of involvement and the UNCRC contains no rights to formal political engagement, such as voting. To be worthwhile, school councils need to be genuine vehicles for children and young people's views to be expressed, with some tangible impacts on decision making.

Conclusion

This chapter has used ideas from governance theories to consider children and young people's participation in schools, particularly through the currently popular formal mechanism of school councils. It demonstrates their potential for deliberative spaces, as well as their current and potential constraints in meeting Cornwall and Coelho's requirements for inclusive and effective participatory institutions.

Carnegie UK's Inquiry into Civil Society (2007) identifies certain threats to civil society, which include the increasing importance of non-institutional forms of civil society associations and the diminishing arenas for public deliberation. Schools could address both these threats, in their continued institutional prominence and their opportunity for deliberative spaces. Cornwall and Coelho (2007) remind us that once participants have a platform for participation, it is a process and there can be a wealth of unintended and unanticipated outcomes. School councils can and could provide just such platforms, if they are freed from narrow preoccupations with representative government and take advantage of the governance potential.

Notes

1. Following the UN Convention on the Rights of the Child (UNCRC), a child is defined as a person under 18, unless national laws recognise the age of majority as being earlier. However, many young people do not want to be labelled as 'children'. The phrase 'children and young people' is thus used, unless other terminology is particularly relevant or used by cited authors.
2. No explanation is given in Whitty and Wisby (2007) as to why the other purposes were not asked for in the second question.
3. The figure for Wales appears to be for children who had been taught about the Convention, rather than simply having heard of it

References

Alderson, P. (2000) 'School students' views on school councils and daily life at school', *Children & Society* 14: 121–34

Barnes, M., Newman, J. and Sullivan, H. (2007) *Power, Participation and Political Renewal*, Bristol: The Policy Press.

Bragg, S. (2007) 'Student voice and governmentality', *Discourse* 28(3): 343–58.

Butler, U. (2008) 'Children's participation in Brazil – A brief genealogy and recent innovations', *International Journal of Children's Rights* 16: 301–12.

Cairns, L. (2006) 'Participation with purpose', in E. K. M. Tisdall, J. Davis, M. Hill, and A. Prout (eds) *Children, Young People and Social Inclusion: Participation for what?* Bristol: The Policy Press.

Carnegie UK (2007) 'The shape of civil society to come', http://democracy.carnegieuktrust.org.uk/civil_society/publications/the shape of_civil_society_to_come, accessed 18 February 2008.

Cockburn, T. and Cleaver, F. (2008) 'How children and young people win friends and influence people: Children and young people's association, their opportunities, strategies and obstacles', unpublished report to Carnegie, UK.

Cornwall, A. and Coelho, V. S. (2007) 'Spaces for change', in A. Cornwall, and V. S. Coelho (eds) *Spaces for Change?*, London: Zed Books.

Cotmore, R. (2003) 'Organisational competence: The study of a school council in action', *Children & Society* 18: 53–65

Crick Report (1998) *Education for Citizenship and the teaching of democracy in schools*, www.qca.org.uk/libraryAssets/media/6123_crick_report_1998.pdf, accessed 17 July 2008.

Cunningham, S. and Lavalette, M. (2004) 'Active citizens or irresponsible truants? School student strikes against the war', *Critical Social Policy* 24(2): 255–69.

Department for Education and Skills (2004) *Working Together: Giving children and young people a say*, www.teachernet.gov.uk/wholeschool/behaviour/participationguidance, accessed 1 July 2007.

Dorrian, L., Tisdall, K. and Hamilton, D. (1999) *Taking the Initiative: Promoting young people's participation in public decision making in Scotland*, London: Carnegie UK Trust and Children in Scotland.

Dworkin, R. (1978) *Taking Rights Seriously*, Cambridge, MA: Harvard University Press.

Faulks, K. (2006) 'Rethinking citizenship education in England', *Education, Citizenship and Social Justice* 1(2): 123–40.

Fielding, M. (2006) 'Leadership, radical student engagement and the necessity of person-centred education', *International Journal of Leadership in Education* 9(4): 299–313.

Fielding, M. (2007) 'Beyond "voice": New roles, relations and contexts in researching with young people', *Discourse* 28(3): 301–10.

Gaventa, J. (2004) *Representation, Community Leadership and Participation: Citizen involvement in neighbourhood renewal and local governance*, London: Neighbourhood Renewal Unit, Office of Deputy Prime Minister.

Hart, R. (1992) *Children's Participation: From tokenism to citizenship*, Florence: UNICEF, Innocenti Centre.

Hinton, R. (2008) 'Children's participation and good governance: Limitations of the theoretical literature', *International Journal of Children's Rights* 16(3): 285–300.

Hirst, P. (1994) *Associative Democracy*, Cambridge: Polity Press.

HMIE (Her Majesty's Inspectorate for Education) (2006) *Education for Citizenship: A portrait of current practice in Scottish schools and pre-school centres*, www.hmie.gov.uk/documents/publication/efcpcp1.pdf, accessed 18 February 2008.

Invernizzi, A. and Milne, B. (2005) 'Introduction: Children's citizenship: a new discourse?' *Journal of Social Sciences* (special issue) 9: 1–6.

Jans, M. (2004) 'Children as citizens. Towards a contemporary notion of child participation', *Childhood* 11(1): 27–44.

Jeffs, T. (2002) 'Schooling, education and children's rights', in B. Franklin (ed.) *The New Handbook of Children's Rights*, London: Routledge.

Kirby, P. with Bryson, S. (2002) *Measuring the Magic? Evaluating and research young people's participation in public decision making*, www.carnegieuktrust.org.uk/cypi/publications/measuring_the_magic, accessed 12 March 2005.

Lewis, J. (2003) 'Responsibilities and rights: The changing balance', in N. Ellison and C. Pierson (eds) *Developments in British Social Policy*, 2nd edn, London: Palgrave Macmillan.

Liebel, M. (2008) 'Citizenship from below: Children's rights and social movements', in A. Invernizzi and J. Williams (eds) *Children and Citizenship*, London: Sage.

Lister, R. (2007) 'Why citizenship: Where, when and how children?', *Theoretical Inquiries in Law* 8: 413–38.

Lovan, W. R., Murray, M., and Shaffer, R. (2004) 'Participatory governance in a changing world', in W. R. Lovan, M. Murray and R. Shaffer (eds) *Participatory Governance: Planning, conflict mediation and public decision-making in civil society*, Aldershot: Ashgate, pp. 1–20.

LTS (Learning and Teaching Scotland) (2002) *Education for Citizenship in Scotland – A Paper for Discussion and Development*, www.ltscotland.org.uk/citizenship/images/ecsp_tcm4–122094.pdf, accessed 17 July 2008.

Marshall, T. H. (1963) 'Citizenship and social class', *Sociology at the Crossroads and Other Essays*, London: Heinemann.

O'Toole, T. and Gale, R. (2008) 'Learning from political sociology: Structure, agency and inclusive governance', *International Journal of Children's Rights* 16: 369–78.

Prior, D., Stewart, J. and Walsh, K. (1995) *Citizenship: Rights, community and participation*, London: Pitman.

Richards, D. and Smith, M. J. (2002) *Governance and Public Policy in the UK*, Oxford: Oxford University Press.

School Councils UK (2008) 'Structures and Definitions', www.schoolcouncils.org/scuk_content/for_free/Structures%20and%20Definitions/scuk_for_free (accessed 12 May 2009).

Shier, H. (2001) 'Pathways to participation: Openings, opportunities and obligations', *Children & Society* 15(2): 107–17.

Smith, A. (2007) 'The children of Loxhica, Mexico: Exploring ideas of childhood and the rules of participation', *Children, Youth and Environments* 17(2): 33–55.

Stalford, H. (2000) 'The citizenship status of children in the European Union', *The International Journal of Children's Rights* 8: 101–31.

Tisdall, E. K. M. (2007) 'School councils and pupil participation in Scottish secondary schools', Glasgow: Scottish Consumer Council, www.scotconsumer.org.uk/publications/reports/reports.htm, accessed 18 February 2008.

Tisdall, E. K. M. (2008) 'Is the honeymoon over? Children and young people's participation in public decision-making', *International Journal of Children's Rights* 16: 419–29.

Tisdall, E. K. M., Davis, J. M., Hill, M. and Prout, A. (eds) (2006) *Children, Young People and Social Inclusion: Participation for what?* Bristol: The Policy Press.

Treseder, P. (1997) *Empowering Children and Young People Training Manual: Promoting involvement in decision-making*, London: Save the Children, UK.

UK Children's Commissioners (2008) *UK Commissioners' Report to the UN Committee on the Rights of the Child*, www.11million.org.uk/resource/31f7xsa2gjgfc3l9t808qfsi.pdf, accessed 17 July 2008.

Whitty, G. and Wisby, E. (2007) 'Real decision making? School councils in action', www.dfes.gov.uk/rsgateway/DB/RRP/u014805/index.shtml, accessed 18 February 2008.

Wyness, M. (2005) 'Regulating participation: The possibilities and limits of children and young people's councils', *Journal of Social Sciences* (special issue) 9: 7–18.

Wyse, D. (2001) 'Felt tip pens and school councils: Children's participation rights in four English schools', *Children & Society* 15: 209–18.

30 After participation

The socio-spatial performance of intergenerational becoming

Greg Mannion

In this chapter I respond to critiques of children and young people's participation that show that a focus on 'voice' and 'listening to children' risks being limited and tokenistic in its reach and purpose. Using theoretical understandings from geography and other post-structural perspectives, I attempt to show how children and young people's participation can be reordered and sustained as a dialogical and spatial practice designed to improve intergenerational spaces and relations. I will argue that research and practice relating to the perceived need to 'listen to children' fails to address a more important purpose – that of improved relations between children and young people and adults through changes to the spaces they separately and together inhabit and the associated identifications.

Participation for what?

The starting point for many people's concern with children's participation is often the perceived lack of opportunity for children and young people to 'have a say' in decision making, and the lack of real opportunity to have a say on social and political matters (see Wyness et al. 2004). In the same vein, Morrow's (2001) study described how children and young people had limited participation in decision making in their communities and schools and argued that there were no consistent channels for children's and young people's views or creativity. The call, logically, goes out to adults and professionals, local authorities and governments and others to 'listen to children' and for new structures of communication to be developed (youth councils, pupil councils and so on) that would afford opportunity for the voices of children and young people to be heard. But what is the *purpose* behind these calls for greater participation by children and young people?

Reasons given for why we should encourage children and young people's participation include (a) it's their right as citizens, (b) it's a legal requirement, (c) it will improve services to children, (d) it's more democratic and leads to better decisions, (e) it ensures children and young people's safety and protection from abuse, and (f) it enhances children and young people's skills, self-esteem and self-efficacy (Sinclair 2000; Mannion 2007). Inherent in this approach is a rationale for children and young people's participation as rights and entitlement but also as *enlightenment* (Warshak 2003): children have something important to tell us (adults) that may change the decisions we make on their behalf.

We might ask if children's participation initiatives could hope to provide such a vast array of outcomes (a–f above). Even if they could, there are other problems. Percy-Smith (cited in Thomas 2007) notes a range of issues with children and young people's participation initiatives, but reminds us that having children and young people participating in structures that are inherently undemocratic will be likely to founder. As practitioners in the field will all know, there are dangers for all adult participation workers: children's voices may be scripted, and adults may be being deluded into thinking that they are really hearing all of what children are trying to say (Mannion 2007). Another rationale put forward for children and young people's participation relates to their *empowerment*. Percy-Smith (cited in Thomas 2007) notes the related tension inherent in the need for children to enjoy their childhood and also bear the burden of decision-making responsibilities. The debate around whether children and young people are 'becomings' or 'beings' relates to this. Tisdall and Davis (2004) reiterate many of the above critiques but add some others: they remind us that in some initiatives only selected types of children get a say, that dialogue with policy makers is usually short-term and that feedback is critical to sustained engagement by children and young people, but is often lacking. Their analysis results in a call to reconsider the positionings of adults and children in so-called participation initiatives. As I will argue later, these altered positionings or identifications for both adults and children are critical considerations and not mere 'background noise'. Three positionings are offered by Tisdall and Davis, although I expect there could be many more, depending on the context:

1   Young participants could be the 'members' of the project while adults could be seen as the 'staff'.
2   The project could be seen as promotional groups 'for' young people rather than seeking to be representative projects 'of' young people.
3   Adults involved could be seen as 'lending' their skills and resources to the young participants, to enhance the young people's status.

(Tisdall and Davis 2004: 140)

What I wish to note here is how important the relational framing between the generations is in this field. The ongoing struggle to create a framework for children's participation (see Thomas 2007) suggests that a more reflexive shift in epistemology and ontology is needed. One starting point comes by noticing how overlooked adults are in all this. Percy-Smith (2006) suggests that this is because children and young people's views are not held in equal terms with adults' views. His more inclusive understanding of participation places children and young people's participation within wider community-based social learning and development. Percy-Smith (2006: 154) argues for participation as *a relational and dialogical process*:

little attention has been paid to the role of adults or the way in which the agenda and values of adults and children are negotiated and power and responsibility are shared. Most frequently, young people tend to 'participate' as a group apart from adults, which reinforces their separation from adults in the everyday spaces of their communities.

The collaborative intergenerational spaces that Percy-Smith envisions reposition adults and decentre their role from one of dominant carer to a co-inquirer or interpretive learner with children and young people. He argues that useful participatory work with children and young people has to be enacted in

> a 'communicative action space' (Kemmis 2001) characterised by flexibility, mutual respect and reciprocity in relationships between young people and adults (Wildemeersch et al. 1998).
>
> (Percy-Smith 2006: 168)

In a related way, whether we see children as potential citizens ('becomings') or as active citizens ('beings') will also determine how children and young people's participation gets played out. In practice, it is less common, however, that children and young people participate *alongside* adults.

Percy-Smith is not alone in arguing that children and young people's participation should have outcomes for *adults* as well as for children. That we do not often surface the outcomes and effects for adults of children's participation is interesting evidence of a lack of reflexivity. As Cockburn notes:

> Adults need to check their own motivations and assess their readiness to work in partnership with children. They need to work on whether they accept the validity of young people's agenda [*sic*] and whether the processes they adopt are more effective and respectful to children. Furthermore, children's views must be placed alongside with [*sic*] other adult stakeholders who may have conflicting agendas.
>
> (Cockburn 2005: 115)

In the next section, I will try to outline some of the consequences of reframing children's participation along these lines, through considering participation as a spatial practice.

Spatial critiques

The idea of children and young people's 'own spaces' for participation is often put forward in projects. A spatial critique of children and young people's participation will reveal that the idea of children's 'own' space of participation is a misrecognition of how spaces come into being and what relations make them possible. Some argue that some children and young people's participation happens, even needs to happen, without adult intervention, away from the gaze and control of adults – that somehow children and young people's participation is purer or less polluted if conducted in this way. (The rhetoric of Roger Hart's ladder of participation may be a case in point, even if it was not intended to be suggestive in that way.) Yet, in my own work, I have yet to see any children and young people's participation project that is not in many ways affected by adults either directly or indirectly (Mannion 2007). Buckingham, analysing the effects of the media on children's lives, notes that 'if children have their own culture, it is a culture which adults have almost entirely created for them – and indeed sold *to* them' (Buckingham 2000: 96).

It is important here to reflect on what notions of space I am working with. A less fixed view of space (Massey 1994; 2005) suggests that it is more than a back-drop or a container for the action. Instead, spaces are *part of* the action, and very consequential in the forms of behaviour they afford and the emergence of the identities that inhabit them. Within this view, the self and space are intertwined in a co-emergent process. Elsewhere, I have argued that spatial and social changes occur in and through the shaping of real and imagined places (see Mannion and I'Anson 2004). With this argument comes the need for a more fluid notion of identity formation as 'becoming'.

Thomson (2007) reminds us that there are many theorists who can help us with the theory of identity here, including Benhabib (1992) and Butler (1990). I find the work of Hall (1996) useful, preferring as he does the notion of ongoing identification to that of identity *per se*. In contrast, behind much of the work on children and young people's participation sits a very modern view of the stable, rational adult self as the active agent. Lee (2001) challenges the view that adults are autonomous and rational, proposing instead the idea that adults as well as children are best seen as human becomings. Within these views of space and identification processes, I am suggesting that child–adult relations and practices are always co-constructed by both children and adults and, reciprocally, affect and are affected by the places and spaces that these groups co-inhabit or inhabit separately. Space is an important factor here because (1) power often resides with those who can act as gatekeepers of places and decision making around how those places might be changed (explored, for example in my own study of school grounds changes, Mannion 2003); (2) because the inclusive and exclusive spaces for children are often managed by non-present adults; and (3) because in many cases young people may want to work *with adults* to co-create new spaces and are acutely aware of the necessary presence of adults to provide support or facilitate the activities. This critique leads me to suggest that the term 'children's spaces for participation' is a misnomer, because 'children's own spaces' or 'children-only spaces' are better understood through the intergenerational relations that give rise to these places in the first instance and how they continue to be maintained and supported by these relations (see Mannion and I'Anson 2004 and Mannion 2007 for empirical examples).

Spatialising 'voices' and its effects

Lundy (2007) is another of a growing number of commentators who are becoming uneasy with the discourse of 'children's voices', their 'right to be heard' and, in educational circles, 'pupil voice'. She argues that the use of such terms is a misrepresentation of the meaning behind Article 12 of the United Nations Convention on the Rights of the Child (UNCRC). For her, 'cosy', conservative readings of the UNCRC mean that sometimes children's right to be heard is seen as a gift of adults where 'what matters' can be constrained by adults; these are in fact legal imperatives. Also, she takes time to point out that it is not up to adults to decide at what *levels* decision making begins to involve children and young people, since the legal requirement is for involvement at all levels, in a consistent and ongoing manner. In response, she advocates a foregrounding of three additional features beyond merely the facilitation of children's views or 'voice', namely:

- space: children must be given the opportunity to express a view
- audience: the view must be listened to
- influence: the view must be acted upon, as appropriate.

By incorporating these features, Lundy (2007) appears to be employing two key strategies: she *spatialises* participation and, in doing so, *stretches* the field of concern across many contexts beyond the local – it is not sufficient, then, for voice to be heard merely in the local domain, though this is clearly a critical element. By requiring participation to have far-reaching effects (through critical *audiences* and *influences*), she forces a more *relational* sense of children and adults collaborating for change. Lundy (2007) further pushes a *relational* view by noting that 'Article 12 must be interpreted in conjunction with Article 5 of the UNCRC (which states that adults' right to provide "appropriate direction and guidance" in the exercise by the child of the rights in the Convention must be carried out in "a manner consistent with the evolving capacities of the child")' (Lundy 2007: 939). We must do more than provide the marginalised with a 'space to speak'. The process must facilitate the sustainability of empowerment beyond the time–space arena of the research or participation project itself.

Fielding (2007) subtly airs similar concerns in relation to participation at school. He suggests that we 'move to a more participatory form of engagement character-ised by an intended mutuality, a disposition to see difference as a potentially crea-tive resource, and more overt commitment to co-construction' and that this shift requires 'quite different relationships and spaces and a quite different conceptual and linguistic schema to frame such aspirations' (p. 307). The argument here, in the context of school, is not about listening to pupils but about reconfiguring the relations between adults and children in and through schooling – a more radical agenda, surely.

Children and young people's empowerment after post-structural critiques?

Other critiques of participation (taken in its wider use, not just with children and young people) come largely from the theoretical paradigm of post-structuralism (see Kesby 1999). These critiques largely relate to efforts to facilitate the partici-pation of marginalised groups in developing countries. Practitioners in the field of adult and community development, particularly in the majority world, have noted that it is dangerous to attempt to describe in one voice what marginalised 'locals' or 'women' may want or have said. Similarly, we need to be careful not to collapse multiple and differentiated views of individuals and sub-groups of children and young people (whether younger or older, from different socio-economic backgrounds and so on). Another critique of participation relates to the need to enable locals to see the limits of their own knowledge – giving people 'a say' when you know little about the topic can give rise to problems rather than empowerment. In turn, children and young people's participation, if treated as an end in itself, may lead us to fail to notice when participation is *not* advancing the cause of inclusion, equity or social justice and may be perpetuating the ills associated with the status quo.

I am acknowledging that children's own perspectives are worth listening to, but that this will not be sufficient for a radical and democratic intergenerational practice. If children's own perspectives are to have any impact, they are likely to need to be aired in the right place and taken on board by those with influence, or by those who may be involved in gatekeeping access to other arenas of influence – or perhaps shared decision making with children and young people. By implication, this means that children and young people's participation is likely to involve adults at some stage in the communication process – in collaborating with children and young people or in working on their behalf to broker children and young people's views and decisions, if not in the local field of the participation project itself (as staff, guides or consultants), then onwards through dissemination and awareness raising. The corollary is also true: children and young people can broker the voices of adults for others, too. This will therefore involve adults and children and young people in taking on new roles, whether that be in standing back, in facilitating dissemination, or in taking part in action arising from intergenerational participatory projects. Critically, however, in taking on board the perspectives of children and young people, in animating this work or as a consequence of it, there must be consequences for all and for their identifications and relations across the generations.

Others have noted that the categories of 'child', 'young person' and 'adult' are far from clearly separated out. Alanen and Mayall (2001) suggest that the subject positions of 'adult' and 'child' are performed, and are by definition interlinked and expressed differently in different locales. This approach rests on a presumption that adults, like children and young people, can be seen as 'becomings' rather than as fully formed, rational individuals. Reflexively, we should note that the potential outcomes for adults have to do with their relations with children and young people, but that it is also these improved relations that may make children and young people's participation possible. Interestingly, this creates a conundrum: the outcomes for adults (their repositioning as reciprocal co-constructors of knowledge and collaborators) are also a useful starting point for intergenerational participatory work. It seems we need to reframe children and young people's participation work more inclusively, as participation between and among various stakeholders in communities (see Percy-Smith 2006), because their identification processes are structurally coupled.

Empowerment and participation after post-structural critiques?

Other critiques of children and young people's participation come from a Foucauldian analysis. Responding to these critiques also suggests that an associational or relational approach is required. Cooke and Kothari's (2001) volume reminds us that participation projects enacted through the use of the microtechnologies of facilitation (focus groups, flipcharts, visual methods etc.) may purport to control the production of knowledge in a fair and equitable manner but are not necessarily so benign and inclusive. As Kesby (2007) outlines (drawing on Allen 2003), we should not hold out the hope that through the deployment of technical facilitative processes we can create a more equal space for engagement by children and young people. This is because there are no power-free spaces that can be created by the routine application of a participatory tool *per se*. Nor can power be redistributed by the mere use of tools and techniques so that participation can be more equitable. This is because power is not a commodity that is concentrated in the hands of some, which can easily be redistributed among participants through some technique.

The post-structural critique starts with a view of power as 'everywhere' and participation always as an *effect* of power. So-called participatory techniques are then seen as enactments of power because they may advance some agenda (perhaps of the facilitator's) through enrolling the participant into predesigned tasks. Participatory approaches are not innocent levellers; some perspectives are always privileged while others are silenced. Participation workers, too, cannot claim to be innocent in how they manage and balance the voices of participants or how their voices get heard beyond the local domain. Mohan (cited in Kesby 2005) has even pointed out that participation in development contexts may privilege the 'local' perspective to the exclusion of outsiders' perspectives. Approaches such as the use of visual methods *per se* do not unproblematically uncover children's own knowledge and views, but are in fact efforts to realign and transform knowledge and to govern respondents and researcher alike, albeit in ways that are counter-hegemonic though still ideologically framed. The argument that 'power is everywhere' and not in the 'hands of folk' seems very devastating to any hope for a viable form of children and young people's participation. Kesby places participation in a relational and complex network of power:

> [P]ower is a more heterogeneous phenomenon, dispersed throughout a network of discourse, practices and relations that are productive of action and effects. These numerous discourses and practices are inherently unstable, requiring constant reproduction and performance just to survive and are continually undergoing mutation and dislocation as they interact and as they respond to resistance. Individuals simultaneously carry and undergo this power. It both enables and conditions their action. Both the dominant and the dominated are implicated in transmitting and reproducing the discourses and practices that constitute the relations between them. Individuals act strategically to manipulate the network of force relations that positions them and others but never fully control it.
>
> (Kesby 1999: web source)

If participation and power are effects, then to act powerfully through participation is to manipulate resources in order to produce effects among others. Again, we see why 'listening to children and young people' is an insufficient aim if it does not watch out and strive for effects. Kesby (2007) tries to reconcile participatory approaches and post-structuralist perspectives and to explore the spatial dimensions of participation and empowerment. His arguments suggest that we can work with a circulating view of power so that new social positionings are made possible for participants as a result of taking part. Kesby draws on Hannah Arendt's idea of 'power with' (Allen cited in Kesby 2007) to recover the participation agenda, but in doing so he also reconfigures participation as an associational process between parties. We may reread Allen with children and adults in mind as the 'agents' he is referring to:

> Allen's (2003) work is useful because it identifies two further modalities of power, this time under the guise of 'associational power' or 'power with' others: negotiation which can take place between agents who have different resources at their disposal, contains no obligation to comply, and is directed towards identifying and achieving common ends; and persuasion which requires an atmosphere of reciprocity and equality and uses strength of argument to produce an effect.
>
> (Kesby 2007: 5)

Kesby (1999; 2007) attempts to recapture some ground for participatory processes through the concept of 'power with'. 'Power with' sees empowerment as emergent within 'lateral' (reciprocal) and not 'vertical' (hierarchical) relationships. For our purposes, these relationships are intergenerational, wherein we can expect the repositioning of all parties as an outcome of true participation, with likely effects for both adults and children. But there are other consequences of taking this post-structural ontological position. Kesby (2007) suggests that we cannot work with a view of the individual as an autonomous rational agent who somehow 'sees the light' and is empowered – this view is not compatible with the post-structural perspective. In response, he reverts to alternative views of the role of self, agency and identification that are seen as reciprocal, lateral and accountable to each other. The empowerment of children within this view ought not to be thought of as the release of each child's or adult's free will, but rather as the social production of their *relational agency* through intergenerational transactions. By the same token, the goals of such agency cannot be determined – by adults or children – in advance.

For Kesby, participatory agency is 'dynamic, strategic, and capable of producing hybridity and the ontologically new yet, at the same time, something that is socially constructed, partial, situated, and achieved through available resources' (Kesby 2007: 7). Potentially, we could imagine the dialogue that would ensue through children and young people's participation as constitutive of various forms of agency and counter-agency, which may at times coexist and or may have oppositional goals – some degree of conflict seems inevitable in lively participation initiatives. This suggests that even for those seeking to achieve 'power with' children and young people, there will be times when 'power against' is felt and worked through. As Kesby (2007) suggests, power and *empowerment* are more alike than we may first think. One wonders how well this view sits with participatory projects that may on occasion set out with predetermined goals (for example, to 'build a play park') and want to 'consult' children and young people on their views.

In line with Kesby, and drawing on post-structural perspectives, I suggest that, through what we call children and young people's participation, knowledge does not emerge from individuals, but rather emerges within intergenerational and interpersonal dialogues within spaces that are also 'part of the action'. This emphasis on the relational interdependence of adults and young people also brings a reciprocal linking of roles that will constantly change (see Fielding 2007). Kesby and others may be salvaging participation from the jaws of strong post-structural critiques. But if they do, only a less definitive and strident form of participation for children and young people is now possible. Now participation is a partial, situated and contestable work-in-progress subject to future challenge and transformation of *all* parties involved, with effects being felt both locally and in more distant contexts. Like Cahill (2007), this approach emphasises the fluidity and multiplicity of subject positions as the basis for personal and social transformation in action projects involving young and old. Fielding (2007) suggests 'dialogue' as one term that might help us to get beyond the limitations of 'voice-led' perspectives, and recognition that there is a radical tradition to draw upon to help us move towards the multi-vocal, spatially informed, action-oriented, intergenerational approach that he and I advocate. But the value of such an outcome may be that it is nonetheless effective at countering oppressive and less self-reflexive forms of power. This form of participation is reconstituted as a form of performance and, like all performances, can be transformed and performed differently, depending on the context.

Conclusion

What I am arguing is that children and young people's participation needs reframing as a relational and spatial practice. (This would include participatory research with children and young people.) Current versions of children and young people's participation offer a limited view of the ways in which participants and spaces reciprocally trigger changes in each other. Clearly, then, the idea of children and young people 'having a say' does not capture everything we wished that it would in the social practices we call children and young people's participation. In advocating a relational and spatial approach we must notice how relations, identifications and space are reciprocally linked: they co-evolve. In effective projects, relations between adults and children, their associated identifications and the spaces they inhabit will likely change. Within this view, participants are embodied, spatially located performers of fluid subject positions, rather than independent rational agents with immobile positions. Identifications for both children and adults are uncertain and destined to co-emerge within the places they actively try to create (separately or together) (see Mannion and I'Anson 2004). Therefore, repositioned roles for adults become the critical and often unseen consequences and processes of children and young people's participation.

Post-structural critiques rehearsed here remind us to be aware of the fact that participation is dialogical, partial, situated and contested. This suggests that what we call children and young people's participation is always unfolding as an inter-generational performance wherein identifications, spaces and power struggles are key. Within these performances, we need to consider *both adults and children* as partial 'becomings' (Lee 2001; Roche 1999). The consequences of participation (with changing levels and experiences of tokenism) will likely be felt differently by different stakeholders, but critically, if they are to be more than tokenistic, the effects will be felt in contexts and times beyond the immediate realm of the participatory work itself. Useful participation will be felt in the way it stretches identifications for all and in the way the effects are felt beyond the participatory initiative itself (in space and time). In this work, the participants (adults and children and young people) in these processes are recursively affected by each other and the spaces they create locally and further afield. Children's participation is not in fact about accessing the silenced voices of children (though this may be a useful starting point). If we take a more relational approach, children and young people's participation projects are always about something that needs to be made more explicit: the creation of new dialogical intergenerational spaces of and for participation, through which new kinds of relationships, identifications and spaces for adults and children emerge and find expression.

A participatory response

In the spirit of the approach taken by the editors of this book, I next want to try to allow some space for a form of participatory and dialogical response. In January 2008, I attended an international conference in Durham entitled 'Connecting People, Participation and Place' organised by the Social Well-Being and Spatial Justice research cluster at Durham University and the Participatory Geographies Working Group of the RGS/IBG. Here were convened theoreticians, practitioners and researchers, mainly in the field of geography, but across other disciplines too. The focus was on participatory approaches to research, learning, action and change in social and environmental science disciplines, voluntary sectors, statutory agencies and community-led organisations around the world. As part of the conference an 'Open Space' event allowed opportunity for a discussion on the topic of participation after post-structuralist critiques. The following notes were generated as a result of the discussion. The small discussion group (see list below) saw value in keeping alive the view that participatory approaches are distinctive and valuable in some way, but after the post-structural critiques (outlined above). The following list of 'Understandings for Action' was created:

Understandings for action after post-structuralism

1   *Inclusion as an aim not as a characteristic of the process*: We defined participatory approaches as those which attempt to more explicitly bring into being the 'new democratic spaces of citizenship' being called for in many arenas. As

such, they set out with the aim of creating greater inclusiveness in society, though critically, the means and ways of getting there may be various and involve actions such as disturbing others' perspectives – so we are not claiming that the processes, practices and journey towards inclusion will be inclusive themselves, but rather fraught with challenges and difficulties, tensions and contradictions. Even the ideal of an inclusive society may be about living within and with these tensions rather than smoothing over them.

2   *Informed participants – making things explicit*: Participatory approaches appear to involve greater degrees of informed consent. We noted that the rules for doing this are socially determined: so it is different for children, since we must gain the consent of their parents, for example. Again, there are degrees of effectiveness here and it may be impossible to fully offer informed consent for all aspects of projects as they unfold. Yet, we sensed that this is a noticeable aspect of the approaches we value as more participatory than others.

3   *Power negotiations made explicit / Negotiating values and principles*: Building on 2 above, here we noted that after the post-structural critique power is every-where (that we are inevitably entangled), participatory approaches could be seen as sustainable and distinguishable from other forms of life if they made the negotiation of this power, values and principles of engagement more explicit. This produces a challenge to be critically reflexive about our roles as facilitators, activists, participation workers. Multiple, shifting and contradic-tory subject positions are likely for all.

4   *Participation is a performative practice*: In some ways, the theoretical problem of 'what is empowerment after post-structuralism?' is solved, to a degree, every day through the local practical and active responses people make to social problems – sometimes through participatory approaches. Here we felt that, because we cannot ever be sure about what is going to work for all participants, we must accept that the tricky practice of taking a participatory approach can be in itself a good enough 'answer' to the theoretical critiques levelled from a post-structural perspective. By practising a 'warts and all' participatory approach, with all the possibilities of failure, we provide a face-valid response that may or may not work; but, critically, this is in itself empowering because it is not accepting that things are impossible. This relates to the idea that embodied performances are responses to injustice.

5   *'Power with' and 'Power over'*: These terms are used first by Hannah Arendt, and picked up by Allen and Kesby in their writing. Empowerment is seen as somehow still possible, despite power being everywhere, because we can have 'power with' participants. We discussed how almost euphoric feelings of inclu-sion and shared engagement – like in a religious group – may well seem like the sort of 'power with' we may think we are after in participatory approaches, but we felt that a more nuanced and less cosy account of what the reality may be was more acceptable after post-structural critiques. We discussed the idea (though this was not entirely agreed upon!) that the 'power with' dynamic was very likely to always exist alongside 'power over', even within groups that seem to have reached consensus of various kinds, and especially as one considers wider arenas within which participatory activities may be occurring.

6   *It's a question of values and diversity*: Finally, the argument can be levelled that since all approaches to engagement with respondents, citizens, community members etc. involve taking part in the world, all aspects of the lifeworld can be seen as participatory in some way (because we participate in family life, work, play etc.). What then makes what we call participation (projects, research etc.) distinctive is a moot point. A locally funded survey could be seen as a participatory research project, as it involves respondents as citizens in constructing databases about the citizenry and this information may be fed back to the respondents – yet is this what we are about? There may also be many elements that many so-called participation projects share: e.g. their voluntary nature, or fully informed consent. We appear to make distinctions between 'good' or more worthwhile approaches, so we set out to describe why.

Perhaps participatory approaches can be seen as 'valued' or 'less valued', appropriate or inappropriate, depending on context. But post-structural critiques mean that we need to be aware of and allow space for the fact that different people will experience participatory approaches differently and value different approaches in different ways. Therefore, there is no once and for all position along a continuum whereon we can place projects and approaches and deem them more or less participatory; and we may just have to live with that.

Discussion participants

Vicky Johnson, Kelvin Mason, Jessie, Katrinka Somdahl, Barbara / BazBorle VanWymendaele, N. D. Schaefer, Greg Mannion (convenor). Thanks to them for their contributions to this last section, and to other participants at the conference who helped move my thinking on in no small way.

References

Alanen, L. and Mayall, B. (eds) (2001) *Conceptualizing Child–Adult Relations*, London: Falmer.

Benhabib, S. (1992) *Situating the Self: gender, community and postmodernism in contemporary ethics*, Cambridge: Polity Press.

Buckingham, D. (2000) *After the Death of Childhood*, Malden, MA: Polity Press.

Butler, J. (1990) *Gender Trouble: Feminism and the subversion of identity*, New York: Routledge.

Cahill, C. (2007) 'The personal is political: Developing new subjectivities through participatory action research', *Gender, Place and Culture* 14(3): 267–92.

Cockburn, T. (2005) 'Children as participative citizens: A radical pluralist case for "child-friendly" public communication', *Journal of Social Science* 9: 19–29.

Cooke, B. and Kothari, U. (eds) (2001) *Participation: The new tyranny?*, London: Zed.

Fielding, M. (2007) 'Beyond "Voice": New roles, relations, and contexts in researching with young people', *Discourse: Studies in the Cultural Politics of Education* 28(3): 301–10.

Hall, S. (1996) 'Introduction: Who needs identity?' in P. du Gay and S. Hall (eds) *Cultural Identity*, London: Sage.

Kesby, M. (1999) 'Beyond the representational impasse? Retheorising power, empowerment and spatiality in PRA praxis', unpublished working paper, University of St Andrews, available online, www.st-andrews.ac.uk/_mgk, accessed July 2008.

Kesby, M. (2005) 'Re-theorising empowerment-through-participation as a performance in space: Beyond tyranny to transformation', *Signs: Journal of Women in Culture and Society* 30(4): 2037–65.

Kesby, M. (2007) 'Spatialising participatory approaches: The contribution of geography to a mature debate', *Environment and Planning A* 39(12): 2813–31.

Lee, N. (2001) *Childhood and Society: Growing up in an age of uncertainty*, Milton Keynes: Oxford University Press.

Lundy, L. (2007) '"Voice" is not enough: Conceptualizing Article 12 of the United Nations Convention on the Rights of the Child', *British Educational Research Journal* 33: 6: 927–42.

Mannion, G. (2003) 'Children's participation in school grounds developments: creating a place for education that promotes children's social inclusion', *International Journal of Inclusive Education* 7(2): 175–92.

Mannion, G. (2007) 'Going spatial, going relational: Why "listening to children" and children's participation needs reframing', *Discourse* 28(3): 405–20.

Mannion, G. and I'Anson, J. (2004) 'Beyond the Disneyesque: Children's participation, spatiality and adult–child relations', *Childhood* 11(3): 303–18.

Massey, D. (1994) *Space, Place and Gender*, Cambridge: Polity Press.

Massey, D. (2005) *For Space*, London: Sage.

Morrow, V. (2001) 'Using qualitative methods to elicit young people's perspectives on their environments: Some ideas for community health initiatives', *Health Education Research: Theory and Practice* 16(3): 255–68.

Percy-Smith, Barry (2006) 'From consultation to social learning in community participation with young people', *Children, Youth and Environments* 16(2): 153–79, available at www.colorado.edu/journals/cye, accessed July 2008.

Roche, J. (1999) 'Children: Rights, participation and citizenship', *Childhood* 6(4): 475–93.

Sinclair, R. with Franklin, A. (2000) *Quality Protects Research Briefing No. 3: Young people's participation*, London: Department of Health.

Thomas, N. (2007) 'Towards a theory of children's participation', *The International Journal of Children's Rights* 15(2): 199–218.

Thomson, F. (2007) 'Are methodologies for children keeping them in their place?', *Children's Geographies* 5(3): 207–18.

Tisdall, E. and Davis, J. (2004) 'Making a difference? Bringing children's and young people's views into policy-making', *Children & Society* 18(2): 131–42.

Warshak, R. (2003) 'Payoffs and pitfalls of listening to children', *Family Relations* 52: 373–84.

Wyness, M., Harrison, L. and Buchanan, I. (2004) 'Childhood, politics and ambiguity: Towards an agenda for children's political inclusion', *Sociology* 38(1): 81–99.

31 Children as active citizens

An agenda for children's civil rights and civic engagement[1]

Joachim Theis

Introduction – limitations in the theory and practice of children's participation

Since the mid 1990s, children's participation has become increasingly popular among child rights and child development agencies. Children are being involved in research, assessments, monitoring and consultations. They work as peer educators, health promoters and young journalists. In many countries, children's clubs, parliaments and youth councils have been formed, and in some cases children have been able to influence public decisions and resource allocations. Despite these investments in children's participation, most children still do not participate in important decisions affecting them. Schools and education are rarely participatory, government decisions are made without children's inputs, and the media continue to broadcast images of children as helpless victims or of adolescents as trouble makers, rather than of children as active contributors to the development of their communities.

Despite its spread and diversity, children's participation has not turned into a broad-based movement in the wider development community.[2] Children's participation remains poorly understood and the field of children's participation is fragmented. Agencies tend to focus on specific forms of children's participation, in relative isolation from other approaches. For example, work done with children in the media is often separate from children's involvement in governance, peer education or environmental activism.

With the spread of children's participation, criticism is increasing. Much of this criticism is based on first-hand experiences of children's participation. Examples from East Asia include children who break down in tears at press conferences or who complain about being misled by the sponsoring agency of a consultation. In the Philippines, some politicians are lobbying to abolish the nationwide children's community councils because some of the councils have been manipulated by local elites for their own political agendas. In Mongolia, efforts to pass a national policy on children and young people's participation are running into resistance in parliament. These examples show that children's participation may in fact face more rather than fewer obstacles, as experience grows.

More generally, the concept of participation has failed to provide a sufficiently strong theoretical basis to forge an agenda for children's participation. Participation simply means 'taking part' – but in what? As a concept, participation is an empty vessel that can be filled with almost anything, which is one of the reasons why it has enjoyed such widespread popularity among development agencies.

As far as children's participation is concerned, the concept does not seem to be able to stand on its own. In order to hold up conceptually, children's participation needs a scaffolding of ladders, degrees, levels, enabling environments and supporting adjectives, such as meaningful and ethical. The discourse on children's participation often lacks theoretical clarity and political astuteness (see critiques by Thomas 2007; Wyness 2001). It is the argument of this chapter that participation can only be understood correctly on a foundation of ideas of *rights* and *citizenship*.

Children as citizens

Repeated efforts have been made to develop theoretically and politically more rigorous approaches to children's participation. Two of the main themes that have emerged from this discourse are 'civil rights' and 'citizenship' (Hart 1992; Hart 1997; O'Kane 2003). Citizenship is the collection of rights and responsibilities that define members of a community. One of the most useful attributes of the citizenship concept is the distinction between *citizenship rights* and *citizenship practice* (Bessell, n.d., following Lister 2003 and Marshall and Bottomore 1992). Citizenship rights are the entitlements and freedoms that enable people to take on public roles and to influence public decisions. Citizenship practice is the active exercise of rights through democratic action and civic responsibility.

Children's participation has focused mainly on children's active performance rather than on their civil rights. The distinction between citizenship rights and citizenship practice has major implications for children's participation. Children's civil rights can be operationalised and the responsibilities of government for civil rights can be identified, just as for any other child right. The CRC is the first human rights treaty to explicitly affirm children's civil rights, including the rights to name and identity, information, expression, association, justice and non-discrimination. These rights are essential instruments that enable children to take part in the life of their community and to influence public decisions.

On the other hand, dominant conceptions of childhood mean that children are routinely denied many of the rights of adults, in particular formal political rights such as the right to vote, or economic rights such as the right to sign contracts or to own property. Children's civil rights and freedoms are often severely curtailed by adults and by the state, for example children's access to justice, freedom of movement, or control over their sexuality. The denial of children's rights as citizens makes children more vulnerable to abuse, exploitation and marginalisation in society.

Children as Active Citizens, a publication by the Inter-Agency Working Group on Children's Participation (2008), identified the following priority list of children's civil rights in East Asia.

- *Birth and civil registration* is an example of a civil right that has already been operationalised by many governments. It is a prerequisite for citizenship, contributes to the fulfilment of the rights to a name and nationality (to some extent) and is essential for the realisation of many other rights, such as access to education, health, protection and the freedom to travel across national borders.

- *Children's expression of opinion and control over decisions* at home and in school is the civil right with the most immediate impact on the majority of children. The foundation for exercising the right to expression is laid during early childhood development. Parenting practices, learning and teaching styles are critically important for developing children's ability to articulate their views and make decisions.

- *Access to information* is a prerequisite for making informed choices and decisions in relation to education, health and protection.

- *Feedback and complaints mechanisms* provide children with essential information and enable them to express their views and to seek help (examples are helplines, student monitors, complaints boxes, student counsellors, and children's ombudspersons). They are particularly important to ensure the protection and survival of children in institutions, and in emergencies and in conflict situations.

- *Justice for children* takes children's civil right to justice and equality before the law beyond traditional approaches to juvenile justice or 'children in conflict with the law'. Justice for children relates to children as witnesses and as plaintiffs. It ensures that children's views are heard and considered in judicial proceedings. More broadly, it relates to children's ability to demand justice.

- *Economic citizenship and equal access to resources for children* refers to children's ability to access the same resources as adults. This is particularly important with respect to children's inheritance rights, control over their earnings and equal access to economic and business services for children who are no longer in school, and the right to social transfers for child-headed households.

While these civil rights are not equivalent to children's participation, they are important prerequisites for enabling children to take on more active roles in their communities and to demand and defend their rights. Moreover, it is easier to define the obligations of governments for specific children's civil rights than to identify and to agree on state responsibilities for children's active participation. In the absence of concrete and specific state accountabilities, children's participation is unlikely ever to become a mainstream development issue. By incorporating and operationalising children's civil rights, it becomes easier to engage governments and development agencies in efforts to promote children's participation.

Developing and practising citizenship

Children's abilities to exercise their citizenship rights and responsibilities evolve as they grow and learn. This is a gradual process that enables older children and adolescents to assume the full range of citizenship rights and responsibilities by the time they become adults. People do not suddenly become citizens on reaching a certain age.[3] Human capacities develop and change throughout life, at different rates, according to individual potential and social environment (Lansdown 2005). Competence as a citizen is not limited to adults, and neither is incompetence restricted to children. Citizenship must be learned through everyday experiences of family and community life, education, civic and political awareness. Access to opportunities in school, media, sports and culture is critical for developing and practising citizenship skills.

Children are making important contributions to their societies. The more they take part in public affairs, the more they learn and develop as citizens. The second decade of life is a time when many adolescents take on increasing responsibilities and greater public roles in their communities. For many others, however, especially for adolescent girls, this is a time when only their responsibilities increase, while their opportunities to participate in public life are becoming increasingly constrained.

The programme and policy guide on *Children as Active Citizens* identifies four main areas for developing opportunities for children to exercise and develop active citizenship.

1   Citizenship competencies and civic engagement

While children are born with certain citizenship rights, citizenship *skills* have to be fostered and learned. Competencies for citizenship include communication and problem-solving skills and an understanding of the ways society works (through civic education). Civic engagement offers children opportunities to practise and develop their citizenship competencies, to contribute to their communities and to develop a sense of responsibility. This can take the form of peer education, community service, community mobilisation and activism (e.g. for the environment or against corruption). Governments, communities, youth networks and child-led organisations play important roles in creating opportunities for children to actively exercise their citizenship.

2   Children as active citizens in the media

The media are related to children's civil rights and citizenship in three different ways. They provide children with access to information and offer opportunities for children to express their views (e.g. for children to develop their own radio productions, newsletters, wall newspapers, TV shows, films and websites). The media can also be powerful tools for projecting positive images of children as active citizens in the public sphere.

3   Children influencing public decisions

This is the most high-profile public role children may take. Children involved in local government councils, policy making and legislative reform, and in international political events push the boundaries of conventional notions of childhood. A possible starting point for children's involvement in political discussions is the monitoring of the CRC and providing feedback on the quality of public services.

4   Child-led associations

These offer children opportunities to develop organisational skills, to get support from other children and to campaign collectively for their rights. Unions of child workers have had significant successes in mobilising children to demand justice and equal treatment in some countries.

Support for children's active citizenship requires specific skills that are more likely to be found in NGOs, youth movements and civil society organisations than in government departments or large international development agencies. Citizenship provides a broader and more concrete conceptual and political framework than participation. It also identifies specific obligations of government and of non-governmental agencies for children's civil rights and active citizenship. This is an ambitious agenda, but only a bold new agenda will move children's participation out of its relative obscurity and bring it into the mainstream of political discourse and development practice.

Ideas for the way forward

Defining children's citizenship and the obligations of governments and development agencies for children's civil rights and civic engagement is an important step. Much more, however, needs to be done to ensure that these rights are realised and that children see some concrete benefits in their daily lives. It took women around the world a hundred years to achieve their voting rights. We can be sure that efforts to demand children's civil rights will encounter significant resistance, aside from the fact that children are facing major barriers to organising themselves to demand their rights.

The rest of this chapter presents various options for moving the agenda of children's citizenship, civil rights and civic engagement forward.

Operationalise children's civil rights

One of the most practical ways forward is to define children's civil rights in relation to education; child protection from abuse, violence and exploitation; health, water and sanitation; the environment; emergency preparedness and response, and other areas typically addressed in international development programmes. This approach promotes children's access to information, opportunities to express their views, to be involved in decisions, and to join and form associations. The focus is on all children in their everyday life – at home, in school, in the community, in institutions, at work – rather than on a few children involved in special events or one-off projects.

Civil rights are instruments that enable children to take a more active part at home, in schools and other institutions, and in their communities. Children learn and develop better if their parents and teachers listen to what they have to say, encourage them to ask questions and involve children in important decisions. Children in institutions are less likely to be abused if they have access to effective complaints mechanisms. Adolescents are better able to protect themselves from sexually transmitted infections or unwanted pregnancies if they have access to sex education and health information. A society that provides children with information and listens to children changes the relationship between adults and children, facilitates communication and understanding between generations, and reduces the unequal power relations between children and adults. It is practical and concrete to convince police officers of the benefits of better communication with children who are in contact with the law, to establish feedback and complaints mechanisms in schools, to put in place child helplines (that link to referral mechanisms), or to publish and broadcast information that helps children to protect themselves from abuse, exploitation and violence. Children who are orphaned or of divorced parents have a higher chance of being protected from abuse if they are involved in decisions about where to live.

Advocate and mobilise for children's civil rights

Beyond the promotion of children's civil rights in the context of education, health, HIV/AIDS or child protection programmes and policies, advocacy for specific civil rights of children can help to raise public awareness and government commitments for children as citizens. The global campaign for universal birth registration is a good example of an initiative that calls for the fulfilment of the civil right of all children to a name and identity. An urgent issue that requires advocacy for children's rights as citizens is the plight of stateless children. This is a largely overlooked concern that affects a surprisingly large number of children, including refugees, migrants and ethnic minorities. The campaign for universal birth registration is an opportunity to raise awareness more generally of children's rights as citizens.

Another potential advocacy issue includes children's right to information. So far, attempts to promote children's access to information have been largely in the context of universal primary education or through information campaigns and programmes on specific issues, such as HIV/AIDS, human rights or civic education. The rapid spread of new technologies makes it easier and cheaper for children even in remote, low-resource areas to access information they need to develop and to lead healthy and productive lives. Current efforts to promote children's right to information tend to lack the vision, scope and ambition that is necessary to make sufficiently large achievements for the majority of children.

Child Helpline International is one of the few NGOs that are attempting to make child helplines accessible for all children. In their most basic form, child helplines provide information and advice for children and young people about problems they are facing or difficult decisions they have to make, including sexual relationships, pregnancy and abortion, HIV and STIs, difficulties with teachers and parents, etc. While many countries have established child helplines, coverage is far from universal. Especially where helplines are telephone-based, access is largely restricted to young people in urban areas with easy access to telephones. They do not reach poorer and younger children and those living in remote areas, speaking languages not understood by those operating the helplines. While helplines may provide useful information, they have to be part of effective complaints mechanisms and referral systems in order to provide children in diffi-culties with concrete support.

Children's civil rights are particularly relevant in relation to efforts to end violence against children, to end child marriage, or to promote children's access to justice and to end impunity for crimes against children. Opportunities to link chil-dren's access to justice with the broader rule-of-law agenda of governments and of international agencies are beginning to be addressed through a joint United Nations Justice for Children approach.

Build common understanding of children's civil rights and civic engagement

Any attempts to build broader constituencies for children's civil rights and civic engagement require a common understanding of what these terms mean, and why it is important for children to exercise civil rights and be actively engaged in their everyday life. 'Participation' has not provided a sufficiently clear and progressive vision for children's active citizenship. A movement for children's civil rights and active citizenship has to overcome the fragmentation of the diverse field of children's participation. There is a need to build a common understanding and common definitions among a broad range of government and non-govern-mental agencies of children's civil rights and civic engagement. Once agencies are convinced of the value of promoting children's civil rights, efforts to promote these rights are less likely to encounter resistance or to be misconstrued.

The process of developing an agenda for children's citizenship is essential in order to build common understanding and commitment among agencies, departments and activists. Priorities for children's civil rights are often region- or country-specific, and require approaches that are sensitive to different political and cultural contexts and that make use of opportunities that exist in a country or region for promoting such rights.

Monitor children's civil rights and civic engagement

Monitoring indicators related to children's information, expression of opinion, justice and civic engagement can raise awareness among governments and devel-opment agencies about children's civil rights. Efforts to monitor children's civil rights could be linked to existing mechanisms for measuring governance, civil liberties and civil society, such as the World Bank's World Governance Indicators, the Gender Empowerment Index or the Civil Society Index that is being compiled by CIVICUS (2006). The programme and policy guide on *Children as Active Citizens* includes a list of suggested indicators and benchmarks for measuring children's civil rights and civic engagement.

Include children in governance

The vast majority of public decisions affecting children are made without consid-ering the views of children, and much of the work of government and civil society is carried out without an explicit recognition of children and young people. Policy making, planning and resource allocation are often viewed as benefiting some 'universal' citizen, without regard to age or gender (Bartlett 2005). Children are not considered as political actors, and they are generally denied the right to vote or to stand for public office. The dominant concept of childhood leaves no role for children in the public political sphere. Children in governance and politics are a contradiction, according to this view of childhood. Children may be junior members of political parties, but they are regarded as apprentices rather than as political actors in their own right.

The CRC, with its primary concern with children's protection, survival and development, largely confirms this dominant childhood paradigm and does not articulate children's roles as political actors. Indeed, the CRC has been used to stress the risks for young political activists and the need to protect and prevent children from becoming involved in political and military struggles (Bainvel, no date).

Children have no formal place at the decision-making table, and adult-controlled mechanisms are always likely to be required for children to represent their own opinions (Van Bueren 1995). Children involved in political processes are often considered as technical actors who can provide useful information, rather than as citizens or political actors with rights to uphold and interests to defend. Many of the activities presented as children's participation in political decisions fall short of their ambitious objectives. Youth parliaments may be little more than debating clubs where children learn about governance and politics. At conferences, adults may listen to children, but, when it comes to the important decisions, children are often excluded. In some cases children present their own resolution or declaration, leaving it up to government delegates to make use of or to ignore their contributions. Adult agencies may use children to present their advocacy agendas, or manipulate children to say what the adults want rather than to present children's own concerns. In some situations it may be safer for children rather than adults to articulate political demands because they are considered to be 'just children' and do not have to be taken seriously.

Another challenge is to move beyond one-off events and consultations. High-profile political events involving children offer brief moments of publicity for small numbers of children, but do little to enable the majority of children to make important decisions. Children taking part in high-profile events require a great deal of support and guidance. During such events a few select children make brief forays into the public, adult-dominated arena. The children are under heavy adult protection, only to be chaperoned safely back into their own world once the event is over and the cameras have gone. More energy is invested in attention-grabbing initiatives for children than in the small, difficult-to-effect organisational changes and tasks that are essential for lasting change (Bartlett 2005).

Building permanent mechanisms for children and young people to influence public planning and budget decisions, and creating a public policy environment where children and young people are being taken seriously, take much time and effort. There are no simple models that are guaranteed to work. Since children are not considered to be part of public decision making, the public arena tends to be hostile to the inclusion of young people. Initiatives that are far removed from children's everyday lives are the least likely to be sustained over long periods of time.

Participation alone is inadequate to improve the performance of government services. Resource constraints, socio-political contexts and political and administrative features of decentralised structures affect government performance. Without accountability and resources, participation can deliver little (Crook and Manor 1998). Children's opportunities to influence public decisions are determined to a large extent by a country's political system and level of democratisation, the degree of decentralisation of political authority, the strength and nature of civil society, and the independence of the media and justice system. Decentralisation may open up new opportunities for children's involvement in governance; on the other hand, local authorities are further removed from international obligations and may feel less bound by the CRC than national authorities.

Children's involvement in governance and politics can be grouped into three overlapping types.

1   Children as political activists and actors outside of the formal governance and political systems. Child activists aim to influence the public decision process from the outside, through lobbying, campaigning and mobilising. Some of the best-known examples include child-led organisations, such as the unions of child workers in India.
2   Children in parallel governance institutions, forums and processes, such as children's parliaments and youth councils.
3   Children as members of decision-making bodies, political institutions and processes. Examples include children as members of management and audit committees or advisory boards. Most of the support by children's rights agencies has focused on children in governance institutions rather than on children's activism outside formal governance structures.

There are many ways to support children in governance and to ensure that decisions are informed and influenced by children's concerns and opinions. The high-profile political events where a few children make public statements may not be the most effective avenues for children's influence over government decisions. Careful research with children and young people can provide a more detailed and more representative account of the views and concerns of children, especially of those who are highly unlikely to be invited to high-profile events. Involving children in the auditing of government services and the review of policies offers opportunities for in-depth discussions and collaboration between children and adults.

What is possible depends to a large extent on the political system and the strength of civil society in a country, and on local context and capacities. In many countries, the space for participatory and democratic forms of governance is severely limited and these constraints are magnified in regard to children's engagement in politics. With so little space for children's political expression, the whole range of opportunities and mechanisms for influencing public discussions has to be considered.

Much can be learned about participatory governance from adult civil society, and more work is needed to link children's involvement in public decisions with the broader governance agenda, for example of UNDP and the World Bank.

There are many challenges, and no approach to the involvement of children in public decision making is guaranteed to succeed. It takes hard work, persistence, innovation, flexibility and attention to detail to build the capacities, commitment, resources, standards and structures needed for children's views to be reflected in policy decisions. Creating space for children's influence on public decisions takes time. Approaches should allow children to assume greater influence over decisions as adults gradually give up some of their control. Some approaches offer the possibility of stepwise progress, but many get stuck at a low level of children's control. Starting low is acceptable, as long as there is movement. Starting high, as in the case of the community youth councils in the Philippines, is no guarantee of success, especially when the environment is not ready to accept and support children's involvement in public decisions.

The following are offered as general principles for children's involvement in public decisions:

1   Place the main emphasis on children's involvement in decisions at community level, rather than the national or international level (see Williams 2004).
2   Ensuring that public decisions are informed and influenced by children's views and concerns is more important than high-profile events that bring children and decision makers together, but that fail to take children's opinions into account.
3   Take a long-term approach to gradually increase children's control over decisions and to strengthen sustainable mechanisms for children's involvement in decision making (Shier 2001).
4   Any large-scale investments for children's involvement in governance should be based on solid evidence and not on political correctness or wishful thinking.
5   Link children's involvement in governance with the broader governance agenda.

Clarify concepts of children's citizenship, civil rights and civic engagement

Any attempt to promote children's civil rights and civic participation in mainstream governance and development work requires a strong theoretical basis. The academic and political discourse on children's citizenship is only in its infancy. Recent publications on the theory of children's citizenship (Lister 2006; Invernizzi and Milne 2005; Cohen 2005; Bessell 2006; Thomas 2007; Wyness 2001; Ennew 2000; Franklin 1986) give an indication of the challenges and contradictions that lie ahead in respect to reconciling concepts of childhood and of citizenship, civil and political rights. Should children be involved and integrated in adult governance and justice mechanisms and processes, or should they have their own special mechanisms, such as juvenile justice and youth councils? A quick scan of initiatives to promote children's voting rights shows wildly diverging views across the political spectrum. Nicaragua and Iran are two of the few countries allowing children (from the ages of 16 and 15) to vote. Neither country is known for its respect of democratic freedoms. Various initiatives are being supported at state level in the USA to grant limited political suffrage to children. Suggestions range from giving children half a vote or a quarter of a vote, to assessing children's political competencies.

The very concept of childhood stands in contradiction to the political, economic and sexual rights associated with adulthood. The CRC and other international treaties, such as the ILO Convention on Minimum Age, with their emphasis on child protection, reinforce children's marginalisation in the worlds of work and of politics. Unravelling the contradictions between childhood and citizenship seems a daunting task, which may explain why most efforts have concentrated on mobilising children – mainly older adolescents – rather than on the political and academic debates.

Children do not exist in isolation from the political, social and cultural context of their societies. The political debate over children's citizenship rights and responsibilities is fought in the context of specific political traditions, such as the civic republican, social, liberal or neoliberal citizenship traditions. We have learned from experiences with children's participation how important the broader context of democracy and the strength of civil society are for enabling children to have their say in public matters that concern them. Most states deny adults any meaningful opportunity to influence political decisions – what realistic chance do children (especially younger children) have to have their views taken into consideration in military dictatorships, theocracies or one-party states that restrict civil society? Equally important are the understanding and practice of citizenship in specific cultures. The position of women, class, caste, ethnic and religious division and dominance give an indication of the potential for children's inclusion and are a predictor for the viability of children's civil rights in a given society (Milne, personal communication).

There is no shortcut to children's civil and political rights. The question is which avenue to take, and which entry point has the greatest potential for yielding results in the foreseeable future. Ideas and debates on their own do not change the world, but they are necessary to inspire concrete action and to define specific areas for policy and legislative change.

Notes

1   This article is based on the work of the Inter-Agency Working Group on Children's Participation (IAWGCP), a group of Bangkok-based children's rights agencies. In early 2007, the IAWGCP began working on an agenda for children's citizenship for the East Asia and Pacific region. This initiative was based on many years of experience with children's participation in the region and drew on experiences in other regions (especially South Asia, Latin America and Western Europe). After a year of discussions and drafts, the group produced a brochure and a programming guide on *Children as Active Citizens*.

2   At the Day of General Discussion on Article 12 in September 2006 in Geneva, dozens of child rights agencies contributed ideas to the deliberations. Only two UN agencies were present: OHCHR and UNICEF.
3   There are great variations in the legal ages at which different countries confer the rights and responsibilities of adulthood on children. These definitions are arbitrary, and do not necessarily reflect the range of capacities of children and adolescents.

References

Bainvel, B. (no date) 'The thin red line: Youth participation in times of human-made crises', n.p.: UNICEF.

Bartlett, S. (2005) 'Special focus: Children and governance', *Children, Youth and Environments* 15(1): www.colorado.edu/journals/cye/15_2/.

Bessell, S. (2006) 'Children, work and citizenship: A framework for policy development and analysis', paper presented to the Asia Pacific Childhoods Conference, National University of Singapore.

Bessell, S. (n.d.) 'Children, human rights and social policy: Is citizenship the way forward?', unpublished manuscript.

CIVICUS (2006) 'CIVICUS Civil Society Index: Preliminary findings phase 2003–2005', www.civicus.org.

Cohen, E. (2005) 'Neither seen nor heard: Children's citizenship in contemporary democracies', *Citizenship Studies* 9(2): 1–20.

Crook, R. C. and Manor, J. (1998) *Democracy and Decentralisation in South Asia and West Africa: Participation, accountability and performance*, Cambridge: Cambridge University Press.

Ennew, J. (2000) 'How can we define citizenship in childhood?', in R. Rajani (ed.) *The Political Participation of Children*, Cambridge, MA: Harvard Center for Population and Development Studies.

Franklin, B. (1986) 'Children's Political Rights', in B. Franklin (ed.) *The Rights of Children*, Oxford: Basil Blackwell.

Hart, R. A. (1992) *Children's Participation: From tokenism to citizenship*, Florence: UNICEF International Child Development Centre.

Hart, R. A. (1997) *Children's Participation: The theory and practice of involving young citizens in community development and environmental care*, London: Earthscan.

Inter-Agency Working Group on Children's Participation (2008) *Children as Active Citizens. Commitments and obligations for children's civil rights and civic engagement in East Asia and the Pacific*, Bangkok: Inter-Agency Working Group on Children's Participation.

Invernizzi, A. and Milne, B. (eds) (2005) 'Children's citizenship: An emergent discourse on the rights of the child?', in *Social Sciences*, Delhi: Kamla-Raj Enterprises.

Lansdown, G. (2005) *The Evolving Capacities of the Child*, London and Florence: Save the Children, UNICEF Innocenti Research Centre.

Lister, R. (2003) *Citizenship. Feminist perspectives*, 2nd edn, New York: New York University Press.

Lister, R. (2006) 'Inclusive citizenship', paper presented at the Annual Canadian Political Science Association Conference, Toronto, Canada.

Marshall, T. H. and Bottomore, T. (1992) *Citizenship and Social Class*, London: Pluto Press.

O'Kane, C. (2003) *Children and Young People as Citizens: Partners for social change*, Kathmandu: Save the Children Alliance (South and Central Asia).

Shier, H. (2001) 'Pathways to participation: openings, opportunities and obligations', *Children & Society* 15(2): 107–17.

Thomas, N. (2007) 'Towards a theory of children's participation', *The International Journal of Children's Rights* 15(2): 199–218.

Van Bueren, G. (1995) *The International Law on the Rights of the Child*, Dordrecht: Martinus Nijhoff Publishers.

Williams, E. (2004) *Children's Participation and Policy Change in South Asia*, Working Paper 6, London: Childhood Poverty Research and Policy Centre (CHIP).

Wyness, M. (2001) 'Children, childhood and political participation: Case studies of young people's councils', *The International Journal of Children's Rights* 9(3): 193–212.

Conclusion

Emerging themes and new directions

Barry Percy-Smith and Nigel Thomas

Drawing together conclusions from the range and diversity of material included in this Handbook is something of a challenge. We could argue that this very diversity is a vindication of the undertaking, and one of the key messages to be drawn from the book. People are working in many different social settings, and many different structural and cultural contexts, to promote children and young people's participation. They are working with diverse groups of children and young people, from babies to young adults, with diverse needs and capacities. They are also working to markedly different agendas and with very different outcomes. It is clear that participation has a wide variety of meanings, for different people and in different contexts. We need to examine and learn from this diversity if we are to achieve a shared understanding of children and young people's participation.

The diversity of experiences reported in Part II of the book also reveal many shared concerns, within which may lie the possibility of talking about children's participation as a whole, as we develop new theories and new practices. In this final chapter we first reflect on what can be learned from these diverse examples of practice, and then on some of the new directions in theory indicated by the contributors to Part III.

Reflections on practice

In the following pages we reflect on some of the issues and questions that have emerged from the chapters in Part II, drawing also on the reflections from our commentary teams. We present this in terms of seven key themes:

1   Participation as a variable construct
2   Participation and protection
3   'Voice' and agency
4   Institutions and communities
5   Self-determination and autonomy
6   Values, processes, learning and outcomes
7   The role of adults.

Participation as a variable construct

In their commentary, Liebel and Saadi note that one cannot simply start with the English term 'participation' and look for semantic equivalents in other languages. Instead we should look at actual practices by and with young people, and try to understand them in their social and cultural settings. This book includes examples of children's participation as contributing to family and community, taking part in associations and activities, identifying and responding to community issues, peer education, building individual and collective capacity, self-help and advocacy, resolving problems in social relationships, as well as having their views represented and active involvement in decision-making and development processes. This diversity highlights the range of meanings given to participation in different settings, and the importance of looking at participation in the context of children and young people's whole lives.

Children and young people's participation cannot be understood in isolation from the social, cultural and political contexts in which it occurs. Whereas interpretations of participation in 'Western' countries have tended to emphasise the expression of views in public sector decision-making, in majority world countries participation often has a wider meaning of 'active contribution to the family and community'. Some of the frustrations and difficulties of developing children's participation in countries such as England and Wales (where we both work) may be partly due to the narrow definitions which have been adopted; for example, merely as 'voice' or consultation. A wider interpretation may provide a more fertile space for more meaningful forms of participation to evolve. Participation can be about formal decision making, of course; but it can also be about ways of being and relating, deciding and acting, which characterise the practice of everyday life. For that reason we think there is value in understanding participation more broadly as a manifestation of individual agency within a social context.

Whereas for some children and young people participation may open up new opportunities and choices, for others, living in circumstances of conflict or poverty, it may be essential for survival. For the latter, participation can be a means by which to access other rights in the daily struggle to meet individual needs. In this way children's participation is inextricably linked to equality and social justice. One of our commentary teams asks how participation can help to alleviate child poverty. One could argue that it is because of problems of poverty and social inequality that participation is imperative, if sustainable solutions to the plight of these children are to be achieved. It may be that fuller participation for children cannot be achieved without structural changes in society as a whole; but the participation of children has to be part of such a process of social and structural transformation. As Ray notes, the participation of children in the most difficult situations is not only a right, but a key strategy in transforming relationships with adults.

Our young commentators from Devon observe how participation may be shaped by history, for example in Rwanda. There is indeed a variety of ways in which social, cultural and historical contexts structure children's ability to participate: dominant constructions of childhood and attitudes to children's rights; strong religious codes or social divisions (such as the caste system); war, conflict and instability. Patterns of participation are structured by cultural values and practices that model social relationships and socialise children into particular ways of being. Corona and colleagues highlight how participation in Mexico is strongly linked to community identity and belonging, giving rise to a form of 'ethnic citizenship'. Expectations of children's status and behaviour regulate relations in the community, for example through subservience to adult elders (Twum-Danso). The form and extent of participation is partly determined by dominant cultural norms which define roles and opportunities for young people, so that traditional values may be a major obstacle to participation (Feinstein and colleagues). Duty to community is often deeply embedded in local culture, defining the social actions and choices of all members of the community; in this respect participation can be an obligation as well as a right. Liebel and Saadi also observe that while paternalism and authoritarianism are incompatible with the participation of children if they have no right to contradict their elders or to demand that adults account for their decisions, deference to adults and obligations to take on responsibility to the community can also be interpreted as expressions of solidarity and interdependence between generations, necessary for the survival of many communities. How, then, can we conceptualise participation within such contexts?

Participation and protection

Tensions emerge in many chapters concerning how to balance protection with participation (Kirby and Laws; Jamieson and Mũkoma; Alderson).[1] Alderson notes that formal participation is often more concerned with provision and protection. On the one hand, adult concerns about protecting children may get in the way of their participation rights, for example by reducing opportunities for them to associate freely or by preventing them from influencing decisions. On the other hand, participation may be an important way for children to achieve provision and protection rights. However, in contrast to assumptions about adults as protectors of children, what is striking in many of our chapters is the extent to which adults are failing children through abuse and neglect, war and poverty, discrimination and prejudice (Ray; Feinstein et al.). Where children cannot rely on adults to act for them we see how, through forms of participation, they can develop their own capacity to act, for example as 'agents of peace' (Feinstein et al.; Austin), as '*promotoras/promotores*' (Shier) or as 'child reporters' (Acharya). It is important to acknowledge the potential for children to contribute directly to social change. One commentary team noted that although child workers are often seen as neglected or vulnerable, several chapters show how these children can be models of the active, competent and participatory child.

Negative expectations of what children and young people can achieve are a significant barrier to their participation. In relation to disabled children, Martin and Franklin argue strongly that a shift in attitudes to their competence is essential if their participation is to move from rhetoric to reality. Twum-Danso shows how paternalism in Ghana results in children being passive because of an expectation that they should rely on their parents to act in their best interests, when there is evidence that parents are actually retreating from their responsibilities.

Recognition of children and young people's capability is essential to counteract their invisibility and powerlessness (Yamashita and Davies). In 'Western' countries children under 10 years are frequently excluded from decision-making situations (Kirby and Laws), although elsewhere in the world children of this age may be heads of households (Pells). We share Liebel and Saadi's assumption that 'a renewal of adults' perspectives on children is necessary in all societies and cultures'.

'Voice' and agency: social participation as active citizenship

Perhaps the most striking theme from this Handbook is the importance of 'social' participation – children as active citizens, making contributions and taking actions within their everyday life settings. To view participation in terms of individual rights to 'have a say' in public decision making – often adult-driven and organisation-based – is only part of the story. The most inspiring accounts in Part II tell of children working as members of a community where roles and responsibilities are shared, where 'agency' rather than 'voice' is the key concept.

Many decisions that shape the lives of individuals and communities are made within the course of everyday life rather than through political structures of government and governance. Social participation within everyday contexts can provide for more ownership and self-determination than is often possible in public decision-making settings (White and Choudhury). Acknowledging social participation in communities can also represent a challenge to models of representative democracy in favour of participatory democratic approaches. As the authors of Commentary 6 note, the need for diverse representation is seen as a stumbling block for children's participation when communities are fragmented into interest groups competing through 'voice' for scarce resources. Instead, they suggest, social diversity can be seen as a basis for 'asset building – building on from skills young people bring and equipping them with the resources they need to be successful'. This reconceptualisation echoes Dewey's account of democracy as based on social cooperation rather than disconnected debate (see Honneth 1998). As Liebel and Saadi note: 'If participation could be conceived of as not only consisting of speaking and being heard, but also of active and routine inclusion in vital social processes, new prospects could be opened up for the situating of children in society.'

Issues have also been raised about the links between individual and collective participation (Dadich; Martin and Franklin). As Batsleer notes, the 'intensely personal and broadly political are intimately entwined'; a sentiment echoed elsewhere, for example by Sotkasiira and colleagues, who argue that effective participation operates at the interface between social interactions and political activity. In order to achieve embedded participation, both individual and collective approaches are needed. Ideas of agency and social participation within communities are important in reorienting children's participation, beyond exercising a right to 'have a say', to a wider concept of active citizenship (Theis). It is arguable that this is a weakness in a solely rights-based case for participation: children may exercise such rights without making a real contribution to social processes, while conversely, other children may have a great deal of responsibility and take an important part in social activities, without being recognised as holders of rights.

Institutions and communities

A fourth theme is the frequent success of projects that start small in communities, contrasted with the more problematic nature of projects that begin at a national level or are based in more formal institutions. Pells expresses this as a difference between 'performed' and 'lived' participation. We can discern a greater emphasis on institutionalised participation and public sector decision making in 'Western' countries, and a stronger orientation to community-based participation in the majority world – where several chapters reveal an element of *sahabagithvaya* ('joining in with others') in a communal and contextual culture of participation (Mason et al.).

Our contributors point to difficulties with participation initiatives that 'mimic' (Thomas 2007) adult-based governance structures, such as the youth council or 'parliament'. Turkie argues that young people need to contest adult structures and decide for themselves how they wish to engage. In the context of English schools, Lewars argues that the scope of participation needs to be widened to permeate every aspect of school life. When embedded within communities, participation seems to acquire a higher level of meaning, effectiveness and sustainability (Austin; Johnson). Within communities the problems of ownership, representation and trust, which plague participation initiatives in Western countries, appear to be lesser (Sancar and Severcan; Shier).

In considering the relative merits of participation within communities or in institutions, it is also useful to consider the different agendas at play, and who benefits. Children's participation in staff recruitment, or consultations about service priorities, may primarily benefit the organisations involved; but the experience of being trusted, having responsibility and opportunities for action, can have massive benefits for young people. Yet, as McGinley and Grieve argue, attempts to further the participation of young people can simply reinforce the status quo as a result of ambiguity in commitment towards young people. However, we want to avoid a false dichotomy between 'political' and 'social' participation, when so many of our chapters suggest that both are necessary. As our first commentary team highlights, in order for participation to be embedded, there must be both 'buy-in' from the top and activism and commitment at the grassroots (see Kränzl-Nagl and Zartler; Austin).

While informal participation methodologies are necessary to build and sustain the participation of children and young people, formal approaches are also essential to create linkage with wider political structures. There is evidence in this book that initiatives which start at a local level before expanding to a regional, national or international level are more likely to be sustainable. Starting small means that young people and communities can develop a sense of ownership and build on resources within the community (Johnson). Sancar and Severcan show the importance of building trust and capacity within the community first, to become more effective at a national level (see also Sotkasiira et al.). Intergenerational collaboration is a natural driving force, and also an outcome, part of a process of building social capital (see Taylor and Percy-Smith 2008).

Self-determination and autonomy

Drawing on perspectives from Aotearoa/New Zealand, commentary team 6 draws our attention to *tino rangatiratanga*, which means 'the ability to make choices and decisions in one's own life'. Many of our contributors provide examples of how children and young people can exercise self-determination. Yet all too frequently adults are not 'letting go' of the process, with the result that participation does not lead to empowerment and self-determination of young people. For many adults working in public services – and who themselves lack power – control and stability are more pressing than change. Although examples of *tino rangatiratanga* do occur in some of our accounts from the West (Dadich; and to a lesser extent Yamashita and Davies), these are exceptions within a generally adult-dominated scene. As Janet Batsleer notes, adults tend to see young people's participation as being about 'shaping the services, policies and institutions that adults have provided'. In contrast, in many of our majority-world examples there appears to be a higher level of trust and belief in young people's abilities, a willingness to let go and take risks, knowing that they can indeed make informed decisions and changes in the community.

Knowing that they can deal with the future is a primary concern for many young people, particularly those in difficult situations who may have experienced loss or discrimination. This is vividly illustrated in the experiences of self-help support groups described by Dadich or the youth organising reported by Sancar and Severcan. For these young people the power of participation as self-advocacy is unquestionably about *tino rangatiratanga* or self-determination, and a developing ability to manage their own lives through reflecting on their situation and transforming their own marginalisation, echoing what Freire (1972) referred to as *conscientização*.

Reflecting on the challenges of monitoring and assessing the impacts of participation (Skeels and Crowley), Batsleer notes that we should exercise care 'not to have a dead hand effect on a potentially life enhancing experience'. Adults have a duty to ensure that spaces are available within which young people can develop their own capacity to participate – increasing their confidence and self-esteem, and their capacity for organising themselves. Commentary team 2 also notes the importance of recognizing the evolving capacities of children and embedding participation in communities at an early age, so that it becomes a part of who children are. Opportunities for participation at an early age enable children to develop and mature through taking on responsibility and learning to make wise choices, to interact and hear different views. As Hart (1992) argued, this comes through practice within everyday environments.

Values, processes, learning and outcomes

Participation is often seen in terms of involvement in change processes, and its value measured by results. However, our contributions show the importance of the *process* of participation, as well as the *outcome*. As commentary team 5 notes, participation is about learning as well as making a difference. Structures alone cannot guarantee success; it is the quality of relationships, and the values shaping them, that emerge as significant. A number of papers recognise the importance of dialogue, interaction and communication, in particular the importance of feedback, follow-up, continual sharing of information, and accountability. For example, Shier's work shows the value of developing a participatory ethos at an early age, through learning and fostering collective responsibility; Johnson highlights the empowering potential of participatory evaluation; and Corona emphasises the critical importance of intergenerational cooperation. Within all of these cases opportunities for social learning are integral to the participation process (see Percy-Smith 2006).

Concerns are often voiced about getting the right structures in place for participation at the start. Yet we see from the contributions to this text that participation is not an idealised process which happens in predefined ways; rather, is it a way of being, an ethic of practice, which informs how individuals and groups respond to issues and problems. A core value for meaningful participation is respect for the individuality of children and young people. Not everyone is, or wants to be, a leader or to be involved in the same way, but there should be scope for all children to make a contribution in whatever way they feel appropriate according to their own inclinations, interests and capacities. At the same time it is important that young people can see the outcomes of their participation. This is more easily achieved at a community level, in contrast to a regional or national level, where inputs can so easily disappear into a black hole of 'governance' (Taylor and Percy-Smith 2008). Participatory practice is not just about including different voices and interests in a particular agenda, but also about acknowledging multiple agendas within a particular initiative; which has implications for assessing outcomes. Crowley and Skeels emphasise the importance of standards and frameworks for monitoring the extent, quality and impact of participation with respect to the four realms of individual, family, community and institution. However, evaluating impact should be undertaken not solely in terms of programme indicators, but in ways that are based on the recognition of meaning, holistically within the context of young people's lives, and according to their own quality criteria.

The role of adults: negotiating new social relations

In many cases the participation of children involves negotiating power and relations with adults. We have already touched on the role of adults, sometimes critically. Yet it is clear from many of the contributions that adults are crucial to children's participation. White and Choudhury argue that children's participation is rarely autonomous and is unlikely to succeed without adults. As Batsleer says, the need is for adults with a 'burning heart', committed to supporting young people's rights and agency in their own lives. Sotkasiira et al., Kirby and Laws, Jamieson and Mũkoma all emphasise the key role of professionals as advocates who can ensure that children's perspectives are represented, and also protect them from undue risk. Their role is to provide an enabling environment where young people can evolve their own means of expression and participation.

We have noted the greater success of participation that is embedded within communities, and we want also to highlight the importance of creating spaces for joint projects of mutual interest to young people and adults. Moss and Petrie (2002: 9) describe 'a domain of social practices and relationships; where values, rights and cultures are created … where there is room for dialogue, confrontation (in the sense of exchanging differing experiences and views), deliberation and critical thinking, where children and others can speak and be heard'. This, it seems to us, is exactly what 'participation work' should be about.

Reflections on theory

Our task in this book was not to produce a theory of participation, but to create a space for some of the work being done to build this.[2] Here we reflect on some of the theoretical ideas raised in the book, alongside some key theoretical perspectives which seem to be important for children's participation.

Much of the reflection on practice in Part II has implications for theory, and we have tried to draw out some of the key strands in this. The contributions in Part III engage directly with different elements of the complex task of theorising children and young people's participation. All recognise the limitations of a theory of participation that involves simply 'listening' to children, and look instead at forms of dialogue between children, young people and adults. Several chapters also highlight the limitations of conventional structures of government, and argue for theories of participation to embrace alternative informal spaces for young people to engage as active citizens.

Fitzgerald and colleagues focus on 'the ways in which we invite, engage and interpret dialogue with children'. They suggest that the development of participation can be seen in terms of three historical moments: a claim based on equality in the 1960s and 1970s, a claim based on difference in the 1980s and 1990s, and a contemporary 'turn to dialogue'. For them the key concept in this is *recognition*, and with it the struggle to achieve intersubjectivity and shared responsibility. This is relevant to participation in both individual and collective settings, because the attention is on interpersonal relationships and, by extension, on group and intergenerational relations too.

Cockburn's focus is more specifically on participation in collective settings, and in particular on public decision making and political processes. In exploring what ideas of 'deliberative democracy' have to offer to young people, he signals the importance of associations as a context for young people's participation and points us to the (largely unused) scope for political theories, especially theories of democracy, to engage with the field of young people's participation. Tisdall also focuses on participation in collective settings, in this case school councils, and also draws on political theories, in this case theories of governance, to look at the potential for deliberative mechanisms.

School councils are a particularly important location for studying children and young people's participation and for thinking about its purpose, potential and limitations. Schools include a full cross-section of children and young people from a wide age range, who come together on a regular basis for shared activity. On the other hand, they are institutions in which children are subject to a high degree of authority and control (commonly including a requirement to be there in the first place). They are therefore a place where *system* meets *lifeworld* in a fairly stark way, as well as being, as Tisdall implies, a point where state meets civil society. Political theory is an important route to an understanding of what goes on in these settings for participation. Social theory, we suggest, can probably also contribute.

Mannion's purpose is to move away from a preoccupation with 'voice' and talking, and to look at the kind of spaces that adults and children can create together and the kind of relationships which they can have in those spaces. While not in contradiction to Cockburn's and Tisdall's concerns with deliberation and discussion, this approach complements their work by putting those processes in their spatial and relational context. Returning to Fitzgerald et al., we see that all our theoretical contributors, from their different disciplinary perspectives, are asking questions about the nature of dialogue in relationships of unequal power and the spaces in which that may happen.

On one level, thinking about children and young people's participation is very simple, if we share certain values. The right to participate is well founded in philosophy, and increasingly in law, and children's agency is now generally accepted in social studies of childhood, and increasingly in social policy concerning children. The complexity comes in with wider questions about what sort of democracy we want and can achieve in our (complex, highly technologised and globally interconnected) contemporary world, with the contested relationship between individual autonomy, obligations to community and demands of wider society (which admittedly varies with culture, but perhaps not as much as we think), and of course with the continuing ambivalence about childhood and youth in all societies.

Theis cuts through some of this in his final contribution, which is located not so much in an academic perspective as in theories of children's rights, combined with the frustration of experience in developing policy and practice in several challenging global settings. His demand for children to be empowered as fellow citizens is a powerful call to go beyond 'participation' to promote children's civil rights and *engagement*.

The theoretical contributions in this Handbook are part of a growing strand of attempts to think more clearly about children and young people's participation and what it means. It is encouraging that this work is beginning, and no doubt it will continue. We are convinced that the ideas around dialogic space represented in these chapters, together with some fundamental questions about democracy and citizenship, will be central to taking this work forward.

What next? Practical steps for the future

We want to conclude by offering some practical steps to promote the participation of children and young people in the directions to which this Handbook is pointing. We do this under six headings.

1   *Supporting the building of participation from the grassroots*

This means ensuring that children and young people have opportunities to participate in meaningful ways in their everyday lives (and working for these opportunities may well be how some young people participate). It means creating informal as well as formal spaces within which children and young people can articulate their own expressions of active citizenship through different forms of participation, but at the same time demanding support and commitment from authorities.

2   *Promoting wider interpretations of participation beyond 'having a say' in decision making*

This means reflecting on where *tino rangatiratanga* (self-determination) can be encouraged, so that children can take on higher levels of responsibility in exercising their agency as active citizens; encouraging reflection, dialogue and social learning within and between groups; inviting contributions from children which may not be just about decision making; supporting the development of peer work among children.

3   *Building capacity with individuals and communities for participation as active citizens*

This means creating enabling environments (at different levels – home, school, community, organisation, city and country) in which possibilities for different forms of participation can be developed; valuing diverse views and contributions; encouraging intergenerational projects which engage children and adults jointly in processes of learning and inquiry around issues of mutual concern; education, training and 'sensitisation' of adults to recognise the importance of children's involvement.

4   *Challenging adult discrimination and negative constructions of childhood*

This means lobbying governments to establish rights in legislation to ensure equal opportunity; safeguarding children against the excesses of adults; challenging adult attitudes experientially through young people developing and articulating their own agency.

5   *Focusing on the role of adults and quality of relationships between adults and children*

This means encouraging adults to think about their role as facilitators and advocates rather than controllers; developing a culture of mutual trust, respect and reciprocity between children and adults and among children; creating opportunities for bringing children and adults together around their joint concerns.

6   *Implementing a framework of civil rights and engagement for children*

This means developing a culturally appropriate understanding of children's civil rights and engagement, which can help to provide a legal imperative and policy framework that will support and enable the 'operationalisation' of children's rights of active citizenship in all spheres of their everyday lives.

Final thoughts

A fundamental starting point for many of our contributors, and for much participatory practice with children and young people, is the UNCRC. In particular, the right in Article 12 for children to have a say in all matters that affect them has been a very important driver for promoting children and young people's participation in many contexts. This has gone hand in hand with an emphasis on children's voice in decision making. Reflecting back on the contributions in this Handbook, and looking forward to the future, we would argue that now is the time to look beyond Article 12, to emphasise other rights in the CRC (for example, to freedom of assembly), and even to go beyond the CRC itself, in two directions. One involves claiming rights for children to play a much fuller part in democratic decision making at all levels and in all areas, rather than merely expressing views in 'matters affecting the child'. The other involves looking much more closely at how rights, equality and justice for children and young people can be met through their active participation in the everyday life of their communities. It seems to us that both are crucially important aspects of real citizenship for children and young people.

Finally, if some of the stories in this book about the lives and experiences of different children and young people around the world may cause sadness or alarm, they also contain some seeds of hope and redemption, as children demonstrate their agency, their creativity and tenacity in overcoming difficult situations. We hope that this Handbook is able to contribute to a shift in thinking about how children's participation can contribute, not only to improving the situation of children, but also to a more healthy, just and democratic world for all.

Notes

1. Mathew and colleagues remind us of Rogers and Wrightsman's (1978) distinction between a 'nurturance' and a 'self-determination' orientation towards children's rights.
2. See, for example, Thomas 2007 and the papers in *International Journal of Children's Rights* 16(3).

References

Freire, P. (1972) *Pedagogy of the Oppressed*, Harmondsworth: Penguin.

Hart, R. (1992) *Children's Participation: From tokenism to citizenship*, Florence: UNICEF.

Honneth, A. (1998) 'Democracy as reflexive cooperation: John Dewey and the theory of democracy today', *Political Theory* 26(6), 763–83.

Moss, P. and Petrie, P. (2002) *From Children's Services to Children's Spaces: Public policy, children and childhood*, London: Routledge.

Percy-Smith, B. (2006) 'From consultation to social learning in community participation with young people', *Children, Youth and Environments* 16(2), 153–79

Rogers, C. M. and Wrightsman, L. S. (1978) 'Attitudes towards children's rights: Nurturance or self-determination', *Journal of Social Issues* 34(2), 59–68.

Taylor, M. and Percy-Smith, B. (2008) 'Children's participation: Learning from community development', *International Journal of Children's Rights* 16(4), 379–94.

Thomas, N. (2007) 'Towards a theory of children's participation', *International Journal of Children's Rights* 15(2), 199–218.

Index

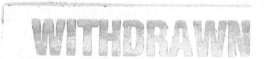